T0215395

Cleft Palate Speech

Cleft Palate Speech: Assessment and Intervention

Sara Howard

University of Sheffield, Department of Human Communication Sciences, Sheffield, UK

Anette Lohmander

Karolinska Institutet, Department of Clinical Science, Intervention and Technique, Division of Speech and Language Pathology, Stockholm, Sweden

⊛WILEY-BLACKWELL

John Wiley & Sons, Ltd., Publication

Library of Congress Cataloging-in-Publication Data

Cleft palate speech : assessment and intervention/ [edited by] Sara Howard and Anette Lohmander.
    p. ; cm.
  Includes bibliographical references and index.
  ISBN 978-0-470-74330-0 (pbk.)
  1. Cleft palate children–Rehabilitation. 2. Articulation disorders in children–Patients–Rehabilitation. 3. Cleft lip–Treatment. 4. Cleft palate–Treatment. 5. Speech therapy. I. Howard, Sara. II. Lohmander, Anette.
  [DNLM: 1. Cleft Lip–rehabilitation. 2. Cleft Palate–rehabilitation. 3. Articulation Disorders–rehabilitation. 4. Speech Therapy–methods. WV 440]
  RJ496.S7C557 2011
  618.92'855–dc23

                                    2011014942

A catalogue record for this book is available from the British Library.

This book is published in the following electronic format: ePDF 9781119998570; ePub: 9781119970644; MOBI: 9781119970651

Set in 9.5/11.5 pt Sabon by Toppan Best-set Premedia Limited

1 2011

Contents

List of Contributors

Martin Atkinson
Martin Atkinson, PhD, is Professor of Dental Anatomy Education in the Academic Division of Oral Pathology, University of Sheffield, UK. He has been involved in teaching anatomy, physiology and neuroscience to Speech and Language therapy students in Sheffield since the inception of the course in Sheffield in 1978 and has won several awards for his teaching innovations. He is co-author of 'Basic Medical Science for Speech and Language Therapy Students' (John Wiley & Sons Ltd).

Lesley Cavalli
Lesley Cavalli, MSc, Cert MRCSLT, currently combines her clinical work at Great Ormond Street Hospital, UK, with a lectureship in voice at University College, London. She has specialised in voice disorders throughout her career, in her clinical work, teaching and research. Her current clinical post involves the tertiary assessment and treatment of children and young people with a wide range of ENT-related conditions. She is the lead Speech and Language Therapist for the Joint Paediatric Voice Clinic at Great Ormond Street Hospital and overall SLT Service for ENT.

Kathy L. Chapman
Kathy L. Chapman, PhD is currently a Professor in the Department of Communication Sciences and Disorders at the University of Utah, USA. She currently teaches courses in phonological disorders in children, cleft palate, and research methods. Her research has focused on children with specific language impairment and language and phonological development of young children with cleft palate. She is especially interested in the impact of clefting on the developing speech sound system. Dr Chapman has numerous database articles and presentations related to these areas of study.

Fiona E. Gibbon
Fiona E. Gibbon, PhD, is a speech and language therapist and Professor and Head of Speech and Hearing Sciences at University College Cork, Ireland. Her research focuses on the use of instrumentation to diagnose and treat speech disorders, particularly those associated with cleft palate. She has published over seventy papers and book chapters, and has been awarded a number of research council and charity funded grants to investigate cleft palate speech. She is a Fellow of the Royal College of Speech and Language Therapists.

Carrie L. Gotzke

Carrie L. Gotzke is currently a Doctoral candidate in the Faculty of Rehabilitation Medicine at the University of Alberta, Canada. Her research interests include paediatric resonance disorders, perceptual-acoustic correlates of speech intelligibility, and measures of speech function and outcome for children with cleft palate.

Anne Harding-Bell

Anne Harding-Bell, PhD, East of England Cleft Lip and Palate Network, UK, and University teacher in the Department of Human Communication Sciences at University of Sheffield, UK. Anne led the first post graduate cleft palate studies course in Cambridge, UK, and now contributes to postgraduate teaching on distance learning courses in cleft palate at the University of Sheffield. Her research interests centre around transcribing, characterising, categorising and treating cleft speech and pre-speech patterns.

Christina Havstam

Christina Persson, SLP, PhD, is a lecturer at the Sahlgrenska academy at Gothenburg University and clinical Speech-Language Pathologist at Sahlgrenska University Hospital, Gothenburg, Sweden. Her main interest in clinical work, teaching and research is speech disorders in patients born with cleft lip and palate or 22q11 deletion syndrome. She has been a member of Gothenburg cleft palate team since 1991 and of the 22q11 deletion syndrome team since 1997.

Gunnilla Henniningsson

Gunilla Henningsson, PhD, is Associate Professor/Senior Lecturer in the Division of Speech and Language Pathology, Department of Clinical Science Intervention and Technology at the Karolinska Institute, Stockholm, Sweden. Her research is in the areas of velopharyngeal function and the development of universal speech samples for reporting speech outcomes in individuals with cleft palate.

Megan Hodge

Megan Hodge, PhD, is currently a Professor and heads the *Children's Speech Intelligibility, Research and Education Laboratory (CSPIRE)* in the Faculty of Rehabilitation Medicine at the University of Alberta, Canada. Her research interests include developmental aspects of normal and disordered speech perception and production and perceptual-acoustic correlates of speech intelligibility.

Sara Howard

Sara Howard, PhD, is currently Reader in Clinical Phonetics in the Department of Human Communication Sciences at the University of Sheffield, UK, and an ESRC Research Fellow. Her research interests span clinical phonetics and phonology (with a particular interest in phonetic transcription and electropalatography) and developmental speech disorders, including cleft palate. She teaches on a series of postgraduate courses in speech disorders and cleft palate and is currently President of the International Clinical Phonetics and Linguistics Association.

Alice Lee

Alice Lee, PhD, is a Lecturer in the Department of Speech and Hearing Sciences, University College Cork, Ireland. Her research interest includes perceptual and instrumental investigations of speech disorders in individuals with structural anomalies and neurological impairment; and listener training for perceptual judgements of speech disorders. Her recent research and publications focus on electropalatographic studies of normal articulation and articulation disorders associated with cleft palate, as well as prosodic disturbance in Cantonese speakers with aphasia.

Anette Lohmander

Anette Lohmander, PhD, is a Professor and Head of the Division of Speech and Language Pathology, Karolinska Institutet, Stockholm, Sweden, and the specialist speech-language pathologist at Karolinska University Hospital. Her research interests in the area of cleft palate focus on the impact of surgical procedure, particularly on speech and language (and hearing) development and the development of efficient intervention procedures.

Brenda Louw

Brenda Louw, DPhil., is currently Professor and Chair of the Department Audiology and Speech-Language Pathology, East Tennessee State University, USA. Her research interests in cleft palate are early intervention, cross-cultural service delivery models and speech assessment. She is the Vice-President of the Pan African Association for Cleft Lip and Palate

Roopa Nagarajan

Roopa Nagarajan, PhD, is currently Professor and Chairperson, Department of Speech, Language and Hearing Sciences, Sri Ramachandra University, Chennai, India. She has been involved in the development of community-based rehabilitation services for individuals with cleft lip and palate in rural India and is currently the President of the Indian Society of Cleft Lip, Palate and Craniofacial Anomalies.

Valerie Pereira

Valerie Pereira is currently undertaking a PhD in the Institute of Child Health, University College London, UK, and is a specialist speech and language therapist with Great Ormond Street Hospital for Children and the North Thames Regional Cleft Service in London. Her clinical and research interests include the instrumental assessment and measurement of speech outcomes, with a particular interest in the impact of orthognathic surgery on speech in cleft lip and palate.

Christina Persson

Christina Persson, SLP, PhD, is a Lecturer at the Sahlgrenska Academy at Gothenburg University and clinical Speech-Language Pathologist at Sahlgrenska University Hospital, Gothenburg, Sweden. Her main interest in clinical work, teaching and research is speech disorders in patients born with cleft lip and palate or 22q11 deletion syndrome. She has been a member of Gothenburg cleft palate team since 1991 and of the 22q11 deletion syndrome team since 1997.

John E. Riski

John E. Riski, PhD, CCC-S, is the Clinical Director of the Center for Craniofacial Disorders and Director of the Speech Pathology Laboratory at Children's Healthcare of Atlanta, USA. His research encompasses speech outcomes of surgical interventions for children born with cleft lip/palate and craniofacial disorders. He is a Fellow of the American Speech Language and Hearing Association and a past-president of the American Cleft Palate-Craniofacial Association.

Nancy Scherer

Nancy Scherer, PhD, is currently Dean of Clinical & Rehabilitative Health Sciences at East Tennessee State University, USA. Her research interests have focused on early developmental milestones of children with cleft lip and/or palate and children with velocardiofacial syndrome. She has been particularly interested in efficacy studies of early speech and language intervention for children with clefts and craniofacial conditions. She is currently Principal Investigator for a comparative study of the effects of a hybrid early intervention model for children with cleft lip and palate funded by the National Institutes of Health.

Debbie Sell

Debbie Sell, PhD, is the Lead Speech and Language Therapist for the North Thames Regional Cleft Service, Head of Department at Great Ormond Street Hospital NHS Trust and is Honorary Senior Lecturer Institute of Child Health, University College London and Visiting Professor at City University, London, UK. She has been an active clinical researcher in the cleft palate field for over 25 years. She has 50 peer-reviewed publications and has co-edited two books in this field. In 2006 she was awarded an OBE for services to the UK National Health Service.

Lotta Sjögreen

Lotta Sjögreen, PhD, is a speech-language pathologist at Mun-H-Center National Orofacial Resource Centre for Rare Diseases, Gothenburg, Sweden. Her doctorate was in medical sciences and her research focuses on evaluation and intervention for orofacial dysfunctions in rare diseases.

Joy Stackhouse

Joy Stackhouse, PhD, is Professor of Human Communication Sciences at the University of Sheffield, UK, where she teaches on the Distance Learning Programmes in Speech Difficulties and Cleft Palate. She is a Fellow of the Royal College of Speech and Language Therapists and a chartered psychologist. Along with Professor Bill Wells, she has developed a psycholinguistic approach to the assessment and management of children with speech and literacy difficulties which is used in research and training.

Triona Sweeney

Triona Sweeney, PhD, is the Senior Clinical Specialist Speech and Language Therapist, The Children's University Hospital, Temple Street, Dublin, Ireland; Lead Speech and Language Therapist on the Dublin Cleft Team; and Adjunct Professor, Speech & Language Therapy Department, University of Limerick, Ireland. Her research interests focus on perceptual and instrumental assessment of nasality and nasal airflow errors, with emphasis on reliability of assessments.

Linda D. Vallino-Napoli
Linda D. Vallino-Napoli, PhD, CCC-SLP/A, FASHA, is Head of the Craniofacial Outcomes Research Laboratory and Senior Research Scientist in the Center for Pediatric Auditory and Speech Sciences at Nemours/Alfred. I. duPont Hospital for Children, Wilmington, Delaware, USA, where she is also a member of the Cleft Palate-Craniofacial team. She is an Adjunct Associate Professor in the Department of Linguistics and Cognitive Science at the University of Delaware. Dr Vallino-Napoli lectures in the area of orofacial anomalies and evidence-based practice and is the author of peer-reviewed articles and book chapters in these areas.

Tara L. Whitehill
Tara L. Whitehill, PhD, is a Professor in the Division of Speech and Hearing Sciences, University of Hong Kong and the specialist speech-language pathologist for the University of Hong Kong/Prince Philip Dental Hospital Cleft Lip and Palate Centre. Her research interests in the area of cleft palate currently focus on speech intelligibility and the relationship between intelligibility and other outcome measures

Mary Wickenden
Mary Wickenden, PhD, has worked in the United Kingdom and India, specialising in work with young children with complex disabilities, and more recently in Sri Lanka, running the first SLT training course there. Subsequently, building on an interest in cultural aspects of health and disability, she has trained as a medical anthropologist. She is a Senior Research Fellow at the Centre for International Health and Development, University College London, UK, teaching and researching on issues related to children and disability in middle and low income countries.

Elisabeth Willadsen
Elisabeth Willadsen, PhD, is currently an Assistant Professor in the Department of Scandinavian Studies and Linguistics at the University of Copenhagen, Denmark. She currently teaches courses in language development of young children, and cleft palate. Her research focuses on pre-speech and early speech and language development of young children with and without cleft palate, with a special interest in the interaction between early phonological and lexical development in children with cleft palate.

Preface

This book emerged out of conversations which we, the editors, enjoyed over a number of years both at conferences and on visits to each other's institutions in Sheffield, Gothenburg and, latterly, Stockholm. Observing current developments in research into speech production in cleft palate, we both recognised the need for a book which reflected the increasing breadth of the research being carried out across the world. Whilst important work was being undertaken in the more traditional areas of speech, there was a growing body of research, which recognised the potential of certain aspects of language, to contribute significantly to the field. We were also keen to recognise the importance of cross-linguistic and cross-cultural issues in cleft speech research. In addition, we wanted to broaden our focus to include both the speaker's own and the listener's perspective on communication. Thus we chose to use the WHO-ICF framework as a backdrop to all of the work contained in this book. Finally, we aimed to include current evidence of best practice (EBP) regarding both assessment and intervention. Our contributing authors were thankfully very receptive to these ideas, and thus the concepts of the WHO-ICF structure and EBP are given specific attention and have been regularly applied throughout the book.

For one of us, there was also a more specific stimulus for this book: coincident with its development, a set of postgraduate courses in cleft palate were being introduced at the University of Sheffield, and this book was designed, in part, with the needs of these students in mind. From this perspective it can be seen as a companion text to Watson, Sell and Grunwell's *Management of Cleft Palate Speech*. Where that book provides a picture of all aspects of the multidisciplinary care of individuals with a cleft, this book focuses specifically on speech, and on assessment and intervention for speech problems associated with a cleft. We have both learnt a lot from conversations with our postgraduate students, who come from all over the world, and hope that this book reflects that learning process and will, in turn, prove useful to all of our future students.

We have clearly been very lucky that such a strong and inspiring set of researchers agreed to collaborate with us on this project. It has been a pleasure and a privilege to work with them. And we have been lucky, also, in having a series of very supportive (and unflappable!) editors at Wiley-Blackwell, who guided us patiently throughout the process, with all its attendant hiccups and delays. Our families should get a mention, too, for their support and forbearance!

Sara Howard and Anette Lohmander

Part One
Speech Production and Development

Sara Howard[1] and Anette Lohmander[2]

[1]University of Sheffield, Department of Human Communication Sciences, Sheffield, S10 2TA, UK
[2]Karolinska Institutet, Department of Clinical Science, Intervention and Technique, Division of Speech and Language Pathology, SE 141 86, Stockholm, Sweden

In this book we examine the nature and impact of speech difficulties associated with cleft. As with all developmental speech impairments, cleft speech problems have experienced a significant broadening of perspective over the last century. Following a long period when all children's speech difficulties were seen as articulatory in origin, and as being wholly interpretable through a medical model (Macbeth, 1967), there has been a gradual but welcome transformation to the current position, where much more emphasis is placed on other potential areas of difficulty (including phonology, language, literacy and interpersonal communication and interaction, as well as psychological and psychosocial implications). Developmental speech impairment is thus now situated within a social context. This fits comfortably with developments over the last decade or so, which have sought to classify and consider speech, language and communication impairments using the ICF (the International Classification of Function, Disability and Health; WHO (World Health Organization), 2001). In this book we use the ICF throughout as a point of reference.

Even a glance at the structure and headings used by the ICF indicates how useful it can be for extending our understanding of the possible impact of a communication

Cleft Palate Speech: Assessment and Intervention, First Edition. Edited by Sara Howard, Anette Lohmander.

impairment associated with cleft palate. There are two main parts ('Functioning and Disability' and 'Contextual Factor') with subcomponents which include, for the former, Body Structures, Body Functions, and Activity and Participation, and for the latter, Environmental Factors and Personal Factors. Such is the value of this framework that in the United Kingdom the Royal College of Speech and Language Therapists, in its manual on commissioning and planning services for cleft palate and velopharyngeal impairment (VPI), provides a detailed description of the impact of a cleft which relates specifically to the ICF classification (RCSLT (Royal College of Speech and Language Therapists), 2009). The ICF provides what McLeod (2006) describes as as 'biopsycho-social view of health' and, thus, of communication impairment.

It is noteworthy, of course, that unlike many types of developmental speech impairment, cleft speech problems do, indeed, have a physical basis, and thus the ICF subcomponent Body Structures is relevant in a way which is not the case for most children with speech difficulties. Thus, we need to understand what the anatomical and functional constraints on speech production are likely to be, as well as being aware of how physical structure and function are likely to be affected, over the lifespan, and over the course of speech and language development, by surgical intervention. Chapters in the following section consider each of these issues and also reflect on current evidence for different methods of assessment and intervention. The ways in which speech development for a child with a cleft palate are likely to be similar to and different from speech development in children without a cleft is clearly a hugely important area, which is also addressed in this section.

To make clinical, diagnostic decisions and to plan effective intervention, we need to be able to distinguish between speech difficulties directly attributable to the cleft and its consequences (including the likelihood of hearing impairment), and the coexistence of more general phonological delay or disorder. Such diagnosis can only take place if we have detailed information about the typical course(s) of speech and language development for children with a cleft. The ICF component 'Body Functions' is relevant here, including, as it does, intellectual and cognitive function, and temperament and personality, as well as specific aspects of speech production, including articulation, voice, fluency and also hearing (McLeod and Bleile, 2004).

In seeking a wider, more holistic perspective on the impact of a speech impairment, the ICF can also help us to understand the effects of a cleft on a child's ability to participate more broadly in social interaction, across different contexts, including vital areas such as education, family and social life. The ICF components remind us that a communication impairment is not just the property of an individual, but is constantly negotiated between different individuals, in different contexts: a child's intelligibility, for example, will differ depending on when, why, where and with whom they are talking. As the title of McCormack et al.'s article (2010) eloquently puts it 'My speech problem, your listening problem and my frustration ...'. Later chapters in this book deal in detail with intelligibility and with the child's ability to participate in society through effective use of communicate.

The second of the main parts of the ICF, Contextual Factors, encourages us to consider the impact of a cleft palate and cleft speech difficulties in terms of the systems, policies, services and attitudes existing in a particular society, country or culture that will exert an influence on the support a child is likely to receive. Taking this perspective, one can quickly see how the impact of a cleft could be very different in the developed versus developing (minority versus majority) world, where infrastructure and attitudes may differ significantly. One of the chapters in the following section addresses this important issue. Personal factors, such as age, gender, race, character and general psychological resilience and well-being, will also need to be taken into account when considering the impact of a cleft. Some children with severe speech disorders will nevertheless prove remarkably resilient in the face of their difficulties, whereas others may need specific help to adapt to even mild speech problems (Nash, 2006).

The ICF, then, provides us with a framework which can extend our thinking about the impact of a speech impairment associated with cleft palate and encourage us to take a more holistic view of individuals thus affected (Ma, Threats and Worrall, 2008). The material we cover in this book endeavours to do just that.

References

Ma, E.P.-M., Threats, T. and Worrall, L. (2008) An introduction to the International Classification of Functioning, Disability and Health (ICF) for speech-language pathology: its past, present and future. *International Journal of Speech-Language Pathology*, **10**, 2–8.

Macbeth, E. (1967) Speech therapy as a paramedical subject. *British Journal of Disorders of Communication*, **2**, 69–72.

McCormack, J., McLeod, S., McAllister, L. and Harrison, L. (2010) My speech problem, your listening problem, and my frustration: the experience of living with childhood speech impairment. *Language, Speech, and Hearing Services in Schools*, **41**, 379–392.

McLeod, S. (2006) An holistic view of a child with unintelligible speech: insights from the ICF and ICF-CY. *Advances in Speech-Language Pathology*, **8**, 293–315.

McLeod, S. and Bleile, K. (2004) The ICF: a framework for setting goals for children with speech impairment. *Child Language, Teaching and Therapy*, **20**, 199–219.

Nash, P. (2006) The assessment and management of psychosocial aspects of reading and language impairments, *Dyslexia, Speech and Language: A Practitioner's Handbook*, 2nd edn (eds M. Snowling and J. Stackhouse), John Wiley & Sons Ltd, pp. 278–301. Chapter 13.

RCSLT (Royal College of Speech and Language Therapists) (2009) RCSLT Resource Manual for Commissioning and Planning Services for SLCS: Cleft Lip/Palate and Velopharyngeal Impairment, RCSLT, London.

WHO (World Health Organization) (2001) ICF: International Classification of Functioning, Disability and Health, WHO, Geneva, Switzerland.

1

Physical Structure and Function and Speech Production Associated with Cleft Palate

Martin Atkinson[1] and Sara Howard[2]

[1] University of Sheffield, School of Clinical Dentistry, Sheffield, S10 2TA, UK
[2] University of Sheffield, Department of Human Communication Sciences, Sheffield, S10 2TA, UK

1.1   Introduction

Speakers with a cleft lip and/or palate contend with unusual structure and function of the vocal organs from birth and physical abnormalities may persist after surgical intervention. (Surgery itself, for many individuals with a cleft, consists of a series of interventions over an extended period, so both structural and functional changes to the speech apparatus may be a feature of the entire period of speech development). These differences and changes may have a profound effect on speech production and speech development, and cleft lip and palate is one area where a significant proportion of the speech difficulties encountered (although not necessarily all) can be traced back in some way to an anatomical or physiological cause. This chapter explores some of the links between atypical vocal organ structure and function in cleft lip and palate, and those many and varied features encountered in speech production associated with cleft palate. Of course, some of these issues are also dealt with in other chapters in this book (Chapters 3, 5, 8, 10, 11 and 12), so the reader is directed, where appropriate, to seek further information from these chapters; this chapter, therefore, focuses on those issues not discussed

Cleft Palate Speech: Assessment and Intervention, First Edition. Edited by Sara Howard, Anette Lohmander.
© 2011 John Wiley & Sons, Ltd. Published 2011 by John Wiley & Sons, Ltd.

elsewhere in the book. More detailed accounts of the physical structures and functions associated with speech production can be found in Atkinson and White (1992) and Atkinson and McHanwell (2002).

1.2   The Hard and Soft Palates and the Velopharynx

1.2.1   Anatomy of the Hard and Soft Plate

The palate comprises the rigid bony hard palate anteriorly and the mobile muscular soft plate (velum) posteriorly. The shape of the hard plate is variable but is usually a concave dome. However it may take on a V-shape with the apex superiorly, which narrows the hard palate. This configuration of the hard palate often accompanies a class II malocclusion (Section1.5.1); as the upper dental arch is narrowed the posterior teeth cannot align along a curved dental arch but follow the V-shape, pushing the anterior teeth forward. The bony plate is formed from components of two pairs of bones; the palatine plates of the maxilla form the anterior two thirds and the horizontal plates of the palatine bones form the remainder. The bones are joined at sutures. A midline suture marks the line of fusion of the two halves of the palate during palatogenesis and terminates anteriorly at the incisive foramen, another landmark relating to the development of the palate. The sutures are, of course, covered in life by the mucosa lining the mouth. However, the site of the incisive foramen is marked by a small incisive papilla visible just behind the central incisor teeth.

The soft palate extends from the posterior border of the hard palate. Four pairs of muscles form the soft palate (Figure 1.1). The tensor veli palatini tenses the velum by exerting a lateral force; these muscles are tendinous within the soft palate and the other muscles are attached to the tendons. The levator veli palatini raises the soft palate. Note that the tensor and levator palatini attach to the Eustachian tube and open it when the velum is raised or tensed, so that fluid drains from the middle ear cavity and air pressure is equalised on the either side of the eardrum. These two muscles are often inefficient in the early stages of cleft palate repair so that the Eustachian tube does not open. Drainage of the middle ear is therefore poor, accounting for the high incidence of 'glue ear' in cleft clients. The palatoglossus and palatophayngeus muscles depress the velum. The soft palate has a backward extension, the uvula which is very variable in shape and size.

1.2.2   Embryology of Palate

In the early embryo, the oral cavity is a slit between the frontonasal process that overlies the developing brain and the first pharyngeal arch. The first arch forms the mandible and associated structures but also the maxilla, including a large component of the palate. The palate develops between the fourth and twelfth week of pregnancy to separate the nasal and oral cavities. It develops from three components that change shape and position from their original location during subsequent growth and development and must fuse together to form the palate. A small triangular component, the primary palate, develops from the frontonasal process as the nasal cavities develop around the fifth week.

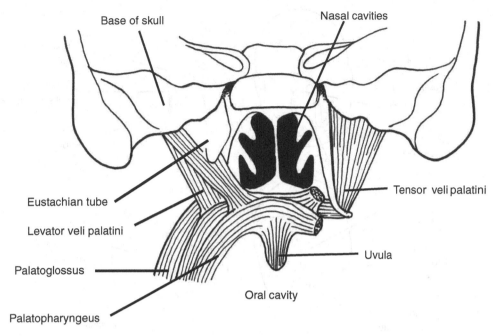

Figure 1.1 The muscles of the soft palate viewed from behind looking into the posterior nasal aperture. (Reproduced with permission from Atkinson & McHanwell, 2002.)

The primary palate forms the area behind the four upper incisor teeth only as far back as the incisive foramen. At six weeks, two palatine processes grow in from either side of the first arch. Logically they would be expected to grow horizontally but they actually grow downwards. The reason for this apparent peculiarity is that the tongue develops very early and fills the developing oral cavity, thus deflecting the palatine processes downwards. Around eight weeks, the mandible widens out and the tongue drops into its conventional position, thus no longer impeding the palatine processes. The palatine processes dramatically 'flip up' into a horizontal position. This change of orientation, palatal elevation, is not simply a consequence of tongue displacement but depends on the build up of hydrophilic (water binding) chemicals that make the processes turgid. At this stage the three processes are separated by quite wide gaps but over the next two weeks the processes grow and converge. Where they make contact, a chain of reactions is triggered within the epithelial cells covering the processes that kill the cells; this process is known as programmed cell death or apoptosis. The death of the epithelial covering allows the underlying tissues to fuse to complete the palate by twelve weeks post-fertilization. The complete palate is invaded by bone anteriorly to form the hard palate and by muscle posteriorly to form the velum; this process is usually complete by about fifteen weeks (Figure 1.2).

From this brief outline of palatogenesis, it is clear that there are several stages where the processes may be disrupted. Essentially, the requisite building blocks may not develop

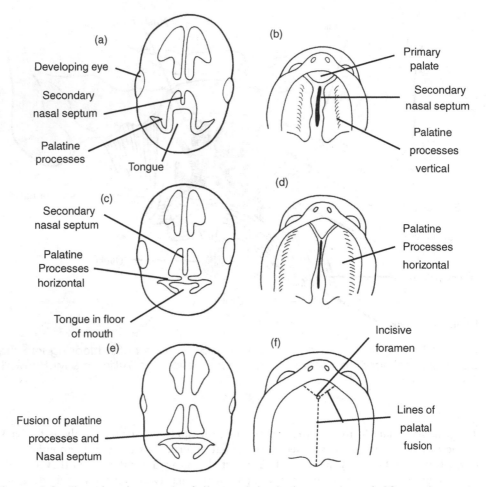

Figure 1.2 The development of the palate between 6 and 12 weeks post-fertilization. (a), (c) and (e) are sections taken through from the top of the head to the mandibular arch. (a) and (b) represent palate formation at about 6–7 weeks, (c) and (d) at 8 weeks as the palate elevates and (e) and (f) at 12 weeks when palatal fusion is complete. (b), (d) and (f) show the sequence of events viewed from the oral aspect of the developing palate. (Reproduced with permission from Atkinson & McHanwell, 2002.)

or may not grow sufficiently; the palatine processes may not elevate if the specific signals to build up the hydrophilic molecules are not given; the processes may not fuse if molecular signals do not trigger apoptosis or if there is any obstruction present. A palatal cleft may manifest anywhere along the Y-shaped lines of fusion between the primary palate and palatine processes (the arms of the Y) and the two palatine processes (the stem of the Y). It can vary from a cleft uvula to a complete bilateral cleft running along the whole extent of the Y and extending into the upper lip.

1.2.3   Velopharyngeal Structure and Function in Relation to Speech Production

Sell and Pereira (Chapter 8) and Sweeney (Chapter 11) provide detailed accounts of the effects of velopharyngeal (VP) problems on speech and on their assessment. Here only a brief account of the main speech production difficulties linked to VP difficulties is given. Because all known spoken languages contain both oral and nasal (and in some cases nasalized) sound segments, the ability to valve air appropriately through the oral and/or nasal cavities in close coordination with phonatory and articulatory activity is a vital component of successful speech production. Where inadequate structure or function of the soft palate and velopharyngeal port do not permit this, as is the case for a speaker with a cleft palate, speech problems are likely to emerge. Interestingly, speech production problems associated with VP insufficiency do not necessarily disappear following surgery and VP function may remain atypical into adulthood (Moon et al., 2007; Mani et al., 2010). Not only range of movement and the ultimate ability to create an adequate seal at the VP port, but also speed and timing of VP movements will affect airflow and resonance (Dotevall, Ejnell and Baker, 2001; Warren, Dalston and Mayo, 1993). Although Kuehn and Moller (2000, p. 351) note that 'excessive nasality or hypernasality is probably the signature characteristic of persons with cleft palate', Peterson-Falzone et al. (2005) state that difficulties achieving velopharyngeal closure can affect not only resonance, but also articulation and phonation, thus providing a reminder of the pervasive consequences of VP difficulties for speech production. Each of the five universal speech parameters proposed by Henningsson et al. (2008) for reporting on the speech of individuals with a cleft palate (hypernasality; hyponasality; audible nasal emission and/or nasal turbulence; consonant production errors; voice disorder) may be traced in some way or another to VP insufficiency.

1.3   The Tonsils and Adenoids

Because speakers with a cleft palate are particularly vulnerable to resonance problems, those structures which may impede velopharyngeal closure are of particular significance for these individuals. The tonsils and adenoids are two such structures, comprising aggregates of lymphoid tissue lying just under the mucosal lining of the pharynx. Lymphoid tissue is involved in defence mechanisms designed to fight bacterial and viral infections, acting as a first line of defence against pathogens entering through the nose or mouth. The paired tonsils (properly termed the palatine tonsils) lie just behind the palatoglossal arch (the anterior pillar of the fauces) that demarcates the junction between the oral cavity and pharynx, and immediately below the lateral attachments of the velum to the tongue and pharynx (Figure 1.3). The adenoids (the pharyngeal tonsils) lie on the posterior wall of the pharynx, behind the nasal cavities, at or just above the point at which the velum makes contact with the pharyngeal wall during elevation and closure.

Although the tonsils do not generally have any effect on articulation, resonance or voice, they may enlarge considerably if they become infected. This, in turn, may cause hypernasality, by obstructing velopharyngeal closure, and has also been linked to the fronting of target velar consonants, by restricting space in the rear of the oral cavity

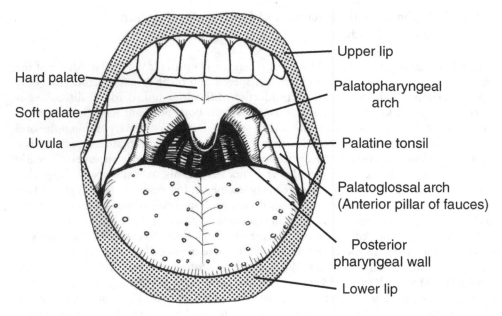

Figure 1.3 A view of the open mouth to show some of the important landmarks. Note the position of the palatine tonsils. (Reproduced with permission from Atkinson & McHanwell, 2002.)

(Maryn *et al.*, 2004). Where a tonsillectomy is performed, significant improvements in speech and voice usually follow (Mora *et al.*, 2009), without any great risk of velopharyngeal inadequacy (Peterson-Falzone, Hardin-Jones and Karnell, 2010).

Compared with the tonsils, the effect of the adenoids on speech production is less clear-cut, due to the fact that for all speakers the adenoids change over time, both in size and in location relative to the other vocal organs. They grow very rapidly after birth to reach their maximum size at about five to six years of age, thereafter decreasing, and they shift from a vertical to a horizontal orientation. Peterson-Falzone, Hardin-Jones and Karnell (2010) provide a reminder that the adenoids are crucial for velopharyngeal (VP) closure in young children, and Maryn *et al.* (2004) suggest that this is so significant that 'veloadenoidal closure' should be added as a fifth category to the different types of VP closure proposed by Skolnick *et al.* (1975). As developmental structural changes take place very gradually, children usually accommodate to them without problems and there is no effect on speech production. However, for children with a submucous cleft or borderline VP inadequacy, the presence of the adenoidal pad may have been critical to achieving adequate VP closure and in these children the normal decrease in size may result in resonance problems. Conversely, enlarged adenoids may cause hyponasality and open mouth breathing, and in some cases therefore surgery may be indicated. However, the sudden structural changes brought about by an adenoidectomy may then cause hypernasality, as the child fails to adjust to the increased velopharyngeal port space (Witzel *et al.*, 1986).

1.4 The Larynx

The larynx plays a key role in speech production, acting as it does as an articulator (for sounds like [h] and [ʔ]), as an airstream initiator (in the production of ejectives and implosives), and as the source of phonation, both at the segmental level, for voiced-voiceless segmental contrasts, and at the level of voice quality and overall vocal settings (Laver, 1994). For normal voicing, the tensed vocal folds vibrate in the egressive airstream. The vocal folds are attached anteriorly very close to the midline of the inner aspect of the thyroid cartilage and posteriorly to the vocal processes of the widely spaced arytenoids cartilages thus forming a V-shaped glottis with the point of the V anteriorly (Figure 1.4). For phonation, the vocal folds must be approximated to build up subglottal pressure and tensed. Approximation (adduction) is achieved by sliding the arytenoid cartilages together on the upper rim of the cricoid cartilage. Tension is created by tilting the anterior part of the cricoid upwards towards the thyroid cartilage ('closing

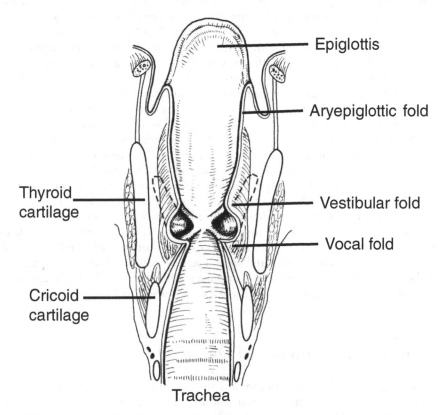

Epiglottis

Aryepiglottic fold

Thyroid cartilage

Vestibular fold

Vocal fold

Cricoid cartilage

Trachea

Figure 1.4 A schematic diagram of the larynx viewed from the posterior aspect. The larynx has been opened to present a clearer view of the positions of the vocal and vestibular folds. Note also the position of the aryepiglottic folds forming the lateral borders of the laryngeal entrance. (Reproduced with permission from Atkinson & McHanwell, 2002.)

the visor'). The cricoid pivots about two thirds of the way back so that the posterior lamina bearing the arytenoids is carried backwards and downwards, thus extending the distance between the anterior and posterior attachments of the vocal folds; the folds are lengthened, tensed and thinned. Tilting the arytenoids forward on the cricoid cartilage has the opposite effects. Because the backward and forward movements are produced by different sets of muscles, they can be varied independently to produce changes in pitch and loudness.

The vestibular folds lie about 2 mm above the vocal folds but are attached more laterally on the arytenoids, so are not normally in the direct egressive air stream. They also lack direct muscle control and therefore cannot be adjusted like the vocal folds. Forced over-contraction of muscles that adduct the vocal folds can tilt the apices of the arytenoids inwards to approximate the vestibular folds and bring them into the air stream. Adduction of the apices of the arytenoid cartilages will also approximate the aryepiglottic folds. The aryepiglottic folds pass from the lateral rim of the epiglottis to the apices of the arytenoids and contribute to the oval profile of the laryngeal entrance. The epiglottis is made of elastic cartilage and moves passively. The flimsy aryepiglottic muscles in the folds cannot overcome the elasticity of the epiglottis but alter the outline of the laryngeal entrance from an oval to a slit during swallowing to minimize the risk of aspiration of foodstuffs. Coupled with extreme adduction of the cartilage apices, these folds could possibly approximate sufficiently to allow some degree of phonation.

Peterson-Falzone, Hardin-Jones and Karnell (2010, p. 240) comment, 'It is clear … that phonation disorders are more common in this population than in individuals without clefts', and Cavalli (Chapter 10) provides an extensive discussion of the voice problems associated with a cleft palate, illustrating how this is largely due to muscle tension disorders, possibly as a compensation for velopharyngeal problems (Chapter 10). There is evidence that laryngeal structures not usually involved in phonation may be recruited in such circumstances (Kawano *et al.*, 1997). In the review of the literature provided by Van Lierde *et al.* (2004) the following voice problems were noted as having been found in the speech production of individuals with cleft palate: breathiness, hoarseness, harshness, aphonia, pitch problems, reduced intensity ('soft voice syndrome') and limited vocal range. As with many speech production features associated with cleft palate, many of these can be seen as stemming from compensatory behaviours aimed at reducing or disguising hypernasality and audible nasal emission. Where vocal fold vibration is associated with the production of specific sound segments (to make distinctions between voiced and voiceless sounds) this does not appear to be a particular problem for speakers with a cleft palate.

1.5   The Jaws, Dentition and Occlusion

In discussing the effect that variations in oral and dental structure might have on speech production in the cleft population, it is important to note that wide variation is also a feature of speakers without a cleft (Beck, 2010). Within the cleft population, it is also the case that many individuals develop and produce speech normally (Peterson-Falzone, Hardin-Jones and Karnell, 2010). These two observations support the long-documented assertion that speakers are able to compensate successfully for variation in the speech apparatus and that unusual oral structure does not inevitably imply unusual speech production (Fairbanks and Lintner, 1951; Nishikubo *et al.*, 2009). Nevertheless, there is also a significant, if equivocal, literature linking some of the misarticulations produced by speakers with cleft lip and palate to atypical palatal morphology, occlusion and dentition: at issue here appears to be the degree to which speakers adapt to unusual structure and function.

1.5.1   The Jaws

The anatomical and dynamic relationships between the mandible and maxilla and the upper and lower teeth are important to ensure correct function for both speech and non-speech activities. In typical speech development, jaw movements appear to stabilize during speech production at an earlier point than either labial or lingual movements (Green, Moore and Reilly, 2002), and this stability is critical for speech production. As Cheng *et al.* (2007, p. 353) suggest 'the jaw provides the foundation necessary for the acquisition of more specialized motor skills', including those of the lips and tongue. Coordination of mandibular and labial movements typically appears to emerge earlier than jaw–tongue coordination and although these are both broadly achieved in infancy, refinement of control and coordination continues throughout early childhood, and perhaps even into adolescence (Green *et al.*, 2002; Smith, 2006). Coordination between the mandible and the tongue is particularly important for tongue-tip sounds, which, of course, have frequently been noted as being especially vulnerable in the speech production of individuals with a cleft palate.

Spatial relationships between the jaws and teeth are also important and are often compromised in individuals with a cleft palate. In a class I dental occlusion, the maxillary arch supporting the upper teeth is wider than the corresponding mandibular arch (Figure 1.5a). The maxilla is positioned such that the upper anterior teeth protrude beyond the lower teeth by about 2 mm when the teeth are brought into occlusion. They also overlap the lower teeth by a similar amount in a vertical dimension. A class II occlusion occurs if the maxilla is too far forward with respect to the mandible: note that this misalignment may be due either to an oversized maxilla or to a reduced mandible (Figure 1.5b). When the converse applies and the mandible is anterior to the maxilla, a class III occlusion is produced in which the lower anterior teeth protrude beyond the upper anterior teeth: this is the most frequently occurring malocclusion in the cleft population (Figure 1.5c).

Dental malocclusions arise when the teeth themselves are malpositioned within dental arches that show a normal relationship. For example, prolonged thumbsucking may displace the upper anterior teeth anteriorly, producing a class II occlusion and/or an anterior open bite. In cleft palate, the teeth are often severely malpositioned as the fusion lines described above pass between the position of upper lateral incisors and canines. The upper dental arch is often narrow, producing a high vaulted palate as the dental arches tend to collapse inward. In many syndromic presentations of cleft palate, there are associated developmental anomalies in the size and position of the maxilla and mandible producing skeletal malocclusions. Repositioning of the teeth and/or jaws can be achieved by orthodontic intervention and/or maxillofacial surgery (Chapter 5).

Johnson and Sandy (1999) suggest that the presence, absence or malpositioning of individual teeth do not appear to have a significant effect on speech sound articulation,

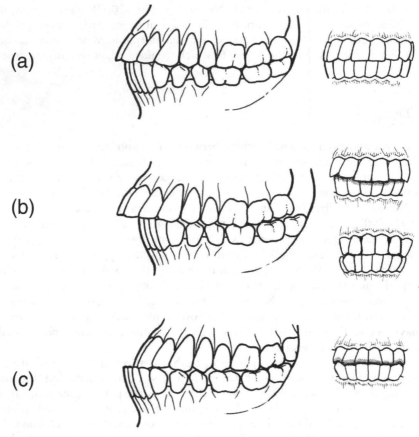

Figure 1.5 A diagram to show the relationship of the teeth in (a). a Class I occlusion, (b) a class II occlusion and (c) a class III occlusion. The left hand diagrams show the relationships of all the teeth. The right hand diagrams show the appearance of the anterior teeth as seen when the client bites together. Note there are two variations in the appearance of the anterior teeth in a Class II occlusion; the incisors may show excess over jet and 'stick out' (division i) or the lateral incisors may override the central incisors, which are pushed back (division ii). (Reproduced with permission from Atkinson & McHanwell, 2002.)

probably because of individual speakers' abilities to compensate for minor structural variation, although Chait *et al.* (2002) suggest that absent lateral teeth may result in misarticulated sibiliant fricative production. A factor which is, however, implicated in sound segment misarticulation is anterior open bite (AOB). Bernstein (1954) was one of the first to note an association between AOB and misarticulation in children's speech, and a specific link to misarticulated fricative and affricates, together with a generally advanced lingual setting for speech has been identified using electropalatography by Suzuki *et al.* (1981), Hiki and Itoh (1986) and Cayley *et al.* (2000).

Malocclusion, however, has also frequently been associated with misarticulation. In Class II and III occlusal relationships, where the maxilla and mandible fall into atypical alignment, the active and passive articulators will consequently also be misaligned. Thus, for example, in a Class II occlusion the bottom lip may fall into a closer vertical relationship with the upper incisors, or even the alveolar ridge, than it does with the upper lip; conversely in the case of a Class III occlusion, the top lip may naturally oppose the lower incisors rather than the bottom lip. Similar misalignments between the tongue tip and blade and the upper teeth and alveolar ridge will also exist. Although it is clear that such minor differences could be compensated for by quite small articulatory adjustments, where the speaker does not actively compensate, atypical articulatory strictures are likely to occur. Some of the unusual places of articulation included in the Extensions to the IPA (Duckworth *et al.*, 1990), including reverse labiodental, labioalveolar, linguolabial, reflect these articulatory patterns in some speakers with cleft lip and palate (Chapter 7). Although Hassan, Naini and Gill (2007, p. 2543) caution that 'there is no clear evidence directly relating malocclusions to speech discrepancies', a series of studies nevertheless point to the potential vulnerability of dental, alveolar and postalveolar segments (particularly the sibilant fricatives) in both Class II and Class III occlusion (Laine, Jaroma and Linnasalo, 1987; Giannini *et al.*, 1995; Laitinen, Ranta and Haapenen, 1999). Where the alignment of maxilla and mandible is corrected by orthognathic surgery some of these misarticulations have been shown by both perceptual and instrumental studies to improve spontaneously and quite rapidly (Vallino, 1990; Wakumoto *et al.*, 1996) although for some speakers these changes may not be maintained a year after surgery (Lee *et al.*, 2002).

Nishikubo *et al.* (2009) question the link between malocclusion and misarticulation, suggesting, on the basis of 3-D palatal imaging, that a more significant predictor of misarticulation in cleft speakers may be the general size and shape of the oral cavity (Chapter 3). Once again, a number of studies seem to support this view, linking relative length and/or shape of palate to various misarticulations of alveolar segments (Hiki and Itoh, 1986; Laine, Jaroma and Linnasalo, 1987; Okazaki, Kato and Onizuka, 1991). It may, however, be not so much structural as sensory anomalies which impact on articulation in speech production associated with cleft palate. Hardcastle (1975) demonstrated changes in lingualpalatal contact patterns for sibilant fricatives in typical speakers where lingual sensation was decreased by application of anaesthesia and, more recently, Premkumar, Venkatesan and Rangachari (2010) have related the misarticulations associated with anterior open bite and tongue-thrusting with an overall reduction in intra-oral sensation. It might also be suspected that any reduction in sensation consequent on post-surgical scarring in the region of the alveolar ridge and hard palate might also affect articulatory patterns in speakers with a repaired cleft palate.

1.6   Symmetry: Structure and Function

Studies have identified significant structural asymmetries in the face (Bugaighis *et al.*, 2010) and the palate and oral cavity (Kilpeläinen and Laine-Avala, 1996) (although not the mandible; Kurt *et al.*, 2010) in individuals with a cleft palate, and structural asymmety has, in turn, been linked to misarticulation (Nishikubo *et al.*, 2009). At the same time, functional asymmetries of labial and lingual articulation have been noted in cleft speakers and speakers with other speech impairments (Howard, 1994; Gibbon, 2004; Cheng *et al.*, 2007). Nevertheless, it is important to note that there is no simple relationship between structural asymmetry and speech production. Minor asymmetries in lingual behaviour are common in typical speech production (Marchal *et al.*, 1988), but it may be the extent of asymmetry which is significant in the perceptual impression of misarticulation (Howard, Clark and Whiteside, 1994).

1.7   The Tongue

The tongue could be described as a bag of muscles, and lingual function, dependent on these muscles, is notoriously challenging to explain (Atkinson and McHanwell, 2002). It is usually straightforward to predict the action of a given muscle, by looking at the bony points to which the two ends of the muscle are attached and anticipating what action contraction of the muscle will have on any joint that the muscle passes over. This is not the case with the tongue: one of the two sets of lingual muscles, the extrinsic muscles, only has one bony attachment, with the other end anchored to other muscles in the tongue. The other set, the intrinsic muscles, has both attachments within the tongue itself (Figure 1.6).

Anatomical textbooks usually suggest that the extrinsic muscles alter the position of the tongue, drawing it towards the anchorage of the extrinsic muscle in question on the mandible or skull, and the intrinsic muscles alter the shape of the tongue. A moment's thought tells us that this is a vast, if convenient, oversimplification. Theoretically, it may be possible to alter tongue position without a change in shape, but it is impossible to alter shape without altering the position of the tongue relative to other articulators. The tongue is, therefore, the best example of the axiom that muscles act as groups rather than as individual entities. This emanates from the processing and control of motor activity in the brain. The brain thinks in terms of overall patterns of activity and sequencing of muscle contractions to produce a given complex movement; the rate, range and force of contraction of the individual muscles required to produce the movement is then superimposed on the overall patterning and movement sequence. When students studying anatomical specimens of the tongue encounter it for the first time, they are usually very surprised by its large size; it is much bigger than they have predicted. The oral, and most mobile, part of the tongue accounts for only about half of the organ; the posterior pharyngeal part is the other 'unseen' half.

Surprisingly, the tongue is usually unaffected by developmental disturbances affecting the face, palate and jaws, even the most severe, as its embryological origins are quite different (Atkinson and McHanwell, 2002) and, consequently, lingual structure and function is generally considered to be unaffected by a cleft palate (Peterson-Falzone, Hardin-Jones and Karnell, 2010). For a small number of individuals with a specific genetic abnormality, however, a cleft palate may be associated with ankyloglossia (tongue tie) (Braybrook *et al.*, 2002), thus potentially affecting the successful elevation of the tongue-tip for alveolar and dental sounds, although how much ankyloglossia affects articulation remains unclear (Suter and Bornstein, 2009). In general, though, the atypical lingualpalatal contact patterns and overall lingual settings reported in the speech of individuals with cleft palate are deemed to be adaptive behaviours which may be linked to velopharyngeal inadequacy and its primary effects on speech. Thus, electropalatog-

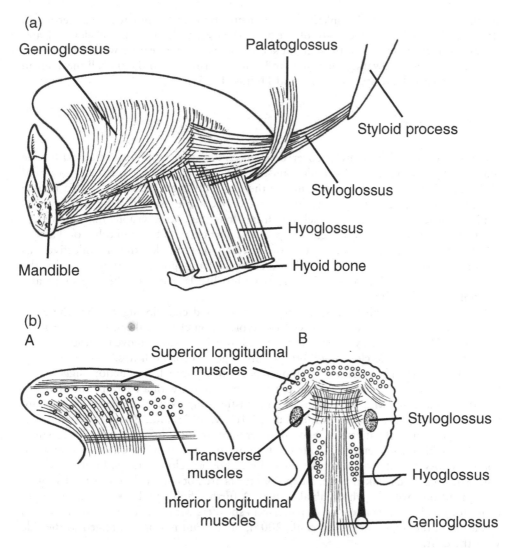

Figure 1.6 The muscles of the tongue. (a) shows the extrinsic muscles and their attachments. (b) shows two views of the intrinsic muscles and their relationship to the extrinsic muscles as seen in a longitudinal section (A) and a cross section of the tongue (B). (Reproduced with permission from Atkinson & McHanwell, 2002.)

raphy has revealed a range of unusual lingualpalatal contact patterns in speakers with cleft palate, including retracted articulation of alveolar and postalveolar consonants, lateralization, palatalization, broad and undifferentiated patterns with overuse of the tongue dorsum, and double articulations, all of which may stem to some extent from articulatory strategies for the prevention or masking of hypernasality and nasal emission (Gibbon, 2004; Howard, 2004; Chapter 12). The retracted patterns of articulation and the tendency to make greater than normal use of the tongue dorsum in segmental articulation seem also to be linked to a frequently observed habitual lingual setting in cleft speakers, whereby the body of the tongue is generally held in an elevated and somewhat retracted position throughout speech production, a feature which it has been argued also aids in elevating the velum and thus contributing to the overall mechanism of velopharyngeal closure (Lawrence and Philips, 1975).

1.8   The Lips

The lips are formed by muscles covered on the outside by non-hairy skin and on the oral side by oral mucosa. A circular muscle, the orbicularis oris, surrounds the oral cavity and is the basis of the structure of the lips. Although anatomically this muscle appears to be a single entity, in reality it is a very complex structure formed by eight semi-independent parts, two in each quadrant. It is these subdivisions that enable the exquisitely precise labial movements in speech in particular, but also in other oral activities. Orbicularis oris is one of a group of subcutaneous muscles known collectively as the muscles of facial expression. Other members of this group exert traction on the upper lip and lower lip, working in concert with orbicularis oris to alter the shape and position of the lips during articulation.

Studies of motor activity in speakers with a repaired cleft lip suggest that there are some significant functional differences from typical non-cleft speakers. For the production of bilabial segments, where the upper and lower lips need to move together to form a stricture of complete closure, differences are reported for both lips. Electromagnetic articulography (EMA) studies of lip movements during speech production suggest that there is more variability in movement patterns in speakers with a cleft lip, and that this variability increases with increases in the linguistic complexity of the utterances examined (Rutjens, Spauwen and van Lieshout, 2001). Van Lieshout, Rutjens and Spauwen (2002) also identified patterns of reduced upper lip movement in speakers with a repaired cleft lip, which complements Trotman, Barlow and Faraway's discussion (2007) of compensatory activity found for the lower lip in bilabial closure tasks. In other words, where lip surgery has taken place, the motor effects are not confined to the site of surgery but spread out over the whole labial system. A further finding which may have significance for the development of speech patterns in speakers with a cleft lip is that of reduced sensation in the upper lip (Essick et al., 2005), once again not only confined to the side with the cleft.

A short and/or tight upper lip, consequent on lip surgery, may affect lip closure for bilabial sounds and also the lip-rounding necessary for vowels such as [ʊ] and [u] (Peterson-Falzone et al., 2005). Interestingly, even where normal labial activity for bilabial sounds is achieved, some speakers with a cleft lip and palate exhibit other unusual articulatory activity during the production of bilabials, in the form of complete lingual-palatal closure patterns concomitant with the lip closure (Gibbon and Crampin, 2002), a pattern which is not found in typical speech production (Gibbon, Lee and Yuen, 2007) and which may, therefore, be a further compensatory pattern associated with the speech production of individuals with a cleft palate.

Although it is generally supposed that speakers with an isolated cleft lip are less likely to have speech output problems than those with a cleft lip and palate or an isolated cleft palate, it cannot be assumed that they will not have any difficulties. A study by Vallino,

Zuker and Napoli (2008) suggests that both articulation and language problems occur at significantly higher rates in individuals with an isolated cleft lip than in the non-cleft population, although they also note, perhaps unsurprisingly, that resonance is generally not a problem.

1.9 Summary: Compensations Across Systems

Although information has been presented here on different articulators and vocal organs and their effect on speech production associated with a cleft palate in a sequence of separate sections, the point cannot be overstated that in speech production no organ or system ever functions in isolation. This is amply illustrated in the literature, where reports of the interrelationship between different subsystems, and of compensations within and across subsystems, serve as a reminder of the complexity of speech production associated with cleft and underscore the heterogeneity of the population of individuals with a cleft lip and/or palate. Different speakers find different solutions to the challenge of producing speech sounds in order to interact with others. It is hoped that this account gives a flavour of the varied features encountered in the speech of individuals with a cleft palate and of some of the reasons for these features, but there will always be a new speaker to be encountered who will offer a slightly different solution to the challenge of being intelligible in the face of structural and functional difficulties.

References

Atkinson, M. and McHanwell, S. (2002) *Basic Medical Science for Speech and Language Therapy Students*, Whurr, London.

Atkinson, M.E. and White, F.H. (1992) *Principles of Anatomy and Oral Anatomy for Dental Students*, Churchill Livingstone, London.

Beck, J. (2010) Organic variation of the vocal apparatus, in *The Handbook of Phonetic Sciences*, 2nd edn (eds W.J. Hardcastle, J. Laver, and F.E. Gibbon), John Wiley & Sons Ltd, Chichester, pp. 155–201.

Bernstein, M. (1954) Speech defects and malocclusion. *American Journal of Orthodontics*, 40, 149–150.

Braybrook, C., Lisgo, S., Doudney, K. *et al.* (2002) Craniofacial expression of human and murine TBX22 correlates with the cleft palate and ankyloglossia phenotype observed in CPX patients. *Human Molecular Genetics*, 11, 2793–2804.

Bugaighis, I., O'Higgins, P., Tiddeman, B. *et al.* (2010) Three-dimensional geometric morphometrics applied to the study of children with cleft lip and/or palate from the North East of England. *European Journal of Orthodontics*, 32 (5), 514–521.

Cayley, A.S., Tindall, A.P., Sampson, W.J. and Butcher, A.R. (2000) Electropalatographic and cephalometric assessment of tongue function in open bite and non-open bite subjects. *European Journal of Orthodontics*, 22, 463–474.

Chait, L., Gavron, G., Graham, C. *et al.* (2002) Modifying the two-stage cleft palate surgical correction. *Cleft Palate-Craniofacial Journal*, 39, 226–232.

Cheng, H.Y., Murdoch, B.E., Goozée, J.V. and Scott, D. (2007) Electropalatographic assessment of tongue-to-palate contact patterns and variability in children, adolescents, and adults. *Journal of Speech, Language, and Hearing Research*, 50, 375–392.

Dotevall, H., Ejnell, H. and Bake, B. (2001) Nasal airflow patterns during the velopharyngeal closing phase in speech in children with and without cleft palate. *Cleft Palate-Craniofacial Journal*, 38, 358–372.

Duckworth, M., Allen, G., Hardcastle, W.J. and Ball, M.J. (1990) Extensions to the International Phonetic Alphabet for the transcription of atypical speech. *Clinical Linguistics & Phonetics*, 4, 273–280.

Essick, G.K., Dorion, C., Rumley, S. *et al.* (2005) Report of altered sensation in patients with cleft lip. *Cleft Palate – Craniofacial Journal*, 42, 178–184.

Fairbanks, G. and Lintner, M.V.H. (1951) A study of minor organic deviations in 'functional' disorders of articulation: 4. The teeth and hard palate. *Journal of Speech and Hearing Disorders*, 16, 273–279.

Giannini, A., Pettorino, M., Savastano, G. *et al.* (1995) Tongue movements in maloccluded subjects. Proceedings of the 13th International Congress of Phonetic Sciences, Vol. 2, 658–661.

Gibbon, F.E. (2004) Abnormal patterns of tongue-palate contact in the speech of individuals with cleft palate. *Clinical Linguistics & Phonetics*, 18, 285–311.

Gibbon, F.E. and Crampin, L. (2002) Labial-lingual double articulations in speakers with cleft palate. *Cleft Palate-Craniofacial Journal*, 39, 40–49.

Gibbon, F.E., Lee, A. and Yuen, I. (2007) Tongue-palate contact during bilabials in normal speech. *Cleft Palate-Craniofacial Journal*, 44, 87–91.

Green, J.R., Moore, C.A. and Reilly, K.J. (2002) The sequential development of jaw and lip control for speech. *Journal of Speech, Language, and Hearing Research*, 45, 66–79.

Hardcastle, W.J. (1975) Some aspects of speech production under controlled conditions of oral anaesthesia and auditory masking. *Journal of Phonetics*, 3, 197–214.

Hassan, T., Naini, F.B. and Gill, D.S. (2007) The effects of orthognathic surgery on speech: a review. *Journal of Oral and Maxillofacial Surgery*, 65 (12), 2536–2543.

Henningsson, G., Kuehn, D., Sell, D. *et al.* (2008) Universal parameters for reporting outcomes in individuals with cleft palate. *Cleft Palate-Craniofacial Journal*, 45, 1–17.

Hiki, S. and Itoh, H. (1986) Influence of palate shape on lingual articulation. *Speech Communication*, 5, 141–158.

Howard, S.J. (1994). Spontaneous phonetic reorganisation following articulation therapy: an electropalatographic study. Proceedings of the 3rd Congress of the International Clinical Phonetics and Linguistics Association, Helsinki (eds R. Aulanko and A.-M. Korpijaakko-Huuhka), University of Helsinki, Helsinki, 67–74.

Howard, S.J. (2004) Compensatory articulatory behaviours in adolescents with cleft palate: comparing the perceptual and instrumental evidence. *Clinical Linguistics and Phonetics*, 18, 313–340.

Howard, S.J., Clark, B. and Whiteside, S. (1994) The perception of sibilant fricatives in typical and atypical speakers. Paper presented at the ASHA (American Speech-Language-Hearing Association) convention, New Orleans, USA (November, 1994).

Johnson, N.C.L. and Sandy, J. (1999) Tooth position and speech – is there a relationship? *The Angle Orthodontist*, 69, 306–310.

Kawano, M., Isshiki, N., Honjo, I. *et al.* (1997) Recent progress in treating patients with cleft palate. *Folia Phoniatrica et Logopaedica*, 49, 117–138.

Kilpeläinen, P.V.J. and Laine-Avala, M.T. (1996) Palatal asymmetry in cleft palate subjects. *Cleft Palate-Craniofacial Journal*, 33, 483–488.

Kuehn, D. and Moller, K. (2000) Speech and language issues in the cleft palate population: the state of the art. *Cleft Palate-Craniofacial Journal*, 37 (4), 348–383.

Kurt, G., Bayram, M., Uysal, T. and Ozer, M. (2010) Mandibular symmetry in cleft lip and palate patients. *European Journal of Orthodontics*, 32, 19–23.

Laine, T., Jaroma, M. and Linnasalo, A.-L. (1987) Relationships between interincisal occlusion and components of speech. *Folia Phoniatrica et Logopedica*, 39, 78–86.

Laitinen, J., Ranta, R. and Haapenen, M.L. (1999) Associations between dental occlusion and misarticulations of Finnish dental consonants in cleft lip/palate children. *European Journal of Oral Sciences*, **107**, 109–113.

Laver, J. (1994) *Principles of Phonetics*, Cambridge University Press, Cambridge.

Lawrence, C.W. and Philips, B.J. (1975) A telefluoroscopic study of lingual contacts. *The Cleft Palate Journal*, **12** (1), 85–94.

Lee, A.S.Y., Whitehill, T., Ciocca, V. and Samman, N. (2002) Acoustic and perceptual analysis of the sibilant sound /s/ before and after orthognathic surgery. *Journal of Oral and Maxillofacial Surgery*, **60**, 364–372.

Mani, M., Morén, S., Thorvardsson, O. *et al.* (2010) Objective assessment of the nasal airway in unilateral cleft lip and palate: a long-term study. *Cleft Palate-Craniofacial Journal*, **47**, 217–224.

Marchal, A., Farnetani, E., Hardcastle, W.J. and Butcher, A. (1988) Cross-language EPG data on lingual asymmetry. *Journal of the Acoustical Society of America*, **84** (S1), 127.

Maryn, Y., Van Lierde, K.M., De Bodt, M. and Van Cauwenberge, P. (2004) The effects of adenoidectomy and tonsillectomy on speech and nasal resonance. *Folia Phoniatrica et Logopaedica*, **56**, 182–191.

Moon, J.B., Kuehn, D.P., Chan, G. and Zhao, L. (2007) Induced velopharyngeal fatigue effects in speakers with repaired palatal clefts. *Cleft Palate-Craniofacial Journal*, **44**, 251–260.

Mora, R., Jankowska, B., Crippa, B. *et al.* (2009) Effects of tonsillectomy on speech and voice. *Journal of Voice*, **23**, 614–618.

Nishikubo, M., Hirihara, N., Gomi, A. *et al.* (2009) 3-D analysis of palatal morphology associated with palatalized articulation in patients with unilateral cleft lip and palate. *Oral Science International*, **6**, 36–45.

Okazaki, K., Kato, M. and Onizuka, T. (1991) Palate morphology in children with cleft palate with palatalized articulation. *Annals of Plastic Surgery*, **26**, 156–163.

Peterson-Falzone, S., Trost-Cardamone, J., Karnell, M. and Hardin-Jones, M. (2005) *The Clinician's Guide to Treating Cleft Palate Speech*, Mosby, St Louis.

Peterson-Falzone, S., Hardin-Jones, M. and Karnell, M. (2010) *Cleft Palate Speech*, 4th edn. Mosby, St Louis.

Premkumar, S., Venkatesan, S.A. and Rangachari, S. (2011) Altered oral sensory perception in tongue thrusters with an anterior open bite. *European Journal of Orthodontics*, **33**, 139–142.

Rutjens, C.A.W., Spauwen, P.H.M. and van Lieshout, P.H.H.M. (2001) Lip movements in patients with a cleft lip and/or palate. *Cleft Lip-Craniofacial Journal*, **38**, 468–475.

Skolnick, M.L., Shprintzen, R.J., McCall, G.N. and Rakoff, S. (1975) Patterns of velopharyngeal closure in subjects with repaired cleft palate and normal speech: a multi-view videofluoroscopic analysis. *Cleft Palate Journal*, **12**, 369–376.

Smith, A. (2006) Speech motor development: integrating muscles, movements and linguistic units. *Journal of Communication Disorders*, **39**, 331–349.

Suter, V.G.A. and Bornstein, M.M. (2009) Ankyloglossia: facts and myths in diagnosis and treatment. *Journal of Periodontology*, **80**, 1204–1219.

Suzuki, N., Sakuma, T., Michi, K.-I. and Ueno, T. (1981) The articulatory characteristics of the tongue in anterior open bite: observation by dynamic palatography. *International Journal of Oral Surgery*, **10** (Suppl. 1), 299–303.

Trotman, C.-A., Barlow, S.M. and Faraway, J. (2007) Functional outcomes of cleft lip surgery. Part III: measurement of lip forces. *Cleft Palate-Craniofacial Journal*, **44**, 617–623.

Vallino, L.D. (1990) Speech, velopharyngeal function, and hearing before and after orthognathic surgery. *Journal of Oral and Maxillofacial Surgery*, **48**, 1274–1281.

Vallino, L.D., Zuker, R. and Napoli, J.A. (2008) A study of speech, language, hearing, and dentition in children with cleft lip only. *Cleft Palate-Craniofacial Journal*, **45**, 485–494.

Van Lierde, K.M., Claeys, S., De Bodt, M. and Van Cauwenberge, P. (2004) Vocal quality characteristics in children with cleft palate: a multiparameter approach. *Journal of Voice*, 18, 354–362.

Van Lieshout, P.H.H.M., Rutjens, C.A.W. and Spauwen, P.H.M. (2002) The dynamics of interlip coupling in speakers with a repaired unilateral cleft-lip history. *Journal of Speech, Language, and Hearing Research*, 45, 5–19.

Wakumoto, M., Isaacson, K.G., Friel, S. *et al.* (1996) Preliminary study of articulatory reorganisation of fricative consonants following osteotomy. *Folia Phoniatrica et Logopaedica*, 48, 275–289.

Warren, D.W., Dalston, R.M. and Mayo, R. (1993) Hypernasality in the presence of 'adequate' velopharyngeal closure. *Cleft Palate-Craniofacial Journal*, 30, 150–154.

Witzel, M.A., Rich, R.H., Margar-Bacal, F. and Cox, C. (1986) Velopharyngeal insufficiency after adenoidectomy: an 8-year review. *International Journal of Pediatric Otorhinolaryngology*, 11, 15–20.

2

The Development of Speech in Children with Cleft Palate

Kathy L. Chapman[1] and Elisabeth Willadsen[2]

[1] University of Utah, Department of Communication Sciences and Disorders, Salt Lake City, UT 84103, USA
[2] University of Copenhagen, Department of Scandinavian Studies and Linguistics, DK-2300 Copenhagen, Denmark

2.1 Overview

The purpose of this chapter is to provide an overview of speech development of children with cleft palate with or without cleft lip.[1] The chapter begins with a discussion of the impact of clefting on speech. Next, a brief description of those factors impacting speech development for this population of children is provided. Finally, research examining various aspects of speech development of infants and young children with cleft palate (birth to age five) is reviewed. This final section is organized by typical stages of speech sound development (e.g. pre-speech, the early word stage, and systematic phonology) and includes a summary of typical characteristics for each stage.

[1] Because speech is not typically impacted for children with cleft lip only, the term cleft palate will be used to refer to children with a cleft of the palate with or without a cleft lip.

Cleft Palate Speech: Assessment and Intervention, First Edition. Edited by Sara Howard, Anette Lohmander.
© 2011 John Wiley & Sons, Ltd. Published 2011 by John Wiley & Sons, Ltd.

2.2   The Impact of Clefting on Speech Production

Palatal clefting impacts speech development for babies with cleft palate (CP). Prior to closure of the palatal cleft, coupling between the oral and nasal cavities will almost inevitably result in hypernasal resonance and difficulty with production of consonants requiring intraoral air pressure (e.g. stops, fricatives and affricates). After the palatal cleft is surgically closed, if the surgery was successful in restoring the velopharyngeal mechanism, the child will continue the task of learning the sound system of his/her language. For some children with cleft palate, however, oral nasal coupling may persist post-surgery due to (i) a two-stage surgery protocol that includes early closure of the soft palate and later closure of the hard palate, (ii) a fistula and/or (iii) velopharyngeal inadequacy (VPI). In the face of VPI, the child may 'choose' either a 'passive' or 'active' strategy. A passive strategy occurs when the child makes no effort to lessen the unavoidable consequences of oral–nasal coupling, resulting in nasalization of vowels and voiced consonants, nasal emission/turbulence and/or reduced intraoral air pressure on obstruent targets. In contrast, an active strategy is when the child seemingly tries to prevent the effects of oral–nasal coupling, typically changing the place and/or manner of articulation, especially for the production of obstruents. The change in place of articulation is most often in the posterior direction to a place below the point of velopharyngeal closure (e.g. glottal stops) or posteriorly but within the oral cavity (e.g. velar fricatives) (Hutters and Brøndsted, 1987).

Trost (1981) provided a description of several backed patterns of articulation (i.e. glottal stop, pharyngeal fricative, pharyngeal affricate etc.) referred to as 'compensatory articulations' (CAs) that were observed in American English-speaking children with CP. These backed productions were referred to as 'compensatory' because it was hypothesized that the speaker was attempting to compensate for VPI.

Researchers in the United Kingdom have provided an alternative term 'cleft type realizations' to refer to the CAs described in Trost (1981) and other 'deviations from the normal developmental patterns' that are seen in the speech of individuals with CP (Harding and Grunwell, 1993, p. 55). They employed the framework of Hutters and Brøndsted (1987) to describe those processes that appeared to be 'subconscious' attempts by the child to create phonological contrasts (active processes) versus those that were natural outcomes of VPI (passive processes) (Harding and Grunwell, 1998).

Production of CAs or active processes/strategies has received a great deal of attention in the cleft palate literature. While most studies of speech outcome comment on the presence or absence of these productions, at least a few investigators have suggested that CAs may be decreasing in the speech of children with cleft palate due to younger ages at time of primary palatal surgery, more aggressive secondary management of VPI (Hardin-Jones and Jones, 2005) or greater access to intervention (Sell *et al.*, 2001). Comparisons of CA use are difficult to make across studies, especially if the investigators are from different countries (discussion of differences in characterization and description of these errors across studies is given in Sell *et al.*, 2001 and Chapter 9). However, it appears that glottal stops are the most frequently occurring CA identified in the speech of children with CP cross-linguistically.

Acquisition of the sound system of a language entails learning (i) articulatory placements and movements for correct sound production (i.e. articulation and motor learning)

(Fey, 1992) and (ii) 'the structure and organization' of the sound system of the target language (i.e. phonological learning) (Gierut and Morrisette, 2005, p. 266). The potential effects of palatal clefting on articulation learning are fairly obvious and have been described above. Less well understood and researched is the impact these structural and functional limitations have on phonological learning for children with CP. As initially suggested by Grunwell and colleagues, although the initial 'cause' of the speech problems of children with CP may be cleft related, as the child is also acquiring the sound system of his/her language, phonological learning may also be impacted. The result may be smaller consonant inventories, collapsing of sound categories, sound preferences and so on (Harding and Grunwell, 1998; Chapter 15). Furthermore, the term 'a cleft-type phonological process' was used by Harding and Grunwell (1998) to describe those active processes where the child treats sounds with similar phonological features in the same way (e.g. alveolars are produced as palatals or velars), suggestive of a phonological rule application or a production constraint. Thanks to these early writings of researchers and clinicians in the United Kingdom, there is a better understanding of the potential impact of clefting on the child's developing sound system.

2.3   Variables Impacting Speech Development for Young Children with Cleft Palate

Prior to beginning a description of the speech development of children with CP, two important points must be made that the readers should consider. Firstly, most of the data reported below are based on group studies; yet, children with CP are heterogeneous. Some children with CP begin to show normal speech development soon after surgical repair of the palatal cleft, others achieve age-appropriate speech after a period of speech intervention and orthodontic and/or surgical intervention, and others may never exhibit 'error-free' speech (Chapman, 2009). A number of variables can influence the course of speech development. Many of these variables are identical to those observed for typically developing children or children with developmental speech sound disorders, and others are specific to children with CP (Table 2.1). While some studies of speech development of children with CP have attempted to 'control' (e.g. only including children with unilateral cleft lip and palate) or at least to provide descriptive information regarding some of these variables (e.g. number of ear infections), most have not, making it difficult to judge the relative impact of each on speech outcome.

Secondly, specific study characteristics should be considered when generalizing the information presented in this chapter to other research or clinical samples of children with CP. For example, it is important to consider when the studies were carried out, as it is expected that changes in management (e.g. timing and type of surgery, earlier speech/language intervention and more aggressive management of otitis media) should have a positive effect on speech development over time, making older studies less relevant. Thirdly, most studies describe the speech development of English, Swedish, Danish or Dutch-speaking children with CP. While it is likely that these findings can be generalized to children with CP who are learning other languages, there are language-specific differences that impact acquisition that we are only beginning to learn about (Chapter 9; this chapter Section 2.4.9). Finally, especially for those studies carried out in the

Table 2.1 Variables impacting speech development.

All children	Children with CP
1. Presence of other conditions (e.g. a syndrome, cognitive delay, learning disability and family history of communication impairment)	1. Cleft type and severity
2. Frequency/Management of otitis media and associated hearing status	2. Timing, type, success of surgical and orthodontic management
3. Access to and frequency and quality of speech/language intervention	3. Status of the velopharyngeal mechanism, presence of fistulae, or a residual cleft in the hard palate, and maxillary deviations
4. Individual differences in child and family characteristics	4. Access to and quality of treatment across all disciplines involved in cleft management and family follow-through with recommendations

United States, clinic or hospital-based samples rather than population-based samples are typically used, which could potentially bias the findings.

2.4   Speech Development: Birth to Age Five

2.4.1   Pre-speech Development: What Is Typical?

The journey of a newborn infant from his/her first cry to production of his/her first meaningful word one year later is complex. During the first year of life, sound productions is influenced by two factors: biological constraints and the language that the baby is hearing spoken around him/her. How each of these impacts early pre-speech development is described below.

2.4.1.1   Biological Constraints   A comparison between the vocal tract of an infant and that of an adult highlights the role of biological constraints on infant vocal production (Kent and Murray, 1982; Kent and Vorperian, 2006). Until approximately three months of age, the vocal tract of an infant is said to resemble that of a lower primate (Liberman, Crelin and Klatt, 1972) (Figure 2.1; Table 2.2). As a result, the infant's early vocalizations are primarily vocalic and, as a consequence of 'engagement of the larynx and velopharynx', the infant's breathing and vocalizations are nasal (Kent and Murray, 1982). When the baby is between four and six months of age, separation of the larynx and velopharynx takes place, enabling the infant to produce oral consonants and 'impound intraoral air pressure' needed for obstruent production (Kent, 1981, p. 164). This ability to separate the oral and nasal cavities during sound production is a very important developmental step as the nasal/oral contrast is present in a vast majority of languages

(Maddieson, 1984). At around this same age, 'supraglottal consonant-like sounds' increase while glottal productions decrease (Holmgren *et al.*, 1986, p. 55) representing another important milestone in the baby's phonetic development (Kent and Hodge, 1991). Oller (1980) labelled this period the *expansion phase*, characterized by 'repetitive sequences of vocalizations' varying systematically on a dimension such as pitch and described as 'squeals', 'vowel-like sounds' and 'growls' (Oller and Griebel, 2008, pp. 146–147).

Perhaps the most talked about accomplishment of the pre-speech period is seen some time between five and ten months of age with the emergence of canonical syllables (e.g. bʌ) or productions that have a fully-resonant vowel, a consonant-like sound, normal phonation and adult-like timing (Oller, 2000). It is the strings of repeated CV syllables (e.g. bʌbʌbʌ) that is typically referred to as 'babbling'.

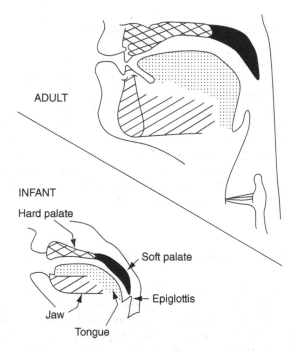

Figure 2.1   The vocal tract of an adult and an infant. (Reproduced from Kent and Murray, (1982), with permission from the American Institute of Physics.)

Table 2.2   Characteristics of the infant vocal tract (Kent and Miolo, 1995).

-Vocal tract (and the pharynx) is shorter
-Oral cavity is broader with the tongue filling almost the entire oral cavity
-The 'right-angle' (characteristic of the adult human vocal tract) is less
    pronounced
-Larynx is higher causing the epiglottis and velum to almost touch (described
    by Kent and colleagues as 'engagement of the larynx and velopharynx'
    (Kent and Miolo, 1995, p. 307)).

2.4.1.2   Influence of the Ambient Language   As the influence of biological constraints on sound production diminishes with age (and growth), influences from the surrounding language increase. For example, it appears that certain sound classes, such as stops, nasals, glides and /h/, are commonly occurring in babbling regardless of the language spoken (Locke, 1983). However, it has also been observed that differences in frequency of occurrence for these sound classes are seen based on the baby's linguistic environment. For example, more stops were noted in the babbling and early words of babies learning Swedish and English compared to those learning French and Japanese (De Boysson-Bardies and Vihman, 1991). As the child acquires the phonology of the language, these language-specific differences are expected to increase. To date, most researchers have been interested in identifying similarities not differences in speech characteristics across languages.

2.4.2   The Importance of Pre-speech Development

Study of pre-speech development is important, as the literature on typically developing babies/toddlers has reported a strong correlation between the sounds and syllable shapes of babbling and early word productions. In support of this proposal, various studies have shown that accomplishments in babbling (e.g. earlier and more frequent and varied babbling) were associated with more advanced speech and/or language development (Stoel-Gammon, 1998a, 1998b). In some cases, these associations were seen as late as three (Vihman and Greenlee, 1987) and even five years of age (Jensen *et al.*, 1988). Interestingly, late onset of canonical babbling is considered a risk factor for hearing disability (Eilers and Oller, 1994) or developmental disabilities including delays in expressive language development (Oller *et al.*, 1999).

2.4.3   Pre-speech Development: Babies with Cleft Palate

Pre-speech development will be disrupted (including acquisition of the oral–nasal contrast, shift in ratio of glottal to supraglottal consonants, onset of canonical babbling etc.) for babies with an unrepaired or partially repaired palate during this important period of development. Further, limitations in pre-speech performance could potentially impact later speech and language learning. The sections below address what is currently known about babbling and early consonant development of babies with CP, and how these early deficits impact later performance.

A number of studies have been interested in the effect of clefting on the baby's ability to produce the rhythmic motor patterns of repeated CV syllables that characterize babbling. Both acoustic (Phillips and Kent, 1984) and perceptual data (Chapman *et al.*, 2001) provide support for the idea that VPI does not interfere with the 'rhythmic pattern of reduplicated babbling' (Phillips and Kent, 1984, p. 148). It also appears to be the case that babies with CP vocalize as much as non-cleft (NC) babies (Scherer, Williams and Proctor-Williams, 2008 (at 6 months); Willadsen and Albrechtsen, 2006), providing them with an equal number (compared to NC babies) of opportunities for vocal practice and stimulation from caregivers (Chapman *et al.*, 2001). At the same time, other aspects of babbling are compromised in babies with CP. Prior to complete closure of the palatal cleft, these babies produce fewer canonical syllables and canonical syllables with oral consonants as early as six months (Scherer, Williams and Proctor-Williams, 2008) and also at nine months of age (Chapman *et al.*, 2001). Additionally, babies with unrepaired CP may be slower in reaching the canonical babbling stage (only 57% of nine-month-old babies with CP had reached this milestone compared to 93% of NC peers; Chapman *et al.*, 2001).

This may not be the case for babies who undergo early veloplasty, however. Two separate studies conducted in Denmark (Willadsen and Albrechtsen, 2006) and Sweden (Lohmander, Olsson and Flynn, 2010) found that almost all babies with and without CP had reached the canonical babbling stage at 11 months of age and 12 months of age, respectively. Because the babies studied by Chapman *et al.* (2001) were younger by two to three months at the time of testing, it is not known if the better performance by the Danish and Swedish babies was because they were older or because early repair of the soft palate facilitated speech development. Based on a follow-up study by Chapman *et al.* (2009), the second explanation seems probable. In that study, the investigators compared babies from Denmark (veloplasty at four months) and babies from the United States (with unrepaired clefts) who were pair-wise matched for age and gender (mean age = 11 months; 7 days). Results indicated that the Danish babies produced a greater number of canonical syllables but not a greater number of true canonical syllables (i.e. syllables that contained supraglottal consonants, but not glides). According to Chapman *et al.* (2009), closure of the soft palate facilitates obstruent production (thus canonical syllable production) posterior to the residual hard palate cleft. This explanation was supported by a high occurrence of velar obstruents in the babbling of babies undergoing early primary veloplasty (see below) (Lohmander, Olsson and Flynn, 2010; Willadsen and Albrechtsen, 2006).

Studies of early speech development of babies with CP have also examined the types of consonants produced (Chapman, 2009). At approximately one year of age, babies with CP produce fewer oral stops compared to babies without CP.[2] This finding is consistent for babies who had completely unrepaired palates (Chapman *et al.*, 2001; Hutters, Bau and Brøndsted, 2001;[3] Konst *et al.*, 1999) and for babies who had the soft palate closed (at four to eight months of age) but still had an unrepaired hard palate at the time of investigation (Lohmander, Olsson and Flynn, 2010; Willadsen and Albrechtsen, 2006). The lower occurrence of oral stops in the pre-speech productions of babies with CP is especially significant because oral stops are considered to be 'easy' and, therefore, are frequent and early developing in the speech of NC babies (Bernhardt and Stemberger, 1998; MacNeilage, 1998). The most straightforward explanation for this finding is that babies with CP actually 'avoid' producing oral stops due to the difficulty impounding sufficient intraoral air pressure. However, an alternative explanation is that the babies are actually attempting to produce stops, but because of nasalization they are heard and transcribed as nasals (Chapman, 1991; Willadsen and Albrechtsen, 2006). Either way, this is probably the most significant difference between babies with CP and NC babies

---

[2] The studies referenced in this section are limited to those including a comparison group of NC babies.

[3] The babies in this study had partial repair of the hard palate (anterior 1/3) at the time of testing (Willadsen, personal communication).

in terms of early speech development. As might be expected, other pressure consonants (e.g. fricatives and affricates) are infrequent in the early productions of babies with CP and NC babies, regardless of the language (Chapman *et al.*, 2001; Willadsen and Albrechtsen, 2006).

Compared to oral stops, other non-pressure consonants, such as nasals, glides and approximates, should be seen more frequently because they are easier to produce for babies with CP (Bernhardt and Stemberger, 1998). Numerous studies have found that nasals were produced more often by babies with CP than by babies without CP, even though this difference was not statistically significant in all studies (Chapman *et al.*, 2001; Hutters, Bau and Brøndsted, 2001; Willadsen and Albrechtsen, 2006). The more frequent use of nasals may be due to a good auditory match between the baby's attempt at these sounds and what is heard in the input (Chapman *et al.*, 2001). The findings regarding other sonorant sound categories are, however, quite diverse, possibly related to differences in the relative occurrence of these sounds among the languages being investigated.

Some interesting findings have also emerged concerning place of articulation of consonants. One-year-old babies with CP produce more sounds with a glottal place of articulation, especially the glottal stop, than babies without CP (Chapman *et al.*, 2001; Hutters, Bau and Brøndsted, 2001; Lohmander, Olsson and Flynn, 2010; Willadsen and Albrechtsen, 2006). Some attribute the high occurrence of glottals in the speech of babies with CP to VPI (Chapman, 1991). However, it is possibly due to a general delay in development. As mentioned above, glottal productions are frequent in the vocalizations of NC babies prior to five to six months of age, but begin to decrease after that age (Holmgren *et al.*, 1986). Glottal productions have also been found to decrease over time in babies with CP, but at a later age (Lohmander-Agerskov *et al.*, 1994; O'Gara, Logemann and Rademaker, 1994).

In contrast to glottal sounds, coronals[4] are produced less frequently by babies with CP than by their NC peers (Chapman *et al.*, 2001; Hutters, Bau and Brøndsted, 2001; Konst *et al.*, 1999; Lohmander, Olsson and Flynn, 2010; Willadsen and Albrechtsen, 2006). One account of this consistent finding is that babies with unrepaired clefts lack an articulatory surface to 'practice' coronals (Trost-Cardamone, 1990). However, in a study by Hutters, Bau and Brøndsted (2001) very few coronal consonants were observed in a group of 13-month-old Danish babies with CP even though closure of the anterior 1/3 of the hard palate at two months of age provided an articulatory surface for consonant production. Similarly, several studies have investigated the impact of infant orthopaedic plates (i.e. a prosthetic plate to cover the cleft until the time of palatal surgery) on consonant development. As a group, these studies concluded that covering the palatal cleft does not promote alveolar productions in babies with CP (Hardin-Jones *et al.*, 2002; Konst *et al.*, 1999; Lohmander, Lillvik and Friede, 2004). Other tenable explanations for a lack of coronal consonants for babies with CP may be insufficient kinaesthetic–tactile feedback in the dental/alveolar area due to scarring, (Hardcastle *et al.*, 1989) or reduced hearing due to middle ear problems; but neither have been tested experimentally.

Babies with an unoperated CP produced very few velar consonants at 9 and 13 months of age, respectively (Chapman *et al.*, 2001; Hutters, Bau and Brøndsted, 2001). In con-

---

[4]Sounds produced with the tongue tip or tongue blade.

Table 2.3 Results of studies comparing size of consonant inventories for babies with CP and NC babies.

CP < NC	CP = NC
Chapman *et al.* (2001)	Chapman (1991)
Lohmander, Lillvik and Friede (2004)	Willadsen and Enemark (2000)
Lohmander, Olsson and Flynn (2010) (at 18 months)	Willadsen and Albrechtsen (2006) (at 12 months)
Willadsen (in press) (at 18 months)*	Scherer, Williams and Proctor-Williams (2008)
	Lohmander *et al.* (in press) (at 12 months)

*Consonants permissible in word-initial position.

trast, babies undergoing early veloplasty produced many velar stops around 12 to 18 months of age, apparently by impounding intraoral air pressure behind the open hard palate (Lohmander, Olsson and Flynn, 2010; Willadsen and Albrechtsen, 2006). Additionally, no difference was found with respect to frequency of occurrence of (bi) labials in babies with and without CP. However, this finding may be due to the fact that babies with CP produce many (bi)labial nasals and approximates (Chapman *et al.*, 2001; Willadsen and Albrechtsen, 2006), while (bi)labial stops are still less frequently seen (Lohmander, Olsson and Flynn, 2010; Willadsen, in press).

Finally, investigators have been interested in comparing size of consonant inventory for babies with CP and NC babies. Although the study findings are conflicting (Table 2.3), all agree that babies with CP show differences in the consonant types that are produced (i.e. fewer oral stops and more nasals as described in the section above).

2.4.4 Relationship between Early Speech and Later Speech: Babies with Cleft Palate

As a result of the research highlighting the relationship between early speech and later speech and language development reported above for NC babies, researchers began to examine how early clefting impacts later speech and language development for babies with CP. Unfortunately, the relationship is not as clear-cut as that observed for NC babies. A summary of that literature suggests that relationships exist, but they are dependent on the age at which the 'predictors' are measured (i.e. pre or post palatal surgery) and what specific outcome variables are measured. A summary of these relationships is given in Table 2.4.

2.4.5 Phonology of Early Words: What Is Typical?

The end of the pre-speech stage is not distinct; rather there is a period when babies produce non-meaningful babbling and early words concurrently. There is also overlap in the characteristics of babbling and first words. Further, these early words may not be

Table 2.4 Summary of studies showing a relationship between early speech and later speech/language performance.

Early speech behaviour	Later speech/language behaviour
Lower babbling frequency	Larger consonant inventory and vocabulary (Scherer, Williams and Proctor-Williams, 2008) Smaller vocabulary (Willadsen, 2007[a])
More syllables and/or different consonants (types) in babbling and early words	Poorer language skills (Chapman, 2004) Larger vocabulary (Chapman, Hardin-Jones and Halter, 2003; Willadsen, 2007[a]) Better speech skills [e.g. stops, number of different sounds, stable sounds (Chapman, Hardin-Jones and Halter, 2003); percent consonants correct (PCC) (Lohmander and Persson, 2008)]
More oral stops	Better speech skills [e.g. number of different sounds, oral stops, stable sounds (Chapman, Hardin-Jones and Halter, 2003)] More intelligible speech (Konst, 2002) Better language skills (Chapman, Hardin-Jones and Halter, 2003; Chapman, 2004; Konst, 2002)
More alveolars	Higher PCC (Lohmander and Persson, 2008; Willadsen, 2007[b]) Fewer cleft-related speech characteristics (Konst, 2002) and 'backed' productions (Russell and Grunwell, 1993)
More velar stops	More retracted productions (Lohmander and Persson, 2008)
Greater number of consonants	Larger vocabulary (Willadsen, 2007[b])

[a]This relationship was noted for children with CP who had complete closure of the hard and soft palate by 12 months.
[b]This relationship was noted for children with CP who had unrepaired clefts of the hard palate.

adult-like in terms of sounds or syllable shapes, and often require contextual information for interpretation (Table 2.5).

2.4.6 Phonology of Early Words: Babies with Cleft Palate[5]

In some countries, decisions regarding timing of primary palatal surgery are based, in part, on the idea that a baby should have a mechanism adequate for speech production prior to onset of the first words (Chapman, Hardin-Jones *et al.*, 2008) or, more recently,

[5]Studies of the early post-surgery period may include babbling only or a mix of babbling and words.

Table 2.5   Characteristics of the first fifty words (Stoel-Gammon and Dunn, 1985; Vihman, 1996).

-Labial or dental stops, nasals, glides are common
-1 or 2 syllables; simplifications (CVC ->CV; CCV ->CV) are common
-Individual differences
-Production variability
-Selectivity/avoidance of words
-Initial consonants are most accurate

---

prior to the onset of canonical babbling (at approximately six months). See Kemp-Fincham, Kuehn and Trost-Cardamone (1990) for a theoretical justification. While there are no developmental studies of babies who have undergone primary palatal surgery at six months, there are studies of babies who had primary palatal surgery at approximately 12 months, which corresponds to the onset of first words in the majority of languages (Slobin, 1985). These studies are important as they provide information about how easily the baby's developing sound system can adapt following palatal repair, as well as having the potential to provide information on 'predictors' of speech outcome.

Only a few studies have examined changes in speech production in the early post-surgery period. Grunwell and Russell (1987) followed three youngsters with CP residing in the United Kingdom prior to primary palatal surgery (at approximately two week intervals) until several months post-surgery. The findings indicated that following a drop in consonant production in the early post-surgery period, babies reached their pre-surgery level between three and seven weeks post-surgery. One of the first areas that appeared to show 'catch up' in the early post-surgery period for English-speaking babies in the United States was frequency (Jones, Chapman and Hardin-Jones, 2003) and variety of syllables produced (Salas-Provance, Kuehn and Marsh, 2003). At the same time, toddlers with CP were slower to 'catch-up' on size of consonant inventory measures (Chapman, Hardin-Jones and Halter, 2003; Jones, Chapman and Hardin-Jones, 2003; Salas-Provance, Kuehn and Marsh, 2003), phonetic diversity, or different vowel or consonant combinations for CV and CVC syllables (Salas-Provance, Kuehn and Marsh, 2003). Additionally, English-speaking toddlers with CP showed less accurate production of oral stops, liquids, labials, dentals and velars in their early words. However, it also appeared to be the case that they were as accurate producing /g/ and /p/ in early words as NC peers by at least seven to nine months post-surgery (Chapman, Hardin-Jones and Halter, 2003; Jones, Chapman and Hardin-Jones, 2003).

2.4.6.1 Lexical Selectivity   Lexical development and phonological development are interrelated in the earliest stages of development; in fact, there is evidence to suggest that toddlers 'select' words to say containing sounds they can easily produce. This phenomenon has been documented for typically developing toddlers (Ferguson and Farwell, 1975), for toddlers with early lexical delays (Leonard *et al.*, 1982) and for toddlers with cleft palate (Estrem and Broen, 1989). For example, compared to NC toddlers of the same age who targeted more words with oral stops, toddlers with CP targeted more words beginning with vowels, nasals or approximates. Additionally, the NC toddlers 'selected' more words containing sounds with an alveolar or dental place of articulation compared to the toddlers with CP who selected more words with sounds 'produced at the periphery of the oral tract' (Estrem and Broen, 1989, p. 16). A recent study of Danish toddlers with CP also found examples of lexical selectivity, that is, these toddlers targeted more words with initial nasals and velars and avoided words containing word initial stop and alveolar targets compared to a group of age-matched peers (Willadsen, 2007).

2.4.7 Systematic Phonology – Toddlers and Pre-school Children: What Is Typical?

As the toddler's vocabulary grows, so does his/her speech production skills. The primary characteristic of this stage is that the young child begins to produce words that resemble the adult target in systematic ways. Of course, children differ in terms of when they begin to develop this *rule-based or systematic phonology* (Menn and Stoel-Gammon, 2005; Vihman, 1996). However, in a few years, the child progresses from numerous mismatches with the adult target to producing all sounds correctly. Age of mastery varies depending on the language the child is learning. McLeod (2007) provided age of speech acquisition data (on 12 dialects of English and 20 other languages) which can be used as a resource in evaluating the progress of children with CP in relation to their NC peers.

2.4.8 Systematic Phonology – Toddlers and Pre-school Children with Cleft Palate

The earliest studies of speech development of children with CP focused on describing articulation patterns of large groups of pre-school children with CP. These classic studies were conducted in the 1950s and 1960s (Bzoch, 1965; Phillips and Harrison, 1969; Spriestersbach, Darley and Rouse, 1956) on English-speaking pre-school children in the United States. While it is hoped that changes in management have resulted in more normal patterns of speech development than was observed then, these studies documented some important characteristics of the speech of children with CP that are still seen in cross-linguistic research reports and clinical practice today (Table 2.6).

A few studies have employed a phonological process framework to describe the rules or processes employed by pre-school children with CP. Studies by Chapman (1993) and Chapman and Hardin (1992) suggested that the processes employed by children with CP were similar to those employed by their NC peers during the pre-school years with one exception – backing. Interestingly, the children with CP did not differ from their NC peers in use of phonological processes at two and five years of age, but they did at three and four years of age. These findings, along with the patterns of errors observed, suggested that toddlers with cleft palate were similar to NC peers when both groups were using processes more frequently (i.e. at two years). However, the documented group differences at age three and four, but not age five, suggested that speech development was protracted for the children with CP (Chapman, 1993; Chapman and Hardin, 1992). Further, it appears that for some children with CP, problems in speech production may be related to other expressive language problems (Powers, Dunn and Erickson, 1990; Morris and Ozanne, 2003) and delays in early pre-literacy skills (Chapman, in press).

Table 2.6 Speech characteristics of children with CP.

1. Delays in speech sound development (pressure and non-pressure consonants)
2. Decreased intelligibility
3. Omissions and substitutions are more frequent than distortions
4. Glottal and pharyngeal substitutions or other 'backed' productions (e.g. alveolars to velars or glottals)
5. Nasal substitutions

2.4.9 Language-Specific 'Cleft' Speech Characteristics

There are many 'cleft' speech characteristics that are seen regardless of the language the child is learning (Brøndsted *et al.*, 1994, Chapter 9). Although less researched, there are also 'cleft' speech characteristics that appear to be language specific. These characteristics are summarized in Table 2.7.

Table 2.7 Language-specific 'cleft' speech characteristics.

	Authors	Findings
Cantonese	Stokes and Whitehill (1996)	-Bilabial fricatives (for /s & f/)
	Whitehill and Stokes (1995)	-Initial consonant deletion
Cantonese	Gibbon *et al.*, (1998)	-Bilabial fricatives (for /s/)
Nepali	Shan (2001)	-Consonant deletion
Arabic	Shahin (2002, 2006)	-Implosive airstream
		-Devoicing of oral stops

2.5 Conclusion

An attempt has been made to summarize what is known about speech development of children with CP. Again the reader must be cautioned that the findings reported here represent group results. Each child with CP is unique; with many children showing normal speech development soon after palatal surgery. What seems to be clear from this review is that clefting impacts babbling and may also influence early word production in terms of lexical selectivity and possibly rate of lexical growth. Although some children with CP exhibit active or passive processes due to continued problems with velopharyngeal function, others follow a more 'typical' but slower trajectory of speech development. More research is needed examining how the child with CP progresses from possessing a limited vocabulary and production constraints, characteristics of the single-word stage, to acquisition of a systematic phonology. Next, there is a need for research describing the speech development of children with CP who speak languages other than those represented in the research studies reviewed here. In addition to providing information about universal as well as language-specific characteristics of CP speech, these data will facilitate international inter-centre comparisons such as those that have been carried out so successfully in Europe. Finally, regardless of what country is lived in or what language is spoken, societies are becoming increasing linguistically and culturally diverse. This information will enable children with CP to receive the best possible care – regardless of their linguistic or their cultural background.

References

Bernhardt, B.H. and Stemberger, J.P. (1998) *Handbook of Phonological Development from the Perspective of Constraint-Based Nonlinear Phonology*, Academic Press, San Diego, CA.

Brøndsted, K., Grunwell, P., Henningsson, G. *et al.* (1994) A phonetic framework for cross-linguistic analysis of cleft palate speech. *Clinical Linguistics & Phonetics*, **8**, 109–125.

Bzoch, K.R. (1965) Articulation proficiency and error patterns of preschool cleft palate and normal children. *Cleft Palate Journal*, **2**, 340–349.

Chapman, K.L. (in press) The relationship between early reading skills and speech and language performance in young children with cleft lip and palate. *Cleft Palate-Craniofacial Journal*.

Chapman, K.L. (1991) Early vocalizations of young children with cleft lip and palate. *Cleft Palate-Craniofacial Journal*, **28**, 172–178.

Chapman, K.L. (1993) Phonologic processes in children with cleft palate. *Cleft Palate-Craniofacial Journal*, **30**, 64–72.

Chapman, K.L. (2004) Is presurgery and early postsurgery performance related to the speech and language outcomes at 3 years of age for children with cleft palate? *Clinical Linguistics & Phonetics*, **18**, 235–257.

Chapman, K.L. (2009) Speech and language of children with cleft palate: interactions and influences, *Cleft Lip and Palate: Interdisciplinary Issues and Treatment*, 2nd edn (eds K.T. Moller and L.E. Glaze), Pro-Ed Publications, Austin, pp. 243–293.

Chapman, K.L. and Hardin, M. (1992) Phonetic and phonologic skills of two-year-olds with cleft palate. *Cleft Palate-Craniofacial Journal*, **29**, 435–443.

Chapman, K.L., Hardin-Jones, M. and Halter, K.A. (2003) The relationship between early speech and later speech and language performance for children with cleft palate. *Clinical Linguistics & Phonetics*, **17**, 173–197.

Chapman, K.L., Hardin-Jones, M., Schulte, J. and Halter, K.A. (2001) Vocal development of 9 month old babies with cleft palate. *Journal of Speech, Language, and Hearing Research*, **44**, 1268–1284.

Chapman, K.L., Hardin-Jones, M., Goldstein, J.A. *et al.* (2008) Timing of palatal surgery and speech outcome. *Cleft Palate-Craniofacial Journal*, **45**, 297–308.

Chapman, K.L., Willadsen, E., Krantz, A. and Hardin-Jones, M.A. (2009) Babbling of babies with cleft palate: the effects of early soft palate closure. Paper presented at the 67th Annual meeting of the American cleft palate-craniofacial association, Scottsdale, AZ, April, 2009.

De Boysson-Bardies, B. and Vihman, M.M. (1991) Adaptation to language: evidence from babbling and first words in four languages. *Language*, **67**, 297–319.

Eilers, R.E. and Oller, D.K. (1994) Infant vocalization and the early diagnosis of severe hearing impairment. *Journal of Pediatrics*, **124**, 199–203.

Estrem, T. and Broen, P.A. (1989) Early speech production of children with cleft palate. *Journal of Speech and Hearing Research*, **32**, 12–23.

Ferguson, C.A. and Farwell, C.B. (1975) Words and sounds in early language acquisition. *Language*, **51**, 419–439.

Fey, M.E. (1992) Clinical forum: articulation and phonology treatment. Articulation and phonology: inextricable constructs in speech pathology. *Language, Speech and Hearing Services in Schools*, 23, 225–232.

Gibbon, F.E., Whitehill, T.L., Hardcastle, W.J. *et al.* (1998) Cross-Language (Cantonese/English) study of articulatory error patterns in cleft palate speech using electropalatography (EPG), in *Clinical Phonetics and Linguistics* (eds W. Ziegler and K. Deger), Whurr, London, pp. 165–176.

Gierut, J.A. and Morrisette, M.L. (2005) The clinical significance of optimality theory for phonological disorders. *Topics in Language Disorders*, 25, 266–280.

Grunwell, P. and Russell, J. (1987) Vocalizations before and after cleft palate surgery: a pilot study. *British Journal of Disorders of Communication*, 22, 1–17.

Hardcastle, W., Jones, W., Knight, C. *et al.* (1989) New developments in electropalatography: a state-of-the-art report. *Clinical Phonetics & Linguistics*, 3, 1–38.

Harding, A. and Grunwell, P. (1993) Relationship between speech and timing of hard palate repair, in *Analysing Cleft Palate Speech* (ed. P. Grunwell), Whurr, London, pp. 48–111.

Harding, A. and Grunwell, P. (1998) Active versus passive cleft-type speech characteristics. *International Journal of Language and Communication Disorders*, 33, 329–352.

Hardin-Jones, M.A. and Jones, D.L. (2005) Speech production patterns of preschoolers with cleft palate. *Cleft Palate-Craniofacial Journal*, 42, 7–13.

Hardin-Jones, M.A., Chapman, K.L., Wright, J. *et al.* (2002) The impact of early palatal obturation on consonant development in babies with unrepaired cleft palate. *Cleft Palate-Craniofacial Journal*, 39, 157–163.

Holmgren, K., Lindblom, B., Aurelius, G. *et al.* (1986) On the phonetics of infant vocalization, in *Precursors of Early Speech* (eds B. Lindblom and R. Zetterstrom), Stockton Press, New York, pp. 51–63.

Hutters, B. and Brøndsted, K. (1987) Strategies in cleft palate speech – with special reference to Danish. *Cleft Palate Journal*, 24, 126–136.

Hutters, B., Bau, A. and Brøndsted, K. (2001) A longitudinal group study of speech development in Danish children born with and without cleft lip and palate. *International Journal of Language and Communication Disorders*, 36, 447–470.

Jensen, T.S., Bøggild-Andersen, B., Schmidt, J. *et al.* (1988) Perinatal risk factors and first year vocalizations: influence on pre-school language and motor performance. *Developmental Medicine and Child Neurology*, 30, 153–161.

Jones, C., Chapman, K.L. and Hardin-Jones, M. (2003) Speech development of children with cleft palate before and after palatal surgery. *Cleft Palate-Craniofacial Journal*, 40, 19–31.

Kemp-Fincham, S.I., Kuehn, D.P. and Trost-Cardamone, J.E. (1990) Speech development and timing of primary palatoplasty, in *Multidisciplinary Management of Cleft Lip and Palate* (eds J. Bardach and H.L. Morris), W.B. Saunders, Philadelphia, pp. 736–745.

Kent, R.D. (1981) Sensorimotor aspects of speech development, in *Development of Perception: Psychobiological Perspectives* (ed. R.N. Aslin, J.R. Alberts and M.R. Peterson), Academic Press, New York, pp. 161–189.

Kent, R.D. and Hodge, M.M. (1991) The biogenesis of speech: continuity and process in early speech development, in *Research on Child Language Disorders: A Decade of Progress* (ed. J. Miller), Pro-Ed, Austin, Texas, pp. 25–54.

Kent, R.D. and Miolo, G. (1995) Phonetic abilities in the first year of life, in *The Handbook of Child Language* (eds P. Fletcher and B. MacWhinney), Blackwell Publishing, Malden, MA, pp. 303–334.

Kent, R.D. and Murray, A. (1982) Acoustic features of infant vocalic utterances at 3, 6, and 9 months. *Journal of the Acoustical Society of America*, 72, 355–365.

Kent, R.D. and Vorperian, H.K. (2006) In the mouths of babes: Anatomic, motor, and sensory foundations of speech development in children, in *Language disorders from a developmental perspective: Essays in Honor of Robin S. Chapman* (ed. R. Paul), Lawrence Erlbaum Associates, Mahwah, NJ, 55–81.

Konst, E.M. (2002) The effects of infant orthopaedics on speech and language development in children with unilateral cleft lip and palate. Doctoral thesis, University of Nijmegen, The Netherlands.

Konst, E.M., Rietveld, T., Peters, H.F.M. and Prahl-Andersen, B. (1999) Phonological development of toddlers with unilateral cleft lip and palate who were treated with and without infant ortho-pedics: a randomized clinical trial. *Cleft Palate-Craniofacial Journal*, 40, 32–39.

Leonard, L.B., Schwartz, R.G., Chapman, K. *et al.* (1982) Early lexical acquisition in children with specific language impairment. *Journal of Speech and Hearing Research*, 25, 554–564.

Liberman, P., Crelin, F.S. and Klatt, D.H. (1972) Phonetic ability and related anatomy of the newborn and adult human, Neanderthal man, and the chimpanzee. *American Anthropologist*, 84, 287–307.

Locke, J.L. (1983) *Phonological Acquisition and Change*, Academic Press, New York.

Lohmander, A. and Persson, C. (2008) A longitudinal study of speech production in Swedish children with cleft palate and two-stage palatal repair. *Cleft Palate-Craniofacial Journal*, 45, 32–41.

Lohmander, A., Lillvik, M. and Friede, H. (2004) The impact of early infant jaw-orthopaedics on early speech production in toddlers with unilateral cleft lip and palate. *Clinical Linguistics & Phonetics*, 18, 259–284.

Lohmander, A., Olsson, M. and Flynn, T. (2010) Early consonant production in Swedish infants with and without unilateral cleft lip and palate and two-stage palatal repair. *Cleft Palate-Craniofacial Journal*. doi: 10.1597/09-105.

Lohmander-Agerskov, A., Söderpalm, E., Friede, H. *et al.* (1994) Pre-speech in children with cleft lip and palate or cleft palate only. Phonetic analysis related to morphologic and functional factors. *Cleft Palate-Craniofacial Journal*, 31, 271–279.

MacNeilage, P.F. (1998) The frame/content theory of evolution of speech production. *Behavioral and Brain Sciences*, 21, 499–546.

Maddieson, I. (1984) *Patterns of Sounds*, Cambridge University Press, Cambridge.

McLeod, S. (ed.) (2007) *The International Guide to Speech Acquisition*, Thomson Delmar Learning, Clifton Park, NY.

Menn, L. and Stoel-Gammon, C. (2005) Phonological development: learning sounds and sound patterns, in *The Development of Language* (ed. J.B. Gleason), Allyn and Bacon, Boston, MA, pp. 62–111.

Morris, H. and Ozanne, A. (2003) Phonetic, phonological, and language skills of children with a cleft palate. *Cleft Palate Craniofacial Journal*, 40, 460–470.

O'Gara, M.M., Logemann, J.A. and Rademaker, A.W. (1994) Phonetic features by babies with unilateral cleft lip and palate. *Cleft Palate-Craniofacial Journal*, 31, 446–451.

Oller, D.K. (1980) The emergence of the sounds of speech in infancy, in *Child Phonology: Vol. 1. Production* (eds G. Yeni-Komshian, J.F. Kavanagh and C.A. Ferguson), Academic Press, New York, pp. 93–112.

Oller, D.K. (2000) *The Emergence of the Speech Capacity*, Lawrence Erlbaum Associates, Mahwah, NJ.

Oller, D.K. and Griebel, U. (2008) Contextual flexibility in infant vocal development and the earli-est steps in the evolution of language, in *Evolution of Communication Flexibility* (eds D.K. Oller and U. Griebel), MIT Press, Cambridge, MA, pp. 141–168.

Oller, D.K., Eilers, R.E., Neal, A.R. and Schwartz, H.K. (1999) Precursors to speech in infancy: the prediction of speech and language disorders. *Journal of Communication Disorders*, 32, 223–246.

Phillips, B.J. and Harrison, R.J. (1969) Articulation patterns of preschool cleft palate children. *Cleft Palate Journal*, 6, 245–253.

Phillips, B.J. and Kent, R.D. (1984) Acoustic-phonetic description of speech productions in speakers with cleft palate and other velopharyngeal disorders, in *Speech and Language: Advances in Basic Research and Practice* 11 (ed. N. Lass), Academic Press, New York, pp. 132–160.

Powers, G.R., Dunn, C. and Erickson, C.B. (1990) Speech analyses of four children with repaired cleft palates. *Journal of Speech and Hearing Disorders*, 55, 542–549.

Russell, J. and Grunwell, P. (1993) Speech development in children with cleft lip and palate, in *Analysing Cleft Palate Speech* (ed. P. Grunwell), Whurr, London, pp. 19–47.

Salas-Provance, M.B., Kuehn, D.P. and Marsh, J.L. (2003) Phonetic repertoire and syllable characteristics of 15-month-old babies with cleft palate. *Journal of Phonetics*, 31, 23–38.

Scherer, N.J., Williams, A.L. and Proctor-Williams, K. (2008) Early and later vocalization skills in children with and without cleft palate. *International Journal of Pediatric Otorhinolaryngology*, 72, 827–840.

Sell, D., Grunwell, P., Mildinhall, S. *et al.* (2001) Cleft lip and palate care in the United Kingdom – The clinical standards advisory group (CSAG) study. Part 3: speech outcomes. *Cleft Palate-Craniofacial Journal*, 38, 30–37.

Shahin, K. (2002) Remarks of the speech of Arabic-speaking children with cleft palate. *California Linguistic Notes*, 27, 1–10.

Shahin, K. (2006) Remarks on the speech of Arabic-speaking children with cleft palate: three case studies. *Journal of Multilingual Communication Disorders*, 4, 1–10.

Shan, L.K. (2001) Analyzing unrepaired cleft palate speech in Nepali: testing the Eurocleft model. BS thesis, University of Hong Kong.

Slobin, D.I. (1985) *The Crosslinguistic Study of Language Acquisition Volume 1: The Data*, Lawrence Erlbaum Associates, Hillsdale, New Jersey.

Spriestersbach, D.C., Darley, F.L. and Rouse, V. (1956) Articulation of a group of children with cleft lips and palates. *Journal of Speech and Hearing Disorders*, 21, 463–445.

Stoel-Gammon, C. (1998a) Sounds and words in early language acquisition. The relationship between lexical and phonological development, in *Exploring the Speech–Language Connection* (ed. R. Paul), Paul H. Brookes Publishing Co., Baltimore, pp. 25–52.

Stoel-Gammon, C. (1998b) Role of babbling and phonology in early linguistic development, in *Transitions in Prelinguistic Communication* (eds A.M. Wetherby, S.F. Warren and J. Reichle), Paul H. Brookes Publishing Co., Baltimore, pp. 87–110.

Stoel-Gammon, C. and Dunn, C. (1985) *Normal and Disordered Phonology in Children*, University Park Press, Baltimore.

Stokes, S. and Whitehill, T. (1996) Speech error patterns in Cantonese speaking children with cleft palate. *European Journal of Disorders of Communication*, 31, 45–64.

Trost, J.E. (1981) Articulatory additions to the classical description of the speech of persons with cleft palate. *Cleft Palate Journal*, 18, 193–203.

Trost-Cardamone, J.E. (1990) Speech in the first year: a perspective on early acquisition, in *Cleft Lip and Palate: A System of Management* (eds D.A. Kernahan and S.N. Rosenstein), Williams & Wilkins, Baltimore, pp. 227–235.

Vihman, M.M. (1996) *Phonological Development: The Origins of Language in the Child*, Blackwell, Oxford.

Vihman, M.M. and Greenlee, M. (1987) Individual differences in phonological development: ages one and three years. *Journal of Speech and Hearing Research*, 30, 503–521.

Whitehill, T. and Stokes, S. (1995) EPG in the description of normal and disordered speech production electropalatographic and perceptual analysis of the speech of Cantonese children with cleft palate. *European Journal of Disorders of Communication*, 30, 193–202.

Willadsen, E. (in press) Influence of timing of hard palate repair in a two-stage procedure on early language development in Danish children with cleft palate. *Cleft Palate-Craniofacial Journal*.

Willadsen, E. (2007) From babbling to meaningful speech in Danish children born with and without cleft lip and palate. PhD thesis, University of Aarhus, Denmark.

Willadsen, E. and Albrechtsen, H. (2006) Phonetic descriptions of babbling in Danish toddlers born with and without unilateral cleft lip and palate. *Cleft Palate-Craniofacial Journal*, 43, 190–200.

Willadsen, E. and Enemark, H. (2000) A comparative study of pre-speech vocalizations in two groups of toddlers with cleft palate and a noncleft group. *Cleft Palate-Craniofacial Journal*, 37, 172–178.

3

The Influence of Related Conditions on Speech and Communication

Christina Persson[1] and Lotta Sjögreen[2]

[1] Sahlgrenska Academy at University of Gothenburg, Department of Speech and Language Pathology, SE 405 30 Gothenburg, Sweden
[2] Mun-H-Center Odontologen, SE 413 90 Gothenburg, Sweden

3.1 Introduction

Children born with a cleft palate is a heterogeneous group, not only due to the different types or extents of clefts but also due to a high frequency of associated anomalies or syndromes, reported in different studies as somewhere between 20 and 60% (Milerad *et al.*, 1997; Shprintzen, Siegel-Sadewitz *et al.*, 1985; Stoll *et al.*, 2000). Possible explanations for the wide range of reported incidence might be differences in definitions of associated anomalies, time after birth, how carefully the patients are examined and the selection of patients. However, one consistent finding is that the frequency of associated anomalies or syndromes is higher among children with clefts in the secondary palate, that is isolated cleft palate, submucous and occult submucous cleft palate (Cohen, 1978; Coleman and Sykes, 2001). Furthermore, total palatal clefts of the secondary palate are more often combined with other birth defects than partial clefts of the secondary palate (Chetpakdeechit *et al.*, 2010).

Cleft Palate Speech: Assessment and Intervention, First Edition. Edited by Sara Howard, Anette Lohmander.
© 2011 John Wiley & Sons, Ltd. Published 2011 by John Wiley & Sons, Ltd.

Several hundreds of syndromes which include clefts are described in the literature. Hence, the aim of this chapter is not to describe all of these syndromes or to provide a comprehensive genetic overview of them, but to discuss some of the ways in which these related conditions can affect speech and some of the consequences this can have for the care of these children. Speech problems related to articulation and velopharyngeal function are not only linked to structural deficits like overt and submucous clefts but also to muscle weakness, hypotonia and cranial nerve palsy, all of which may result in dysarthria. Another possible cause of speech problems in this population is deficits in the motor planning process, leading to childhood apraxia of speech (CAS).

Trost (1981) used a classification of suggested etiologies, which included velopharyngeal impairment, structural etiologies (i.e. unrepaired clefts, post-surgical insufficiency), neurogenic etiologies (i.e. cerebral palsy, difficulties with motor association /motor programming) and velopharyngeal mislearning (i.e. phoneme-specific nasal emission, hearing impairment). In this chapter, a similar framework is used to describe how related conditions, including a variety of syndromes, might have an impact on structure and function, and thus on speech production. Conditions related to structural etiologies, conditions related to neurological etiologies and conditions related to a combination of the two are described. Finally, some clinical implications on assessment and intervention are discussed.

3.1.1   Related Conditions

When two or more anomalies occur together, it could be suspected that they are related, either as a syndrome, sequence, or an association. All of these have a presence of multiple anomalies in the same individual; the difference is the aetiology. In a syndrome all of the multiple anomalies have a single cause, for example genetic or teratogenic, while in a sequence some of the anomalies are secondary to a primary anomaly, which causes a chain reaction. Finally, in an association the aetiology is unknown. Many of these conditions are multisystemic diseases and, therefore, speech and communication may be impaired not only by velopharyngeal impairment (VPI) but also by developmental speech and language disorders, oral motor dysfunction, hearing impairment and pragmatic deficits related to neuropsychiatric diagnoses. In this chapter the main focus is on articulation and velopharyngeal function but other aspects of speech, language and communication are briefly described.

3.2   Conditions Related to Structural Etiologies

Several structural deviations, apart from cleft palate, can interfere with speech development. Examples of this include unusual shapes and sizes of the pharynx: larger or smaller than usual, or asymmetric. Other structural differences, including the overall structure of the oral cavity, the size and shape of the tonsils, dentition and occlusion, might also have an impact on speech (Chapter 1). Other less common anomalies are choanal atresia and absent velum. The latter is a larger palatal anomaly than cleft palate, while choanal atresia is a rare condition that is present from birth, where the nasal passages are blocked on one or both sides by bone or tissue. This is not a comprehensive list of possible structural deviations; a summary of a range of important features is now discussed further in relation to the speech development.

3.2.1   Wide and Deep Pharynx

Several decades ago, a number of investigators described that individuals with clefts of the secondary palate have a wider pharynx than expected. Furthermore, abnormalities of the cervical spine and a flattened cranial base angle may cause an abnormally deep pharynx; that is, the posterior pharyngeal wall will be moved backwards. (A more extensive review of this literature is given in Peterson-Falzone, Hardin-Jones and Karnell, 2001, pp. 200–201.) Craniofacial syndromes often exhibit an alteration of the bony structures (e.g. maxilla, basicranium and upper cervical spine) underlying the soft tissues composing the velopharyngeal port, adenoids, lateral and pharyngeal walls, and velum. For example, Oto-palato-digital syndrome, Robinow syndrome and Van der Woude syndrome have all been reported to have a wide pharynx (Shprintzen, 1982).

22q11 deletion syndrome (22q11 DS) is a good example of a common syndrome with increased pharyngeal airway space. Besides the wide pharynx, platybasia (i.e. flattening of the skull base) has also been found in this population, resulting in an atypically deep pharynx (Arvystas and Shprintzen, 1984). More recent studies have confirmed the high prevalence of a wide and deep pharynx and a short hard palate in 22q11DS (Ruotolo *et al.*, 2006), as well as a variety of upper cervical spine abnormalities (Hultman *et al.*, 2000). A consequence of this is a large ratio between the depth of the pharynx and the length of velum. Thus, alterations in cranial base anatomy have been suggested to be the most important factor leading to VPI and can explain why 22q11DS has been described as the most common genetic cause of VPI (McDonald-McGinn *et al.*, 1999). 22q11DS has an extensive and variable phenotype (McDonald-McGinn *et al.*, 1999; Óskarsdóttir *et al.*, 2005). Some of the most common features are congenital heart disease, immunodeficiency, hypocalcemia, feeding difficulties, behavioural problems, psychiatric disorders and several types of malformations and deformities. Over half of the affected individuals have a cleft palate with or without cleft lip or a submucous cleft, while the majority have VPI irrespective of a cleft or not. Specifically, a high prevalence of severe hypernasality and compensatory articulation is common. In summary, this syndrome has two structural deficits that might affect speech: palate anomalies and the overall morphology of the velopharyngeal port.

Furthermore, the neurological deficit pharyngeal hypotonia may have an additional impact on velopharyngeal function. Speech and language development are characterized by delayed language onset, with delays in expressive language suggested to be beyond what is expected for their general developmental level (Scherer, D'Antonio and Kalbfleisch, 1999): a large proportion of three-year-olds are still non-oral or just use words or simple phrases (Solot *et al.*, 2001). However, there is a developmental progression and children normally develop speech successfully, although language disorders may persist longer (Persson *et al.*, 2006). The severe VPI requires surgery in many patients. Although the outcome is not always a normalized velopharyngeal function, the improvement in function can still be important for speech outcome. Reduced intelligibility is common in pre-school and early school age children with 22q11 DS (Persson *et al.*, 2003) but will be improved by age.

3.2.2 Narrow Pharynx

In contrast to the wide and deep pharynx found in some conditions, others have a narrowing of the nasal and pharyngeal airway caused by an acute cranial base angle that moves the posterior pharyngeal wall forward, by posterior displacement of the tongue and/or by hypoplastic pharyngeal musculature (Shprintzen, 1997, pp. 131–135; Vallino, Peterson-Falzone and Napoli, 2006). This narrowing of the nasal and pharyngeal airways can cause airway obstruction and hyponasal speech. Crouzon syndrome, Nager Acrofacial Dysostosis and Treacher Collins syndrome are examples of syndromes with a narrow pharynx.

Another example is *Apert syndrome,* which is characterized by an irregular craniosynostosis, mid-face hypoplasia and bilateral syndactyly of the hands and feet. Other skeletal structures of the body can be affected as well. The inheritance is autosomal dominant, although most cases are new mutations and the incidence rate is 1:100 000 (Shipster *et al.*, 2002). Cognitive impairment has been reported to be a part of the syndrome but the prevalence is uncertain. The palate is often narrow and high arched and in about 30% of the cases a cleft palate or a submucous cleft palate occurs. Severe malocclusion is common and choanal stenosis/atresia has also been described. Articulation errors and hyponasal/denasal resonance related to the structural defects are common. Besides the articulation errors, phonological errors related to language development, receptive language impairment and voice problems have been described (Shipster *et al.*, 2002). The structurally-related articulation errors can probably not be treated successfully until the relationship between the maxilla and the mandible is improved by mid-face advancement surgery or orthodontic treatment, but the phonological language-based errors can be addressed earlier, which may improve intelligibility (Shipster *et al.*, 2002).

3.2.3 Asymmetric Pharynx

Facial asymmetries as well as other asymmetric body parts may be due, for example, to syndromes, *in utero* deformities and trauma. Although not all facial asymmetries will cause speech problems, when the pharyngeal and palatal structures are asymmetric both articulation and velopharyngeal function will probably be affected (Chapter 1). Oculo-Auriculo-Vertebral Spectrum (OAVS) is a typical example of a condition that can include these features. Because of its variable expression this broad spectrum of malformations has been given a variety of names, including Goldenhar syndrome, craniofacial dysplasia, Facio-Auriculo-Vertebral Malformation Complex and Hemifacial microsomia, and it can include a range of congenital abnormalities of the head and neck. Mostly these are asymmetric and they often involve ear anomalies (ranging from minor ear anomalies or pre-auricular tags to anotia), mandibular and maxillar hypoplasia, ocular malformations and cervical spine anomalies. Besides these, congenital heart disease and malformations of the renal tract, the skeleton, the central nervous system and other organs may also be involved.

Speech evaluations have revealed velopharyngeal impairment (hypernasality, nasal emissions) and voice and articulation problems (Shprintzen *et al.*, 1980; D'Antonio, Rice and Fink, 1998). The structural and functional etiologies of the speech symptoms are related to palatal, pharyngeal and laryngeal abnormalities. Overt palatal clefts and submucous clefts have been described, as well as unilateral palatal paresis/unilateral hypodynamic palate, an asymmetry of the palate/lack of soft tissue and asymmetry of the lateral and the posterior pharyngeal wall. An association between VPI and a more severe soft tissue deficiency, mandibular hypoplasia, macrostomia and the presence of learning disabilities has been suggested (Funayama *et al.*, 2007). Patients with VPI often have a lateral impairment with the gap on the microsomic side of the face. An asymmetric movement of the velum toward the unaffected side has been described, as well as a reduced movement of the lateral wall on the affected side (Shprintzen *et al.*, 1980). An important implication for assessment and treatment planning of the velopharyngeal function is that it cannot be assumed that these patients have a midline gap as is often seen in other patients and a careful assessment of the velopharyngeal function is needed.

Nasendoscopy gives important information about the structure and function of the palate and the lateral walls, as well as the frontal view of videofluoroscopy (Chapter 8). However, it is important to be aware that the lateral view of videofluoroscopy only shows the closure between the velum and the posterior pharyngeal wall in the midline, hence the lateral gap will not be demonstrated on this view. A careful diagnosis is important for treatment planning and specially tailored surgery can be required. In this population, a high prevalence of abnormalities of laryngeal structures has also been reported (D'Antonio, Rice and Fink, 1998), including small, asymmetric larynx and also narrowed airway dimensions, which are thought to contribute to the high prevalence of airway symptoms in this population.

3.2.4   Absent Velum

A severe form of palatal anomaly is agenesis of the soft palate, that is an absent velum. This condition is commonly described in *Nager Acrofacial Dysostosis*, a rare syndrome characterized by upper and lower limb deformities, short stature, hearing loss (as a result of external and middle ear anomalies), severe micrognathia, restricted jaw opening, and a small and narrow pharynx. The craniofacial abnormalities may cause serious airway obstruction and problems with feeding, dental occlusion and appearance, as well as speech and language impairment (Vallino, Peterson-Falzone and Napoli, 2006). Receptive and expressive language delay has been reported as well as reduced intelligibility (Meyerson and Nisbet, 1987). The severely distorted articulation associated with this condition could be related to malocclusion and crowding of the oral cavity, together with compensatory articulation (glottal stops) related to velopharyngeal impairment. Hypernasality is present because of the absent velum, but may be lessened because of nasal obstruction and other structural abnormalities. This means that the resonance is not always as hypernasal as would be expected with an absent velum, and has instead sometimes been described as muffled.

3.2.5 Micrognathia

Mandibular micrognathia (an abnormally small lower jaw) is a condition that can affect feeding in infancy and in later development may influence the alignment of the teeth. An association of micrognathia and upper airway obstruction caused by glossoptosis (a downward displacement of the tongue) in newborns was described by the French stomatologist Pierre Robin in 1923. Later he added the presence of cleft palate to the symptoms that have historically been known as Pierre Robin Syndrome (Shprintzen, 1988). Thus, the classic triad of symptoms for this condition (which have attracted some debate and disagreement) include micrognathia, upper airway obstruction and a wide U-shaped cleft palate. Today it is agreed that this condition does not constitute a syndrome, with a single primary cause, but rather a sequence, (thus *Pierre Robin sequence*, also called Robin sequence) with micrognathia described as the primary anomaly that, in turn, causes the cleft palate and upper airway obstruction (Shprintzen, 1992). However, micrognathia has multiple etiologies and may be caused by genetic syndromes, chromosomal syndromes, teratogenic influences, mechanically induced factors and multifactorial contributions (Shprintzen, 1992). This means that many of the patients with Pierre Robin sequence do have the sequence as a part of a syndrome, for example Stickler syndrome, 22q11 deletion syndrome, Fetal Alcohol Syndrome or Treacher Collins syndrome (Evans *et al.*, 2006; Shprintzen, 1992). In the non-syndromic group it is thought that the growth of the mandible *in utero* is prevented by mechanical factors, such as uterine compression, or an abnormally small amount of amniotic fluid.

Irrespective of the aetiology, the small mandible prevents the tongue from descending between the two palatal shelves. This makes the fusion of the shelves in the midline impossible, leading to a wide U-shaped palatal cleft (Shprintzen, 1997, pp. 76–79). The high association with syndromes calls for careful and thorough diagnosis of children with Pierre Robin sequence. The heterogeneity of the Pierre Robin group makes it difficult to provide a general description of the speech and language in children with Pierre Robin sequence, which should, rather, be described in relation to the underlying aetiology.

3.2.6 Choanal Atresia

Choanal atresia is a congenital constriction (unilateral or bilateral) of the passage between the nose and throat in the posterior nasal cavities. In bilateral cases the airway requires support immediately after birth, since newborns are obligate nose breathers. Bilateral choanal atresia can be associated with a number of related conditions, including Treacher Collins syndrome and Apert syndrome, and it is a key symptom in *CHARGE syndrome* (Burrow *et al.*, 2009). The acronym stands for the symptoms associated with the condition: Coloboma (C), Heart defect (H), Atresia of the choanae (A), Retardation of growth and/or mental development (R), Genital hypoplasia (G) and Ear anomalies (E). Cleft lip and palate (bilateral or unilateral) is also a frequent finding, as is unilateral facial weakness. A combination of severe visual impairment and sensorineural hearing loss is common, such that some affected individuals are candidates for cochlear implants.

The cause in the majority of cases is a mutation on the CHD7 gene on chromosome 8 (Zentner *et al.*, 2010).

Communication is severely affected in some individuals with CHARGE syndrome due for the most part to a combination of profound hearing and visual impairment. Other symptoms that can have an influence on communication and speech include cognitive deficits, neuropsychiatric disorders and craniofacial anomalies (Strömland *et al.*, 2005). In children with choanal atresia the nasopharyngeal airway is corrected by surgery soon after birth. Recurrent choanal atresia might, however, cause hypo/denasality and repeated dilatations are sometimes necessary during childhood. If a child with choanal atresia also has velopharyngeal impairment the speech problems related to the VPI may sometimes be reduced due to the choanal atresia, but mixed resonance may result.

3.3   Conditions Related to Neurological Aetiology

Muscle weakness and impaired motor function are primary symptoms in cerebral palsy but are also frequent findings in many congenital syndromes and diseases. If the orofacial and velopharyngeal muscles are involved there is a risk for dysarthria, dysphagia, impaired facial expression and poor saliva control. It is common that muscle weakness and deviant motor function have a secondary effect on growth pattern and joint mobility. In the orofacial area this might lead to malocclusion and restricted jaw opening (Kiliaridis and Katsaros, 1998; Botteron *et al.*, 2009). This interrelationship between form and function will aggravate the orofacial problems. An important issue to bear in mind in this regard is that motor deficits are likely to complicate the ability to compensate for structural deficits. For example, a child with typical oral motor development will, in general, have little difficulty compensating for a high palate, but for someone with impaired tongue mobility this unfavourable combination of symptoms might lead to atypical speech production for some consonants. Furthermore, some neurological and neuromuscular diseases have a progressive course that must also be considered when planning therapy (Voet *et al.*, 2010).

Another group of patients has difficulties with sensorimotor planning, rather than motor execution for speech. These are the children with childhood apraxia of speech (CAS). CAS can be an isolated symptom, can accompany other neurological signs or can be part of a syndrome. Significantly, sensorimotor planning deficits can also affect velopharyngeal function (Sealey and Giddens, 2010). CAS can be found in combination with other diagnoses affecting communication, such as language delay, dysarthria and compensatory articulation due to craniofacial anomalies (McCauley and Strand, 2008).

3.3.1   Neuromuscular Diseases

Neuromuscular diseases have their primary defect in the motor neuron, in neuromuscular transmission or in the muscle. They are characterized by muscle weakness and some have a progressive course. Respiratory insufficiency is common due to weak respiratory muscles. A description of the neuromuscular disease *myotonic dystrophy type 1* will serve as an example of a diagnosis where muscle weakness may result in a dysarthria with hypernasal speech.

Myotonic dystrophy type 1 (DM1) is a disease with autosomal dominant inheritance caused by a trinucleotide repeat expansion on chromosome 19q13. There are four subtypes of DM1 defined by age at onset and predominant symptoms: congenital, childhood, classical (or adult) and mild (Koch *et al.*, 1991). It is a multisystemic disease affecting skeletal muscle, smooth muscle, the heart and brain, endocrine regulation and the skin. Distal muscles, including the orofacial area, are generally more affected than proximal muscles. Muscle weakness and wasting is slowly progressive in DM1. Myotonia in the hands, tongue and jaw muscles is a common symptom in adults with DM1 (Harper, 2004, pp. 3–13). In children, clinical myotonia usually becomes successively more common with age (Kroksmark *et al.*, 2005). Most children with DM1 have a developmental delay and cognitive deficits; in some children, DM1 is associated with a neuropsychiatric diagnosis (Roig *et al.*, 1994; Ekström *et al.*, 2009). Another sign of central nervous system involvement is excessive tiredness. Orofacial weakness will interfere with the development of speech and feeding. Speech development is delayed in children with congenital DM1 but the majority will attain acceptable speech skills eventually. Weak facial muscles lead to weak or deviant articulation of labial speech sounds, as well as limited facial expression. In cases of a more general oral motor deficiency, articulation might be imprecise and intelligibility is affected to various degrees. Some children have severe VPI but in many cases this is a symptom that follows the progression of the disease and becomes worse with age (Sjögreen *et al.*, 2007).

3.3.2 Congenital Syndromes

Hypotonia (low muscle tone) is a primary symptom in Down syndrome and many other congenital syndromes. Hypotonic muscles can cause a variety of problems, such as feeding impairment, flaccid dysarthria (including hypernasality) and obstructed airways. *Prader–Willie syndrome* is presented here as an example of a multisystemic disorder with generalized hypotonia in order to show how speech development might be affected.

Prader–Willie syndrome (PWS) is caused by the absence of normally active paternally inherited genes on chromosome 15q11–13. Infantile hypotonia and feeding difficulties are common. When children with PWS are two to four years old, they start to overeat and must be on a constant diet in order to avoid becoming overweight. Short stature and learning disability are other symptoms associated with the disorder. Language development follows the cognitive development. In addition, some have a neuropsychiatric diagnosis. Muscle tone improves as the children grow older but seldom to a fully functional level (Åkefeldt and Gillberg, 1999; Chen *et al.*, 2007). Hypotonia has a negative effect on speech intelligibility, especially if the velopharyngeal muscles are affected, as is often the case in this diagnosis. As muscle tone improves with age hypernasality can resolve simultaneously. Therefore, caution is advised in relation to the recommendation of velopharyngeal surgery for young children with PWS (Shprintzen, 1997). Conversely, some individuals with PWS have hyponasal speech because of narrowing in the nasal and oro-pharyngeal area (Kleppe *et al.*, 1990; Åkefeldt, Åkefeldt and Gillberg, 1997).

3.3.3 Upper and Lower Motor Neuron Lesions

Dysarthria can be due to palsy or paresis of the muscle groups activated in speech. If the Genioglossus (N IX) and Vagus (N X) cranial nerves are involved there is a risk for hypernasal speech as part of the dysarthria. Among children, suprabulbar lesions are typically found in cerebral palsy and in bilateral congenital perisylvian syndrome (Worster Drought syndrome, operculum syndrome) (Clark and Neville, 2008). Traumatic brain injury can be another cause. Möbius syndrome is a diagnosis characterized by multiple cranial nerve defects, often in combination with craniofacial and limb anomalies.

3.4 Conditions Related to a Combination of Structural and Neurological Aetiology

The potential complexity of speech problems is particularly highlighted in syndromes with a combination of structural and neurological aetiology. *Möbius syndrome and 22q11DS* can exemplify the complex picture of a combination of neurological and structural deficiencies.

Möbius syndrome is a rare congenital syndrome, the cause of which is not yet fully understood, although an early insult to the embryo has been suggested. Diagnostic criteria include palsy of the congenital facial (N VII) and abducent (N VI) cranial nerves, caused by hypoplastic lower motor neurons in the brain stem. Other cranial nerves may also be affected, most often the hypoglossus (N XII), glossopharyngeus (N IX) and vagus (N X). Other conditions associated with Möbius syndrome are the Pierre Robin sequence and limb anomaly (Möbius, 2008). Orofacial dysfunctions such as difficulties with feeding/eating, facial expression and saliva control, as well as speech production problems, are common. Some children with Möbius syndrome have cognitive and neuropsychiatric dysfunctions. However, most will have typical development and no language delay. Bilateral facial palsy interferes with the production of labial speech sounds and, in case of total paralysis, compensatory articulation is necessary. Severe dysarthria results if tongue mobility is also impaired. About 20% of individuals with Möbius syndrome have isolated or submucous cleft palate. Some have hypernasal speech as a consequence of glossopharyngeal and vagus nerve palsy (Sjögreen, Andersson-Norinder et al., 2001).

Another example where hypotonia may occur is in 22q11DS. In addition to the structural deficits described earlier, pharyngeal hypotonia has also been reported. An investigation of the superior pharyngeal constrictor (SPC) muscle suggests that this muscle has significantly decreased thickness in patients with 22q11DS and that it contains a significantly greater proportion of type 1 fibres in patients with 22q11DS than in adults without 22q11DS. It was also found that the fibres were more loosely packed. These differences are thought to offer insight into the cause of pharyngeal hypotonia in individuals with 22q11DS (Zim et al., 2003). Furthermore, cranial nerve defects have been observed, with the N Vagus most often involved, which is thought to explain the velar paresis identified in many patients with 22q11DS (Hultman et al., 2000).

3.5   Clinical Implications

Speech assessment and intervention are discussed in detail in later chapters in this book. However, as demonstrated here, many conditions related to cleft palate can have an extensive impact on speech and language. This underlines the importance of obtaining a correct genetic diagnosis, undertaking a comprehensive assessment of speech (in relation to both the structural, neurological and functional findings) and to taking all of this information into consideration when assessing and treating these patients. It is of crucial importance for intervention decisions, in order to differentiate between articulation problems related to structural etiologies like retrognate maxilla, malocclusion or VPI, articulation problems related to a neurological condition and phonological problems related to language delays and disorders (Chapter 15). It is also important to relate the child's speech and language development to their cognitive level.

In assessment and treatment planning for VPI the structures need to be carefully assessed in relation to the specific structural defect, using effective assessment techniques (Chapters 8 and 11). It can also be necessary to tailor velopharyngeal surgery carefully when structures are deviant. Patients with related conditions who are in need of velopharyngeal surgery might have symptoms that could negatively affect the outcome of the surgical procedure (e.g. muscle hypotonia and/or a wide and deep pharynx). For this group it is important in planning surgery to give serious attention, pre-operatively, to the possibility of a less successful outcome than might be expected for patients with normal muscle function and a normal pharynx. However, in such a discussion it would be important to note that although the velopharyngeal function may not be completely normalized by surgical intervention, speech production and intelligibility may still be improved. In relation to velopharyngeal function it is also important to remember that symptoms of VPI may be lessened or may produce mixed nasality in patients with choanal atresia, nasal septum deviation or other constrictions in this area. If the constriction is treated, the VPI may become more obvious and may have a more negative effect on speech production. Even so, of course, it may still be necessary to treat the constriction for other reasons. Thus, for example, an adenoidectomy in patients with cleft palate can potentially risk creating VPI. In conditions with a deep pharynx (for example 22q11DS) and those with generalized hypotonia (e.g. Down syndrome) the risk of developing VPI after adenoidectomy is increased and this surgery should thus be avoided if at all possible. This chapter has thus demonstrated that patients with related conditions are a heterogeneous and challenging group that cannot be treated by a single profession, but needs careful assessment and treatment by a multidisciplinary team.

References

Arvystas, M. and Shprintzen, R.J. (1984) Craniofacial morphology in the velo-cardio-facial syndrome. *Journal of Craniofacial Genetics and Development Biology*, 4, 39–45.

Botteron, S., Verdebout, C.M., Jeannet, P.Y. and Kiliaridis, S. (2009) Orofacial dysfunction in Duchenne muscular dystrophy. *Archives of Oral Biology*, 54, 26–31.

Burrow, T.A., Saal, H.M., de Alarcon, A. *et al.* (2009) Characterization of congenital anomalies in individuals with choanal atresia. *Archives of Otolaryngology Head and Neck Surgery*, 135, 543–547.

Chen, C., Visootsak, J., Dills, S. and Graham, J.M. Jr (2007) Prader-Willi syndrome: an update and review for the primary paediatrician. *Clinical Pediatrics (Phila)*, **46**, 580–591.

Chetpakdeechit, W., Mohlin, B., Persson, C. and Hagberg, C. (2010) Cleft extension and risks of other birth defects in children with isolated cleft palate. *Acta Odontologica Scandinavica*, **68**, 86–90.

Clark, M. and Neville, B.G. (2008) Familial and genetic associations in Worster-Drought syndrome and perisylvian disorders. *American Journal of Medical Genetics*, **146A**, 35–42.

Cohen, M.M. (1978) Syndromes with cleft lip and cleft palate. *Cleft Palate Journal*, **15**, 306–328.

Coleman, J.R. and Sykes, J.M. (2001) The embryology, classification, epidemiology, and genetics of facial clefting. *Facial Plastic Surgery Clinics of North America*, **9**, 1–13.

D'Antonio, L.L., Rice, R.D. and Fink, S.C. (1998) Evaluation of pharyngeal and laryngeal structure and function in patients with oculo-auriculo-vertebral spectrum. *Cleft Palate-Craniofacial Journal*, **35**, 333–341.

Ekström, A.B., Hakenäs-Plate, L., Tulinius, M. and Wentz, E. (2009) Cognition and adaptive skills in mytonic dystrophy type 1: a study of 55 individuals with congenital and childhood forms. *Developmental Medicine and Child Neurology*, **51**, 982–990.

Evans, A.K., Rahbar, R., Rogers, G.F. *et al.* (2006) Robin sequence: a retrospective review of 115 patients. *International Journal of Pediatric Otorhinolaryngology*, **70**, 973–980.

Funayama, E., Igawa, H.H., Nishizawa, N. *et al.* (2007) Velopharyngeal insufficiency in hemifacial microsomia analysis of correlated factors. *Otolaryngology – Head and Neck Surgery*, **136**, 33–37.

Harper, P.S. (2004) Myotonic dystrophy: a multisystemic disorder, in *Myotonic Dystrophy, Present Management, Future Therapy* (eds P.S. Harper, B.G.M. van Engelen, B. Eymard and D.E. Wilcox), Oxford University Press, New York, pp. 135–149.

Hultman, C.S., Riski, J.E., Cohen, S.R. *et al.* (2000) Chiari malformation, cervical spine anomalies, and neurologic deficits in velocardiofacial syndrome. *Plastic and Reconstructive Surgery*, **106**, 16–24.

Kiliaridis, S. and Katsaros, C. (1998) The effects of myotonic dystrophy and Duchenne muscular dystrophy on the orofacial muscles and dentofacial morphology. *Acta Odontologica Scandinavica*, **56**, 369–374.

Kleppe, S.A., Katayama, K.M., Shipley, K.G. and Foushee, D.R. (1990) The speech and language characteristics of children with Prader-Willi syndrome. *Speech and Hearing Disorders*, **55**, 300–309.

Koch, M.C., Grimm, T., Harley, H.G. and Harper, P.S. (1991) Genetic risks for children of women with myotonic dystrophy. *American Journal of Human Genetics*, **48**, 1084–1091.

Kroksmark, A.K., Ekström, A.B., Björk, E. and Tulinius, M. (2005) Myotonic dystrophy: muscle involvement in relation to disease type and size of expanded CTG repeat sequence. *Developmental Medicine and Child Neurology*, **47**, 478–485.

McCauley, R.J. and Strand, E.A. (2008) Treatment of childhood apraxia of speech: clinical decision making in the use of nonspeech oral motor exercises. *Seminars in Speech and Language*, **29**, 284–293.

McDonald-McGinn, D.M., Kirschner, R., Goldmuntz, E. *et al.* (1999) The Philadelphia story: the 22q11.2 deletion: report on 250 patients. *Genetic Counseling*, **10**, 11–24.

Meyerson, M.D. and Nisbet, J.B. (1987) Nager syndrome: an update of speech and hearing characteristics. *Cleft Palate Journal*, **24**, 142–151.

Milerad, J., Larson, O., Hagberg, C. and Ideberg, M. (1997) Associated malformations in infants with cleft lip and palate: a prospective population-based study. *Pediatrics*, **100**, 180–186.

Möbius, P.J. (2008) About congenital bilateral abducens and facial palsy (1888). *Strabismus*, **16**, 39–44.

Óskarsdóttir, S., Persson, C., Eriksson, B.O. and Fasth, A. (2005) Presenting phenotype in 100 children with the 22q11 deletion syndrome. *European Journal of Pediatrics*, **164**, 146–153.

Persson, C., Lohmander, A., Jönsson, R. *et al.* (2003) A prospective cross-sectional study of speech in patients with the 22q11 deletion syndrome. *Journal of Communication Disorders*, **36**, 13–47.

Persson, C., Niklasson, L., Óskarsdótir, S. *et al.* (2006) Language skills in five to eight year-old children with 22q11 deletion syndrome. *International Journal of Language and Communication Disorders*, **41**, 313–333.

Peterson-Falzone, S.J., Hardin-Jones, M.A. and Karnell, M.P. (2001) *Cleft Palate Speech*, 3rd Edn, Mosby, Inc., St Louis, MO.

Roig, M., Ballliu, P.R., Navarro, C. *et al.* (1994) Presentation, clinical course, and outcome of the congenital form of myotonic dystrophy. *Pediatric neurology*, **11**, 208–213.

Ruotolo, R.A., Veitia, N.A., Corbin, A. *et al.* (2006) Velopharyngeal anatomy in 22q11.2 deletion syndrome: a three-dimensional cephalometric analysis. *Cleft Palate-Craniofacial Journal*, **43**, 446–456.

Scherer, N.J., D'Antonio, L.L. and Kalbfleisch, J.H. (1999) Early speech and language development in children with velocardiofacial syndrome. *American Journal of Medical Genetics (Neuropsychiatric Genetics)*, **88**, 714–723.

Sealey, L.R. and Giddens, C.L. (2010) Aerodynamic indicies of velopharyngeal function in childhood apraxia of speech. *Clinical Linguistics & Phonetics*, **24**, 417–430.

Shipster, C., Hearst, D., Dockrell, J.E. *et al.* (2002) Speech and language skills and cognitive functioning in children with Apert syndrome: a pilot study. *International Journal of Language and Communication Disorders*, **37**, 325–343.

Shprintzen, R.J. (1982) Palatal and pharyngeal anomalies in craniofacial syndromes. *Birth Defects*, **18** (1), 53–78.

Shprintzen, R.J. (1988) Pierre Robin, micrognathia, and airway obstruction: the dependency of treatment on accurate diagnosis. *International Anesthesiology Clinics*, **26**, 64–71.

Shprintzen, R.J. (1992) The implication of the diagnosis of Robin sequence. *Cleft Palate-Craniofacial Journal*, **29**, 205–209.

Shprintzen, R.J. (1997) *Genetics, Syndromes, and Communication Disorders*, Singular Publishing Group, Inc., San Diego, CA, USA.

Shprintzen, R.J., Croft, C.B., Berkman, M.D. and Rakoff, S.J. (1980) Velopharyngeal insufficiency in the Facio-Auriculo-Vertebral Malformation Complex. *Cleft Palate Journal*, **17**, 132–137.

Shprintzen, R.J., Siegel-Sadewitz, V.L., Amato, J. and Goldberg, R.B. (1985) Anomalies associated with cleft lip, cleft palate, or both. *American Journal of Medical Genetics*, **20**, 585–595.

Sjögreen, L., Andersson-Norinder, J. and Jacobsson, C. (2001) Development of speech, feeding, eating and facial expression in Möbius sequence. *International Journal of Pediatric Otorhinolaryngology*, **60**, 197–204.

Sjögreen, L., Engvall, M., Ekström, A.B. *et al.* (2007) Orofacial dysfunction in children and adolescents with mytonic dystrophy. *Developmental Medicine and Child Neurology*, **49**, 18–22.

Solot, C.B., Gerdes, M., Kirschner, R.E. *et al.* (2001) Communication issues in 22q11.2 deletion syndrome: children at risk. *Genetics in Medicine*, **3**, 67–71.

Stoll, C., Alembik, Y., Dott, B. and Roth, M.P. (2000) Associated malformations in cases with oral clefts. *Cleft Palate-Craniofacial Journal*, **37**, 41–47.

Strömland, K., Sjögreen, L., Johansson, M. *et al.* (2005) CHARGE association in Sweden: malformations and functional deficits. *American Journal of Medical Genetics*, **133A**, 331–339.

Trost, J.E. (1981) Articulatory additions to the classical description of the speech of persons with cleft palate. *Cleft Palate Journal*, **18**, 193–203.

Vallino, L.D., Peterson-Falzone, S.J. and Napoli, J.A. (2006) The syndromes of Treacher Collins and Nager. *Advances in Speech-Language Pathology*, **8**, 34–44.

Voet, N.B., van der Kooi, E.L., Riphagen, I.I. *et al.* (2010) Strength training and aerobic exercise training for muscle disease. *Cochrane Database of Systematic Reviews*, (1), CD003907.

Zentner, G.E., Layman, W.S., Martin, D.M. and Scacheri, P.C. (2010) Molecular and phenotypic aspects of CHD7 mutation in CHARGE syndrome. *American Journal of Medical Genetics*, **152A** (3), 674–686.

Zim, S., Schelper, R., Kellman, R. *et al.* (2003) Thickness and histologic and histochemical properties of the superior pharyngeal constrictor muscle in velocardiofacial syndrome. *Archives of Facial Plastic Surgery*, **5**, 503–510.

Åkefeldt, A. and Gillberg, C. (1999) Behavior and personality characteristics of children and young adults with Prader-Willi syndrome: a controlled study. *Journal of the American Academy of Child and Adolescent Psychiatry*, **38**, 761–769.

Åkefeldt, A., Åkefeldt, B. and Gillberg, C. (1997) Voice, speech and language characteristics of children with Prader-Willi syndrome. *Intellectual Disability Research*, **41**, 302–311.

4

Surgical Intervention and Speech Outcomes in Cleft Lip and Palate

Anette Lohmander

Karolinska Institutet, Department of Clinical Science, Intervention and Technique, Division of Speech and Language Pathology, SE 141 86, Stockholm, Sweden

4.1 Introduction

'Despite the relatively long history of palatal surgery, little consensus has been reached regarding the best surgical techniques, and even less regarding optimal timing' (Peterson-Falzone, Hardin-Jones and Karnell, 2010, p 149). 'There are still no standard protocols to address the issues of ideal timing for cleft palate repair to attain optimal speech and to avoid abnormal maxillofacial growth after repair' (Leow and Lo, 2008, p. 341). The reason for these opinions is that the scientific basis for intervention of cleft lip and palate (CLP) is inadequate. The huge diversity of practises is a reality – originally reported in 2000 by Shaw et al. in the survey of European cleft services, where 201 teams reported 194 different surgical protocols for unilateral CLP alone (Shaw et al., 2000), it is still the position a decade later. Virtually no elements of treatment, that is surgical technique, timing and sequencing, orthodontics and speech therapy, are based on scientific evidence (Roberts, Semb and Shaw, 1991; Shaw et al., 2000; Friede, 2009). The most likely factors

Cleft Palate Speech: Assessment and Intervention, First Edition. Edited by Sara Howard, Anette Lohmander.

guiding a surgeon's choice of protocol might be their own previous experience or learning from mentors.

The continuing and controversial debate on optimal age for palatal closure has been based on unclear comparisons regarding timing, staging, sequence and techniques. From the theoretical perspective of speech–language development and the particularly sensitive period or state of readiness for speech development between the ages of four and six months, there is no controversy that an early, complete palatal closure is preferable, as advocated by, for example, Kemp-Fincham, Kuehn and Trost-Cardamone (1990).

All palatal repairs have, however, the potential to disturb midfacial growth to a greater or smaller degree, perhaps with the exception of repair after facial growth has been completed, as in post-puberty (Ortiz-Monasterio *et al.*, 1959; Mars and Houston, 1990). The controversy regarding timing of palatal closure is related to the goal of achieving both adequate facial growth and normal speech development. Since an unoperated cleft maxilla exhibits near normal or even exuberant (according to Mars) growth (Mars and Houston, 1990), but is associated with extremely poor speech (Chapter 6), it has been logical to claim that delaying hard palatal repair until maxillary growth is completed would be a desirable approach (Kuijpers-Jagtman and Long, 2000). Delayed surgery *per se* has not been proven always to result in better growth than early procedures (Ross, 1987). Nevertheless, examples of favourable growth results after delaying repair of the hard palate have been reported from two European centres, one of them from Zurich, Switzerland (Gnoinsky and Haubensak, 1997) and the other one from Gothenburg, Sweden (Friede and Enemark, 2001; Lilja *et al.*, 2006). After comparison of various protocols for two-stage palate repair, it has been pointed out that this surgery does not actually form a single approach to improvement of maxillary growth. Different surgical methods for repair might lead to a great variation in growth outcome, irrespective of timing of the procedure (Friede, 2009).

The benefit of early palate closure for speech development was hypothesized decades ago (Jolleys, 1954; Lindsay, LeMesurier and Farmer, 1962; Evans and Renfrew, 1974) but the opinion was based solely on chart reviews. Even in the 1980s the scientific evidence for ideal age at palatal repair was weak, with only clinical reviews as the basis for choosing three to seven months as the ideal age for surgery (Kaplan, 1981; Randal *et al.*, 1983). A delay of repair to twelve to eighteen months, which still seems to be the most commonly used age range, was considered a worse alternative than two-stage repair with early soft palate closure (Kaplan, 1981). This latter protocol was considered as the second best alternative and has since then been supported by, for example, Rohrich *et al.* (2000). They claimed that a sequenced procedure with early velar closure at around three to six months and a delayed hard palate repair at age fifteen to eighteen months would provide the best opportunities for favourable maxillary growth as well as normal speech development. In terms of practice, however, this approach has not taken off. Instead, one-stage repair between six and eighteen months is the common practice.

Presently, diversity of surgical techniques for palatal repair might more or less mirror the variation found in timing of surgery. For instance, procedures described as examples of early or late palatal repair might also be examples of different techniques, which make it difficult to get a clear view of the impact of timing of surgery on speech. This chapter reviews current evidence regarding speech outcome after different surgical protocols.

Specifically, attempts are made to answer questions such as, what is the evidence regarding speech development after currently practised surgical regimens, and what other considerations have to be made?

4.2 Basics of Surgery on Cleft Palate

By its location a cleft palate has an impact on structure and function for feeding, hearing and speech. For patients born with a CLP malformation, maxillary growth and midfacial appearance might also be affected, particularly after palatal surgery. The purpose of cleft palate repair is to establish a separation between the oral and nasal cavities in the area of the hard palate and to restore a functioning velopharyngeal closure mechanism primarily by soft palate repair. A further purpose is to establish good Eustachian tube function.

During the nineteenth century there were important inventions of new surgical methods for palatal repair, such as the Von Langenbeck repair and the Wardill-Kilner push-back closure. During the twentieth century further development occurred with the creation of new procedures as well as refinement of existing methods. Today, the main objective of cleft palate surgery is to enhance speech development without jeopardizing maxillary growth.

After a brief exposition of commonly used surgical procedures, current knowledge about speech outcome is presented here. This is followed by a discussion about the shortcomings of certain protocols as well as needs for future improvements. In addition to the timing issue, surgical closure of palatal clefts can be divided into one- and two-stage repairs. Regarding the latter, the sequence of the palatal procedures must also be considered.

4.2.1 One-Stage Procedures

With respect to one-stage procedures there are two major techniques for closure of the hard palate, both of them developed a long time ago. The *Von Langenbeck repair* was introduced in the early 1860s but the method is still widely practised, often with some modifications. Almost always the method involves use of a *vomer flap* to repair the nasal mucosa. To close the palatal side of the cleft, mucoperiosteal flaps are moved medially and sutured in the midline. This leaves areas laterally on each side of the hard palate, where bone is exposed resulting in growth-restricting scar tissue. The procedure is traditionally performed without levator reconstruction. The other major method for one-stage palatal repair is the *Wardill-Kilner push-back closure,* developed in 1937. This technique is also still practised by many surgeons. The push-back of palatal mucosa was introduced with the intention of lengthening the soft palate, which would supposedly facilitate velopharyngeal closure for speech. It was not taken into consideration that large patches of denuded bone were created anteriorly as well as laterally in the hard palate. This resulted in extensive areas of scar tissue with great risks for severe impairment of maxillary growth. A narrow cleft in the palate might be repaired without the lateral releasing incisions, thereby reducing the negative effect of scaring on growth (Sommerlad, 2008) (Figure 4.1).

There are also two major techniques for soft palate repair in one-stage procedures. The *intravelar veloplasty* (IVV) consists of a radical dissection of the muscles of the soft palate, allowing for reconstruction of the normal levator sling in the posterior part of the soft palate (Kriens, 1969). This principle of radical dissection of the levator palati muscles has been further modified by Sommerlad in his palate repair technique (Sommerlad, 2008). The combined procedures of both von Langenbeck with IVV and Wardill-Kilner with IVV are illustrated in Figures 4.2 and 4.3. *Furlow double-opposing Z-plasty* (Figure 4.4) was developed in the 1980s, allowing radical realignment of the levator sling as well as lengthening of the soft palate.

Thus, the one-stage procedures consist of different techniques for repair of the hard and soft palate cleft, respectively, but they are carried out in the same operation. It should be noted, however, that in some surgical protocols the vomer flap repair of the anterior palate is undertaken at the time of the lip repair in complete cleft lip and palate, most usually three months of age, thus being a two-stage procedure (Sommerlad, 2008).

4.2.2 Two-Stage Procedures and Their Sequence

For most clinicians a two-stage protocol for palatal surgery means soft palate repair first, followed by hard palate closure to at some later time (Figure 4.5), though a reverse order of the procedures is not uncommon. The same or similar techniques as described for one-stage palatal repair might be used in two-stage regimens as well. However, new procedures have also been developed (Friede, 2009). At closure of the soft palate, common practice today is to separate the velar mucosa and the abnormally positioned muscles from the posterior hard palate. This will achieve a longer velum after the repair, which will enhance possibilities for adequate velopharyngeal function. From the point of view of future maxillary growth, it is crucial that the dissections are made in such a way that only minor areas of palatal bone are left exposed after surgery. Also, repair of the hard palate should be accomplished with minimal or no palatal bone left denuded after surgery to minimize the risk for later maxillary growth impairments.

4.2.3 Timing

The timing of cleft palate surgery relates to age at repair in both one-stage procedures and both operations in two-stage procedures. Palatal repairs are often described as early or late closure with unclear definition of 'early' and 'late'. It becomes even more confusing when timing of one-stage procedures is compared to timing of two-stage procedures without clarifying which of the three possible operations is referred to.

Early one-stage procedures are usually performed between six and eighteen months of age. In a two-stage procedure, early soft palate closure is usually carried out between three and nine months, whereas age for hard palate repair can vary between twelve

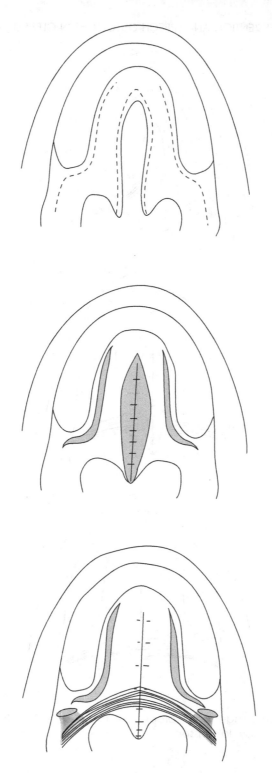

Figure 4.1 A one-stage repair with intravelar veloplasty without releasing incisions (Image courtesy of May Johansson).

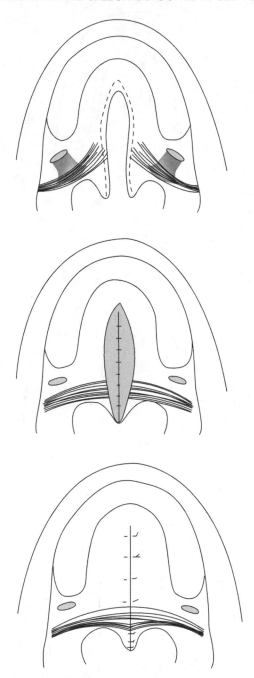

Figure 4.2 The von Langenbeck procedure modified with intravelar veloplasty (Image courtesy of May Johansson).

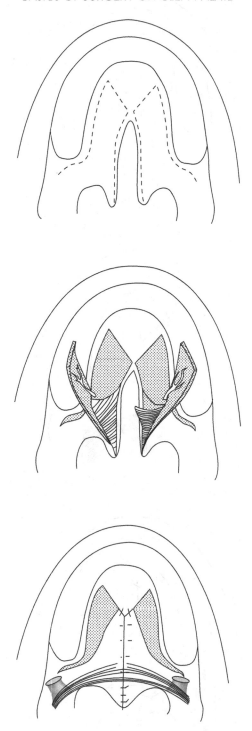

Figure 4.3 The Wardill-Kilner procedure modified with intravelar veloplasty (Image courtesy of May Johansson).

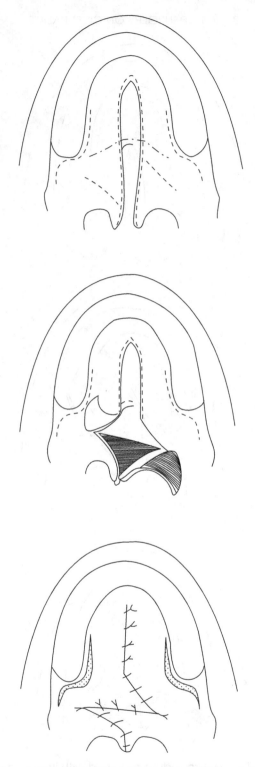

Figure 4.4 The Furlow procedure (Image courtesy of May Johansson).

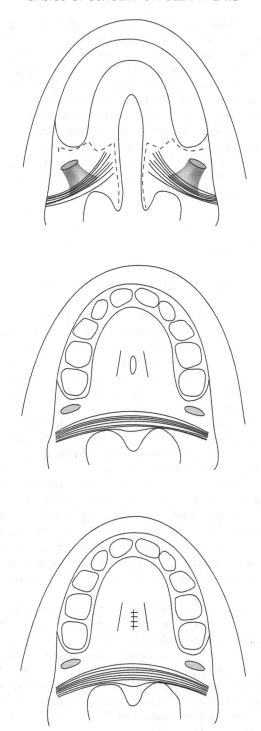

Figure 4.5 A two-stage closure with soft palate repair first and hard palate closure later (Image courtesy of May Johansson).

months and adolescence. A later age for hard palate repair (delayed hard palate closure, DHPC) has been thought to enhance maxillary growth (Friede, 2009).

For decades there have been controversies about the effect of age at surgery. It is easy to imagine that palatal repair at different ages would affect speech development differently. According to clinical opinion and generally supported by literature, some types of palatal surgery will enhance speech development but might restrict maxillary growth. Other techniques might result in more normal maxillary growth but will increase the risk of poor speech development. However, and as shown later in this chapter, the evidence base for speech outcome related to different surgical procedures is weak. Regarding palatal surgery from a historical perspective, the reader is referred to a comprehensive review by Peterson-Falzone, Hardin-Jones and Karnell (2010). For secondary outcomes, the reader is referred to Chapter 5).

4.3 Basics of Outcomes

There are many types of bias in clinical outcome research for patients with CLP. These include, for example, different susceptibility for poor or favourable results due to differences in patients' cleft severity, in a small group of patients perhaps familial facial growth patterns; differing skills of surgeons; the conscientiousness of record keeping; different rules for retrospective patient exclusions; absence of agreed-upon rating scales of outcome; likeliness to report positive findings rather than negative ones. In this chapter sources of bias are addressed regarding current evidence for speech outcome after different primary surgical practices. In addition, different hierarchies of evidence (Chapter 18) are considered.

The importance of longitudinal data was highlighted decades ago. Such information would, for instance, show possible changes in ability for velopharyngeal closure as the child grows. This will be missed in studies only relying on one-time post-operative assessments (Hardin-Jones *et al.*, 1993; Karnell and Van Demark, 1986). Fifteen years ago, Peterson-Falzone (1996) was confident that future studies would report evidence from longitudinal data since more treatment centres were collecting longitudinal outcome data on babies operated before twelve months of age (Barimo *et al.*, 1987; Grunwell and Russell, 1987; Copeland, 1990). Unfortunately, even today, neither studies frequently referred to in the literature, nor more recent reports include any (or only sparse) longitudinal data. In addition, many speech outcome investigations are based on chart reviews or live assessments without reliability data and the possibility of checking or replicating the study.

To review the evidence of speech outcome after primary surgery in individuals born with CLP, the focus of this chapter is primarily on those longitudinal and cross-sectional studies in which speech outcomes are based on speech recordings, thereby fulfilling the requirement of repeatability. However, those studies, based on chart reviews and live assessments, that are often referenced to in the literature will also be referred to. The review is based on the minimum methodological requirements as stated by the American Cleft Palate Association as early as 1993 (American Cleft Palate–Craniofacial Association, 1993) and updated in 2000 by Lohmander and Olsson (2004) in their critical review of the literature, and by Sell (2005).

4.4   Speech Outcomes

A total of 34 articles based on assessment from recordings (audio or video) including speech data from children to young adults were found. They were published in English language Journals over the 25 year period (1984–2010) and represented nine different languages. The articles are presented in Appendix 4.A and are included in the reference list. Because the only criterion was being based on recordings, a number of biases were found in the studies, of which all but two were retrospective. This needs to be taken this into account when interpreting the information below.

4.4.1 Degree of Evidence

From Appendix 4.A it could be summarized that no study fulfilled the requirements for evidence level I (i.e. high quality, randomized controlled trial (RCT) with adequate power or systematic review of these studies) (Chapter 18). Only two studies were found that fulfilled the requirements for evidence level II (lesser quality RCT, prospective cohort study or systematic review). Both of them contained very small numbers and in the RCT there were mixed cleft types and no reliability figures reported. Ten studies were comparative retrospective studies, that is previously recorded material was used for comparison of speech outcome. Nine of these reported comparison of procedure and/or timing of cleft palate surgery, one reported timing of palatal surgery and lexical development, and one considered pre-surgical orthopaedics. Ten studies were retrospective longitudinal case series and 12 were cross-sectional.

4.4.2 Bias

The bias in these studies included small sample sizes (only eight studies included 50–100 subjects and only five more than 100), selection bias, comparison bias, lack of reporting of reliability, and in most studies only internal raters were used, that is, the Speech–Language Pathologists normally working with the patients were also performing the ratings. A summary of the bias found is given in Table 4.1.

Table 4.1   A summary of the bias found in 34 studies reviewed for speech outcome.

Bias	Number (%)
Small group (<50)	16 (47)
Selection or exclusion	22 (65)
Listener (single or no external)	21 (62)
Reliability not reported	8 (24)

4.4.3 The ICF[1]

Only two of the 34 studies included aspects of function, activity and participation in the outcome of the study. In 16 articles only aspects of function were reported; in 11 papers aspects of function and activity; in six articles aspects of function (with or without activity) and contextual factors (personal in five and environmental in one); and in one study activity and contextual environmental were reported. It can be assumed that, until recently, aspects of participation and contextual factors have been more often included in articles in other areas of the discipline, for example psychology (Chapter 17).

4.4.4 Ages

Each cross-sectional study often covered a large age range, for example 6–16 or 7–20 years of age. In three studies the range covered ages from children to adults. In five studies only adults were included. In studies of children, typically one age level between three and twelve years of age was used. There were nine longitudinal investigations, which included between two and five ages within the subjects and typically covered ages between three and ten years. In two studies the early ages 1– 1.5 years were included, and one study covered the ages from five to nineteen years of age. In summary, there are most data on speech (both cross-sectional and longitudinal) available from the ages between five and ten years of age.

4.4.5 Cleft Types

In 15 articles only one cleft type was investigated.Thirteen articles included a mix of different cleft types but separately reported on. In the six remaining studies the information on cleft type was missing or they reported on all cleft types as a group.

4.4.6 Surgical Method

A one-stage operation had been used in 15 studies and a two-stage procedure in 14. The Wardill-Kilner (WK) and von Langenbeck (vL) techniques were most commonly used in one-stage procedures and were often compared regarding their speech outcome. Two studies compared one-stage versus two-stage procedures, and in three studies there was no information on surgical technique.

---

[1]See Introduction and Chapter 17

4.4.7 Summary of Speech Outcomes

A summary of speech outcomes reported in the reviewed articles was categorized in terms of speech accuracy, that is prevalence of absence of nasal emission, hypernasality, articulation errors and *good* intelligibility. In addition, the occurrence of secondary pharyngeal surgery was noted (Appendix 4.A), although the problems of using this as an outcome measure have been highlighted by Sommerlad (2008). The data confirm that the less severe the cleft (i.e. in the soft palate only), the better the speech outcome. The most common surgical procedures used were WK, vL and a two-stage procedure with DHPC. In four studies speech outcome after vL and WK was compared, three of which related to adults and to different cleft types (Becker *et al.*, 2000; Farzaneh *et al.*, 2008; Farzaneh *et al.*, 2009) and one to five-year-olds with unilateral cleft lip and palate (UCLP) (Pigott *et al.*, 2002). No obvious differences in outcome between the two procedures were found. The outcome after the Furlow procedure (F) was compared with vL in two studies. The first was a small RCT with outcome reported at 3.5 years of age, with best results after the Furlow procedure (Spauwen, Goorhuis-Brouwer and Schutte, 1992). The other reported outcome retrospectively in adults (Van Lierde *et al.*, 2004).

In the remaining studies speech outcome was compared following different surgical procedures or timing (early versus late) in one-stage or two-stage procedures. It is therefore impossible to detect the significant factor, if any, for speech outcome. It is, however, worth noticing that the speech outcome reported after two-stage procedures could be at least as good as or even better than reported after one-stage procedures (Van Demark *et al.*, 1989; Persson *et al.*, 2002; Lohmander *et al.*, 2006). This is true even at ages when the cleft in the hard palate was still unoperated. This has been explained by the combination of a good velar function after early successful veloplasty and a reduction of the residual cleft size in the hard palate. Although no obvious relationship between size of the residual cleft and speech outcome has been found, this is presumably due to the difficulties measuring the size from the oral side of the cleft (Lohmander, Persson and Owman-Moll, 2002).

One further interesting comparison can be made. Two recent studies on isolated cleft palate, both comparing Swedish-speaking children with a cleft in the hard as well the soft palate (HCP) and children with a cleft in the soft palate only (SCP) at five years of age, have included acceptable sample sizes (Persson *et al.*, 2002; Nyberg *et al.*, 2010). Both studies were carried out with sufficient and similar methodology. A two-stage palatal repair with soft palate closure at eight months and hard palate repair at four years of age was performed in the study by Persson *et al.* (2002). That means that the individuals born with a SCP had the whole palate closed at eight months of age. In the other study the palatal cleft was closed in children with HCP and SCP in a one-stage procedure at 12 to 15 months of age. The results revealed a favourable outcome for both HCP and SCP with the soft palate repaired at eight months of age. Not only was speech accuracy lower in the children who had their palates closed at 12 to 15 months, but 27% of the group had received pharyngeal flaps compared to 2% in the group who had a two-stage repair. When comparing the outcome in children with a SCP the differences become even more striking. All or close to all children had no nasal emission or hypernasality at five years of age after soft palate closure at eight months compared to 50% in the group who had the palate closed at 12 to 15 months of age. It is reasonable to believe that the timing of soft palate repair (8 versus 12 to 15 months) but also the technique contributed to the highly significant differences.

The Appendix also indicates that the number of secondary pharyngeal surgeries (flaps), performed in order to improve speech, increased with age. In the studies of adults a mean of 23% of the individuals had been treated with a pharyngeal flap. The lowest figure (11%) was found in the study of individuals born with UCLP treated with a two-stage procedure with DHPC. The highest figures were found in individuals born with bilateral cleft lip and palate (BCLP), thus confirming larger difficulties with velopharyngeal function and speech in the most severe cleft type.

A comparison was also made with results reported in frequently referenced studies, although performed from live ratings of chart reviews. Interestingly, there were, with few exceptions, no major differences in the results presented in these articles; however, they focused on articulation. There was most information available on five-year-olds with reported articulation proficiency in the 26–66% range (Park *et al.*, 2000; Hardin-Jones and Jones, 2005; Dalston, 1990; Peterson-Falzone, 1990). These were all longitudinal chart reviews. Two studies differed, though. One was by Copeland (1990), who reported 91% articulation accuracy in the five-year-olds age group and who also reported over 90% normal resonance. No obvious reason for these favourable results could be detected. The other study is at the other end of the scale with 0% articulation accuracy at age four years and only 17% at age six years (Pradel *et al.*, 2009). The results were based on clinical live assessments. The longitudinal chart reviews revealed a mean articulation proficiency at 10–16 years of age of 84% and a follow up at young adulthood of 80% (Hardin-Jones *et al.*, 1993). The figures are, with few exceptions, similar to the ones obtained in the current studies chosen for review.

Based on the speech outcome reviewed for different age groups and compared with reported outcome from chart reviews and live assessments, it is concluded that 50–60% of three-year-olds could be expected to have good speech. At four to five years of age the expected figure is about 60 to 70% and at age six to eight years about 70 to 80% of children should have normal speech. Between 10 and 16 years of age around 80% could be expected to have good speech and in young adulthood 90–100%, with remaining s-distortions as the most commonly reported problem. The lower figures are reported for individuals with BCLP and the higher ones for individuals with SCP.

Even though possible differences related to timing and technique are not yet clarified there are observations that need further attention. Whereas some studies report on glottal misarticulations as the main articulation problem during pre-school/early school ages (Hardin-Jones and Jones, 2005), other papers report only backing or oral retraction as the main problem (Van Demark *et al.*, 1989; Lohmander *et al.*, 2006; Lohmander, Friede and Lilja, 2009). These differences were presumably related to the surgical procedure and/or their timing, with velopharyngeal closure possible in spite of a remaining unoperated cleft in the hard palate. One-stage closure at around 12 to 18 months was most common in studies reporting glottal misarticulations as the main problem, while two-stage procedures with early soft palate closure were practised in the studies reporting retracted oral articulation as the main problem. This also holds true for the early development of speech, where a two-stage procedure with early soft palate closure at around six months of age has been shown to lead to a higher occurrence of oral plosives, even if the cleft in the hard palate is unoperated and uncovered (Lohmander, Lillvik and Friede, 2004; Willadsen and Albrechtsen, 2006), than a one-stage procedure at around 12 months (Jones, Chapman and Hardin-Jones, 2003; Scherer, Williams and Proctor-Williams, 2008). The development from early speech production in pre-speech to speech is currently the subject of considerable interest. For information of the early development of speech the reader is referred to Chapter 2.

Another interesting issue, which was not highlighted until results of longitudinal studies were published, is *the effect of time* – that is, that speech improves with increasing age. '... time was an even more important variable than timing of palatoplasty for the acquisition of desirable phonetics articulation features.' (O'Gara, Logemann and Rademaker, 1994, p. 450). A similar conclusion was drawn in a study of the effect of different delays of hard palate closure where age at study, but not age at closure of the cleft in the hard palate, could explain improvement of speech (Lohmander *et al.*, 2006). This needs further attention in more longitudinal studies: there is the possibility of some clarification of the impact of surgical technique and timing through a large RCT which is currently running (the Scandcleft project). The initial report from this project will deal with speech and maxillary growth at age five years. The effect on speech from three different surgical procedures for palatal repair will be tested against a fourth method, which actually is the main protocol under investigation (Lohmander *et al.*, 2009). Another large RCT (Timing of Primary Surgery in cleft palate, TOPS) on the effect of timing of palatal surgery (six or twelve months of age) on speech in individuals born with CPO was initiated in 2010. Accordingly, in the coming years, a much better basis for decisions about optimal procedure and timing for palatal surgery will be available. Preferably, the information will also include information on case-load volume and/or surgical skill, which is thought to be an important variable but which has not been very much discussed in relation to outcome.

4.5   Conclusions

A brief summary of the most reliable studies of speech in individuals born with CLP revealed 'expected speech outcomes' at different ages. These have to be interpreted with caution since considerable heterogeneity exists within the study groups. More comparative studies of surgical methods for cleft palate closure are needed, as well as longitudinal ones. Careful data collection and collaboration between centers will enhance this research. There will, however, always be possible differences related to the surgeon, since operative techniques are difficult to reproduce (Sommerlad, 2008). The best practice for speech outcome is the surgical procedure that is safe and provides the optimal basis for speech development for each individual as well as for the group of babies born with CLP as a whole.

We need to expand our knowledge regarding which surgical method or methods give the best speech outcome both in early speech development and in the longer term. However, since speech development is also influenced by factors other than the cleft itself and the surgical method adopted, and it is well known that not all children born with CLP develop speech disorders, we also need to increase our understanding of the additional factors that have an impact on the speech development. This will increase the potential for efficient intervention in babies born with CLP.

Appendix 4.A Review of Evidence and Methodology in Studies of Speech Outcome in Individuals Born with Cleft Lip and Palate

Reference (Language)	Design	ICF level (WHO, 2001)	Level of evidence[a]	Cleft Type	Selection No. included/ Out of possible	Ages for speech assessment (SA) and operation	No. of surgeons
Spauwen, Goorhuis-Brouwer and Schutte, 1992 (Dutch)	Randomized controlled trial (procedure)	Function	II	BCLP: 4 UCLP: 5 CPO: 11	20/NI	SA: 3.5 years *One-stage* vL: NI Furlow: NI	2
Lohmander and Persson, 2008 (Swedish)	Prospective cohort (longitudinal)	Function and activity	II	UCLP Controls:10	20/NI	SA: (18 months), 3,5,7 years *Two-stage* SPC: 6 months HPC 3–4 years	2
Harding and Campbell, 1989 (British English)	Retrospective comparative, cross-sectional, (Procedure/ Timing)	Function and contextual environmental	III	BCLP: 6 UCLP: 20 HCP: 8 SCP: 15	48/NI	SA: 6–8.4 and 14 years respectively *One-stage* (n = 20) 15 months (WK) *Two-stage* (n = 28) SPC: 18 months HPC: 7–8 years	1
Henningsson, Karling and Larsson, 1990 (Swedish)	Retrospective comparative, cross-sectional, (Procedure/ Timing)	Function and activity	III	UCLP: 36 BCLP: 9	45/NI	SA: 3–5.5 years *One-stage* 18 months 'Early' *Two-stage* NI 'Late'	NI
Karling et al., 1993 (Swedish)	Retrospective comparative, cross-sectional, (pre-surgical orthopedics, PSO)	Function and activity	III	BCLP: 19 UCLP: 84 Controls: 40	103/NI	SA: 7–20 years *One-stage* (WK) 13–35 months PSO: no difference	NI

Method for documentation and assessment	Bias	Speech outcome (%)				Secondary Phar. flap surgery (%)
		Absence of nasal emission	Absence of hypernasality	Absence of artic. errors	Good intelligibility	
Audio recordings Multiple raters (2)	Small group Comparison bias Blinding? No reliability	vL: 70 F: 100	50 100	70 60	NI NI	NI NI
Audio recordings Randomized Identity blinded multiple raters (2) External rater (1) Inter- and intra-rater reliability	Small group	3Y[b]: 60 5Y: 90 7Y: 90	43 70 90	42 83 81	NI 82 NI	0 0 0
Audio recordings Multiple blinded (?) raters SLT (4) Surgeons (2) Lay listeners (3)	Small group Selection bias No reliability Listener bias?	6–8Y: 48 6Y[b]: 40 14Y: 75	80 50 80	25 45 50	NI NI NI	NI NI NI
Audio recordings	Small group Selection bias Comparison bias Randomization? Listener bias No inter- and intra-rater reliability No external rater	NI	NI	E: 61 L: 56	NI	NI
Audio recordings Multiple blinded (?) raters (3) + live assessment (2) Inter- and intra-rater reliability	Selection bias Randomization? No external rater	NI prevalence	64	NI prevalence	86	UCLP: 24 BCLP: 42

(Continued)

Appendix 4.A (*Continued*)

Reference (Language)	Design	ICF level (WHO, 2001)	Level of evidence[a]	Cleft Type	Selection		Ages for speech assessment (SA) and operation	No. of surgeons
					No. included/ Out of possible			
Becker et al., 2000 Swedish	Retrospective comparative, cross-sectional (Procedure/ Timing)	Function and contextual personal	III	CPO	66/80 randomly selected from 160		SA: >18 y *One-stage* 7 months (vL) 18 months (WK)	NI
Pigott et al., 2002 (British English)	Retrospective comparative, cross-sectional (Procedure)	Function	III	UCLP	66/139		SA: 5 years *One-stage* 6 months (CV, vL, ML)	1
Van Lierde et al., 2004 (Flemish)	Retrospective comparative, cross-sectional (Procedure/ Timing)	Function and activity	III	NI	37/103		SA: 16–30 years *One-stage* (n = 20) (WK) 1–2 years *Two-stage* (n = 17) (F) SPC: 13–28 months HPC: 8–12 years	2
Chapman et al., 2008 (American English)	Retrospective comparative cross-sectional, (Timing/ Lexical development)	Function	III	BCLP: 8 UCLP: 24 HCP: 4 SCP: 4 Controls: 40	40/NI		SA: 3 years *One-stage* Early (n = 20) 7–14 months Late (n = 20) 12–23 months[c]	10
Farzaneh et al., 2008 (Swedish)	Retrospective comparative, cross-sectional (Procedure/ Timing)	Function	III	UCLP	61/ Randomly from 181		SA: 'adults' *One-stage* 8 months (vL) (n = 34) 18 months (WK) (n = 27)	NI
Farzaneh et al., 2009 (Swedish)	Retrospective comparative, cross-sectional (Procedure/ Timing)	Function, activity, and contextual personal	III	BCLP	36/69		SA: 'adults' *One-stage* 8 months (vL) (n = 26) 18 months (WK) (n = 10)	NI

Method for documentation and assessment	Bias	Speech outcome (%)				Secondary Phar. flap surgery (%)
		Absence of nasal emission	Absence of hypernasality	Absence of artic. errors	Good intelligibility	
Audio recordings Multiple raters (3) Blinded Inter- and intra-rater reliability	Selection bias No external rater Randomization?	WK: NI vL: NI	68 84	88 88	NI NI	36 48
Audio recordings Multiple raters (2) Blinded? Inter-rater reliability	Selection bias Randomization? No external rater No intra-rater reliability	CV: 68 vL: 77 ML: 54	54 64 59	23 46 68	NI NI NI	9 9 9
Audio recordings Multiple raters (2) Consensus transcription Inter-rater reliability	Selection bias Comparison bias Randomization? No external rater No intra-rater reliability	WK:NI F: NI	76 43	s-distort. only	82 79	NI NI
Audio recordings Multiple raters (2) Blinding? Inter- and intra-rater reliability	Small group Selection bias Comparison bias Randomization? No external rater	E: NI L: NI	NI NI	61 56	NI NI	NI NI
Audio recordings Multiple blinded (?) raters (2) Inter- and intra-rater reliability	Randomization? No external rater	WK: 74 vL: 94	67 79	s-distort. only	100 97	15 26
Audio recordings Multiple blinded (?) raters (2) Inter- and intra-rater reliability	Small group Selection bias Randomization? No external rater	WK: 80 vL: 89	40 50	s-distort. only	100 79	40 35

(Continued)

Appendix 4.A   (*Continued*)

Reference (Language)	Design	ICF level (WHO, 2001)	Level of evidence[a]	Cleft Type	Selection		Ages for speech assessment (SA) and operation	No. of surgeons
					No. included/ Out of possible			
Nyberg *et al.*, 2010 (Swedish)	Retrospective comparative, cross-sectional (Procedure/ Cleft type)	Function	III	HCP: 53 SCP: 33 Controls: 18	86/133		SA: 5 years *One-stage* 12–15 months (MIT, n = 60) (MITmr, n = 26) Procedure: No difference	NI
Riski and DeLong, 1984 (American English)	Retrospective case series, *longitudinal*	Function	IV	All cleft types	108/NI		SA: 3–8 years No information on operation	1
Lohmander-Agerskov *et al.*, 1995 (Swedish)	Retrospective case series, *longitudinal*	Function and activity	IV	BCLP: 5 UCLP: 10	15/18		SA: 5,7,8.5,10 years *Two-stage* SPC: 6–8 months HPC: 8–9 years	NI
Lohmander-Agerskov *et al.*, 1998 (Swedish)	Retrospective case series, *longitudinal*	Function and activity	IV	BCLP: 5 UCLP: 13 HCP: 3	21/35		13 mos, 3, 5 years *Two-stage* SPC: 8 months HPC: 8–9 years	NI
Pulkkinen *et al.*, 2001 (Finnish)	Retrospective case series, *longitudinal*	Function	IV	UCLP: 30 CPO: 35	65/NI		SA: 4,6,8 years *One-stage* 1–2 years (WK or Cronin)	NI
Zansi, Cheroillod and Hohlfeld 2002 (French)	Retrospective case series *longitudinal*	Function	IV	BCLP: 7 UCLP: 11	18/18		SA: 3.5–7 years *Two-stage* SPC: 3 months HPC: 6 months (Malek proc) edure	1

Method for documentation and assessment	Bias	Speech outcome (%)				Secondary Phar. flap surgery (%)
		Absence of nasal emission	Absence of hypernasality	Absence of artic. errors	Good intelligibility	
Audio recordings Randomized Multiple, blinded raters (2), external raters (2) Inter- and intra-rater reliability	Selection bias	HCP: 61 SCP: 53	51 50	81 87	NI NI	27/4$_{mr}$ 0
Audio recordings	Selection bias Single rater Inter-rater reliability on training sample No intra-rater reliability	3Y:NI 4Y:NI 5Y:NI 6Y:NI 7Y:NI 8Y:NI	NI NI NI NI NI NI	10 21 36 53 67 74	NI NI NI NI NI NI	43
Audio recordings Randomized Identity blinded multiple raters (2) Inter- and intra-rater reliability	Small group No external rater	5Y^b: 67 7Y^b: 67 10Y: 93	53 87 93	53 60 80	NI 60 100	13 27
Audio recordings Multiple raters (2) Randomized, identity blinded	Exclusion bias Small group No external rater	3Y^b: 53 5Y^b: 76	60 78	50 72	NI 79	0 0
Audio recordings, Multiple listeners (2) Blinded? Inter- and intra-rater reliability	Small group Selection bias Randomization? No external rater	3Y: 41 6Y: 60 8Y: 82	67 59 72	90 94 100	NI NI NI	13 13 13
Video recordings Multiple blinded(?) raters (2)	Small group Comparison bias No external rater No reliability	60 (VPC)		NI	94	17

(Continued)

Appendix 4.A   (*Continued*)

Reference (Language)	Design	ICF level (WHO, 2001)	Level of evidence[a]	Selection		Ages for speech assessment (SA) and operation	No. of surgeons
				Cleft Type	No. included/ Out of possible		
Lohmander, Persson and Owman-Moll, 2002 (Swedish)	Retrospective case series, *longitudinal*	Function and activity	IV	UCLP: 22	22/22	SA: 5,7 y *Two-stage* SPC: 2–12 months HPC: 8–9 years	NI
Lohmander et al., 2006 (Swedish)	Retrospective case series, *longitudinal*	Function and activity	IV	UCLP: 26	26/26	SA: 5,7,10 years *Two-stage* SPC: 7 months HPC: 3–7 years	2
Persson, Lohmander and Elander, 2006 (Swedish)	Retrospective case series, *longitudinal*	Function	IV	HCP: 11 SCP: 15	26/32	SA: 3,5,7,10 years *Two-stage* SPC: 6 months HPC: 4 years	NI
Lohmander, Friede and Lilja 2009 (Swedish)	Retrospective case series *longitudinal*	Function and activity	IV	UCLP	55/65	SA: 5,7,10,16,19 years *Two-stage* SPC: 8 months HPC: 8 years	NI
Havstam, Dahlgren Sandberg and Lohmander, 2011 (Swedish)	Retrospective case series, *longitudinal*	Function, activity, and contextual personal	IV	BCLP: 8 UCLP: 20 HCP: 18 SCP: 8	54/68	SA: 5,7,10 years No information on operation	NI
Bardach, Morris and Olin, 1984 (German)	Retrospective case series, cross-sectional	Function	IV	UCLP Controls: 8	43/NI (Random selection)	SA: 12–23 years *Two-stage* SPC: 6–18 months HPC: 8–22 years	1

Method for documentation and assessment	Bias	Speech outcome (%)				Secondary Phar. flap surgery (%)
		Absence of nasal emission	Absence of hypernasality	Absence of artic. errors	Good intelligibility	
Audio recordings Randomized Identity blinded multiple raters (2) Inter- and intra-rater reliability	Small group No external rater	5Y[b]:40 7Y[b]: 67	72 74	75 82	NI NI	0 0
Audio recordings Randomized Identity blinded multiple raters (2), external rater (1) Inter- and intra-rater reliability	Small group	5Y: 36 7Y: 68 10Y: 79	72 72 79	75 75 97	55 80 100	12 20
Audio recordings Randomized, identity blinded external, multiple listeners (3)	Small group Selection bias	3Y: 70 5Y: 62 7Y: 65 10Y: 60	75 72 71 84	70 71 87 100	NI NI NI NI	0 0 12 20
Audio recordings Randomized Identity blinded multiple raters (2), external rater (1) Inter- and intra-rater reliability	Exclusion bias?	5Y[a]: 68 7Y[a]: 88 10Y: 92 16Y: 96 19Y: 98	72 91 92 91 100	60 78 96 97 99	82 98 100 100 100	0 11 11 11 11
Audio recordings Randomized Identity blinded multiple raters (2), external rater (1) Inter- and intra-rater reliability	Selection bias	5Y: 72 (VPC) 7Y: 82 (VPC) 10Y: 83 (VPC)		59 80 88	70 88 94	NI NI NI
Live vs Audio recordings Multiple raters (3) Inter-rater reliability	Selection bias No intra-rater reliability	12–23Y: NI	30	14	NI	5

(Continued)

Appendix 4.A (*Continued*)

Reference (Language)	Design	ICF level (WHO, 2001)	Level of evidence[a]	Cleft Type	Selection		Ages for speech assessment (SA) and operation	No. of surgeons
					No. included/ Out of possible			
Myklebust and Åbyholm, 1989 (Norwegian)	Retrospective case series, cross-sectional	Function	IV	CLP: 107 CPO: 78 (CL:18)	185/NI		SA: 6 years *One-stage* 11–55 months (vL)	1
Van Demark et al., 1989 (German)	Retrospective case series, cross-sectional	Function	IV	UCLP	37/54		SA: 6–16 years *Two-stage* SPC: 15–34 months HPC: 6 years	1
Lohmander-Agerskov and Söderpalm, 1993 (Swedish)	Retrospective case series, cross-sectional	Function	IV	BCLP:14 UCLP:16	30/38		SA: 7–13 years *Two-stage* SPC: 8 months HPC: 8 years	NI
Lohmander-Agerskov et al., 1993 (Swedish)	Retrospective case series, cross-sectional	Function and contextual personal	IV	CPO	31		SA: 10–14 years *One-stage* 8 months (WK)	NI
Sell et al., 2001 (British English)	Retrospective case series, cross-sectional	Function and activity	IV	UCLP	238/326 218/321		SA: 5 or 12 years Different types in the UK	NI
Timmons, Wyatt and Murphy, 2001 (British English)	Retrospective case series, cross-sectional	Function and activity	IV	UCLP: 21 CPO: 33	44/54		SA: 5 or 12 years *One-stage* 5–14 months (IVV)	1

Method for documentation and assessment	Bias	Speech outcome (%)				Secondary Phar. flap surgery (%)
		Absence of nasal emission	Absence of hypernasality	Absence of artic. errors	Good intelligibility	
Audio recordings Random selection for inter- and intra-reliability	Single rater No external rater	NI	80	86	NI	15
Audio recordings Identity blinded external rater (1) multiple raters (2) inter- and intra-reliability	Selection bias	94,6 (VPC)		70	NI	0
Audio recordings Randomized Identity blinded multiple raters (2) Inter-and intra-rater reliability	Small group Selection bias No external rater	97	94	77	90	10
Audio recordings Randomized Identity blinded multiple raters (2) Inter-and intra-rater reliability	Small group No external rater	NI	77	97	NI	26
Audio recordings Randomized Identity blinded multiple raters (2) Inter- and intra-rater reliability	Selection bias	5Y: 67 12Y: 94	70 70	66 83	49 81	16 20
Video recordings Identity blinded multiple raters (2) Inter-rater reliability	Selection bias No intra-rater reliability	5–12Y: CPO: 80 UCLP: 78	90 75	74 76	37 53	37 0

(Continued)

Appendix 4.A   (*Continued*)

Reference (Language)	Design	ICF level (WHO, 2001)	Level of evidence[a]	Cleft Type	Selection — No. included/ Out of possible	Ages for speech assessment (SA) and operation	No. of surgeons
Dotevall et al., 2002 (Swedish)	Retrospective comparative, cross-sectional	Function	IV	BCLP: 5 UCLP: 3 HCP: 3 SCP: 3 Controls: 15	14/NI	SD: 7, 10 years *Two-stage* SPC: 7 months HPC: 8 years	NI
Persson et al., 2002 (Swedish)	Retrospective, case series, cross-sectional	Function	IV	HCP: 26 SCP: 25	51/85	SA: 5 years *Two-stage* SPC: 8 months HPC: 4 years	NI
Brunnegård and Lohmander, 2007 (Swedish)	Retrospective case series, cross-sectional	Function	IV	UCLP: 12 CPO: 26	38/39	SA: 9–11 years *Two-stage* SPC: 9 months HPC: 2–3 years	NI
Havstam, Lohmander and Dahlgren Sandberg, 2008 (Swedish)	Retrospective case series, cross-sectional	Function and contextual personal	IV	BCLP: 10 UCLP: 25	35/63	SA: 22–32 years *One-stage* 9 months (WK)	NI
Van Lierde et al., 2010 (Dutch)	Retrospective case series, cross-sectional	Activity Contextual environmental	IV	UCLP	43/53	SA: 2.5–7.6 years *One-stage* 11–24 months	NI

NI = No Information; SA = Speech Assessment; WK = Wardill-Kilner; vL = von Langenbeck; MMI = Minimal Incision Technique ($_{mr}$ = muscle reconstruction); ML = Medial Langenbeck; CV = Cuthbert-Veau-Wardill-Kilner; IVV = Intra Velar Veloplasty; VPC = Velopharyngeal Competence; W = Words; S = Sentences; E = Early; L = Late.
[a]Chapter 18
[b]Unoperated hard palate cleft.
[c]Including three with two-stage palatal repair.
Comparison bias = groups not comparable due to heterogeneity in cleft types, ages at operation, ages at speech assessment.
UCLP = Unilateral Cleft Lip and Palate; BCLP = Bilateral Cleft Lip and Palate; CPO = Cleft Palate Only; HCP = Hard Cleft Palate; SCP = Soft Cleft Palate; SPC = Soft Palate Closure; HPC = Hard Palate Closure.

Method for documentation and assessment	Bias	Speech outcome (%)				Secondary Phar. flap surgery (%)
		Absence of nasal emission	Absence of hypernasality	Absence of artic. errors	Good intelligibility	
Audio recordings Randomized Blinded multiple raters (2) Inter- and intra-rater reliability	Small group Selection bias No external rater	79	64	93	NI	NI
Audio recordings Randomized Identity blinded multiple raters (2) Inter- and intra-rater reliability	Selection bias No external rater	HCP: 67 SCP: 100	69 94	100 100	NI NI	2 0
Audio recordings Randomized Identity blinded external multiple raters (2 Inter-and intra-rater reliability	Small group	72	66	75	NI	17
Audio recordings Randomized Identity blinded multiple raters (2) Inter- and intra-rater reliability	Selection bias	86	77	97	NI	20
Audio recordings	Selection bias Listener bias	2.5–5Y:NI 5–7.6Y:NI	NI NI	NI NI	W:73; S:54 W:89; S:85	NI

References

American Cleft Palate–Craniofacial Association (1993) Parameters for evaluation and treatment of patients with cleft lip/palate or other craniofacial anomalies. *Cleft Palate-Craniofacial Journal*, 30 (Suppl.): S1–S16.

Bardach, J., Morris, H.L. and Olin, W.H. (1984) Late results of primary veloplasty: the marburg project. *Plastic and Reconstructive Surgery*, 73, 207–215.

Barimo, J.P., Habal, M.B., Scheuerle, J. and Ritterman, S.I. (1987) Postnatal palatoplasty, implications for normal speech articulation – a preliminary report. *Scandinavian Journal of Plastic and Reconstructive Surgery*, 21, 139–143.

Becker, M., Svensson, H., Sarnäs, K.V. and Jacobsson, S. (2000) Von Langenbeck or Wardill procedures for primary palatal repair in patients with isolated cleft palate – speech results. *Scandinavian Journal of Plastic and Reconstructive Surgery and Hand Surgery*, 34, 27–32.

Brunnegård, K. and Lohmander, A. (2007) A cross-sectional study of speech in 10 year old children with cleft palate: results and issues of rater reliability. *Cleft Palate-Craniofacial Journal*, 44, 33–44.

Chapman, K.L., Hardin-Jones, M.A., Goldstein, J.A. *et al.* (2008) Timing of palatal surgery and speech outcome. *Cleft Palate-Craniofacial Journal*, 45, 297–308.

Copeland, M. (1990) The effects of very early palatal repair on speech. *British Journal of Plastic Surgery*, 43, 676–682.

Dalston, R.M. (1990) Communication skills of children with cleft lip and palate: a status report, in *Multidisciplinary Management of Cleft Lip and Palate* (eds J. Bardach and H.L. Morris), WB Saunders, Philadalphia, pp. 746–749.

Dotevall, H., Lohmander-Agerskov, A., Ejnell, H. and Bake, B. (2002) Perceptual evaluation of speech and velopharyngel function in children with and without cleft palate and the relationship to nasal airflow patterns. *Cleft Palate-Craniofacial Journal*, 39, 409–424.

Evans, D. and Renfrew, C. (1974) The timing of primary cleft palate repair. *Scandinavian Journal of Plastic and Reconstructive Surgery*, 8, 153–155.

Farzaneh, F., Becker, M., Peterson, A.M. and Svensson, H. (2008) Speech results in adult Swedish patients born with unilateral complete cleft lip and palate. *Scandinavian Journal of Plastic and Reconstructive Surgery and Hand Surgery*, 42, 7–13.

Farzaneh, F., Becker, M., Peterson, A.M. and Svensson, H. (2009) Speech results in adult Swedish patients born with bilateral complete cleft lip and palate. *Scandinavian Journal of Plastic and Reconstructive Surgery and Hand Surgery*, 43, 207–213.

Friede, H. (2009) Two-stage palate repair, in *Comprehensive Cleft Care* (eds J.E. Losee and R.E. Kirschner), McGraw Hill, pp. 413–429.

Friede, H. and Enemark, H. (2001) Long-term evidence for favorable midfacial growth after delayed hard repair in UCLP patients. *Cleft Palate-Craniofacial Journal*, 38, 323–329.

Gnoinsky, W.M. and Haubensak, R.R. (1997) Facial pattern and long-term growth in pateints with complete unilateral cleft lip and palate, in *Transactions 8th International Congress on Cleft Palate and Related Craniofacial Anomalies* (ed. S.T. Lee), Academy of Medicine, Singapore, p. 764.

Grunwell, P. and Russell, J. (1987) Vocalizations before and after cleft palate surgery: a pilot study. *British Journal of Disordered Communication*, 22, 1–17.

Harding, A. and Campbell, R.C. (1989) A comparison of the speech results after early and delayed hard palate closure: a preliminary report. *British Journal of Plastic Surgery*, 42, 187–192.

Hardin-Jones, M.A. and Jones, D.L. (2005) Speech production of preschoolers with cleft palate. *Cleft Palate-Craniofacial Journal*, 42, 7–13.

Hardin-Jones, M.A., Brown, C.K., Van Demark, D.R. and Morris, H.L. (1993) Long-term speech results of cleft palate patients with primary palatoplasty. *Cleft Palate-Craniofacial Journal*, 30, 55–63.

Havstam, C., Lohmander, A., Dahlgren Sandberg, A. and Elander, A. (2008) Speech and satisfaction with treatment in young adults with unilateral or bilateral complete clefts: answers to a patient questionnaire compared to speech assessments. *Scandinavian Journal of Plastic and Reconstructive Surgery and Hand Surgery*, **42**, 182–189.

Havstam, C., Dahlgren Sandberg, A. and Lohmander, A. (2011) Communication attitude compared to speech assessments in 10-year-old children with cleft palate. *International Journal of Speech-Language Pathology*, **13**, 156–164.

Henningsson, G., Karling, J. and Larsson, O. (1990) Early or late surgery of the hard palate? A preliminary report on comparison of speech results, in *Cleft Lip and Palate, Long-Term Results and Future Prospects. Proceedings of the First International Meeting of the Craniofacial Society of Great Britain* (eds A.G. Huddart and M.L.W. Ferguson), Manchester University Press, pp. 402–411.

Jolleys, A. (1954) A review of the results of operations on cleft palates with reference to maxillary growth and speech function. *British Journal of Plastic Surgery*, **7**, 229–241.

Jones, C., Chapman, K. and Hardin-Jones, M. (2003) Speech development of children with cleft palate before and after palatal surgery. *Cleft Palate-Craniofacial Journal*, **40**, 19–31.

Kaplan, E.N. (1981) Cleft palate repair at three months? *Annals of Plastic Surgery*, **7**, 179–190.

Karling, J., Larsson, O., Leanderson, R. and Henningsson, G. (1993) Speech in unilateral and bilateral cleft palate patients from Stockholm. *Cleft Palate-Craniofacial Journal*, **30**, 73–77.

Karnell, M. and Van Demark, D. (1986) Longitudinal speech performance in patients with cleft palate: comparison based on secondary management. *Cleft Palate Journal*, **23**, 278–288.

Kemp-Fincham, S.I., Kuehn, D.P. and Trost-Cardamone, J.E. (1990) Speech development and the timing of primary palatoplasty, in *Multidisciplinary Management of Cleft Lip and Palate* (eds J. Bardach and H.L. Morris), WB Saunders, Philadelphia, pp. 736–745.

Kriens, O. (1969) An anatomical approach to veloplasty. *Plastic and Reconstructive Surgery*, **43**, 29–41.

Kuijpers-Jagtman, A.M. and Long, R.E. (2000) The influence of surgery and orthopedic treatment on maxillofacial growth and maxillary arch development in patients treated for orofacial clefts. *Cleft Palate-Craniofacial Journal*, **37**, 527. 1–12.

Leow, A.M. and Lo, L.J. (2008) Palatoplasty: evolution and controversies. *Chang Gung Medical Journal*, **31**, 335–344.

Lilja, J., Mars, M., Elander, A. *et al.* (2006) Analysis of dental arch relationships in Swedish unilateral cleft lip and palate subjects: 20-year longitudinal consecutive series treated with delayed hard palate closure. *Cleft Palate-Craniofacial Journal*, **43**, 606–611.

Lindsay, W.K., LeMesurier, A.B. and Farmer, A.W. (1962) A study of the speech results of a large series of cleft palate patients. *Annals of Otology, Rhinology, and Laryngology*, **29**, 273–288.

Lohmander, A. and Olsson, M. (2004) Perceptual assessment of speech in patients with cleft palate: a critical review. *Cleft Palate-Craniofacial Journal*, **41**, 64–70.

Lohmander, A. and Persson, C. (2008) A longitudinal study of speech production in Swedish children with cleft palate and two-stage palatal repair. *Cleft Palate-Craniofacial Journal*, **45**, 32–41.

Lohmander, A., Friede, H. and Lilja, J. (2009) Long-term, longitudinal follow-up of speech in individuals with UCLP after the Gothenburg primary early veloplasty and delayed hard palate closure. Presentation at the 11th international conference on cleft palate and related craniofacial anomalies, Fortaleza, Brazil (September 2009).

Lohmander, A., Lillvik, M. and Friede, H. (2004) The impact of early infant jaw-orthopaedics on early speech production in toddlers with unilateral cleft lip and palate. *Clinical Linguistics and Phonetics*, **18**, 259–285.

Lohmander, A., Persson, C. and Owman-Moll, P. (2002) Unoperated clefts in the hard palate speech deficits at age 5 and 7 years and the relationship to cleft size. *Scandinavian Journal of Plastic and Reconstructive Surgery and Hand Surgery*, 36, 332–339.

Lohmander, A., Friede, H., Elander, A. *et al.* (2006) Speech development in patients with unilateral cleft lip and palate treated with different delays of hard palate closure after early velar repair: a longitudinal perspective. *Scandinavian Journal of Plastic and Reconstructive Surgery and Hand Surgery*, 46, 267–274.

Lohmander, A., Willadsen, E., Bowden, M. *et al.* (2009) Methodology for speech assessment in the Scandcleft project – An international randomised clinical trial on palatal surgery: experiences from a pilot study. *Cleft Palate-Craniofacial Journal*, 46, 347–362.

Lohmander-Agerskov, A. and Söderpalm, E. (1993) Evaluation of speech after completed late closure of the hard palate. *Folia Phoniatrica*, 45, 25–30.

Lohmander-Agerskov, A., Havstam, C., Söderpalm, E. *et al.* (1993) Speech assessment in children with an operated isolated cleft palate. *Scandinavian Journal of Plastic and Reconstructive Surgery and Hand Surgery*, 27, 307–310.

Lohmander-Agerskov, A., Söderpalm, E., Friede, H. and Lilja, J. (1995) A longitudinal study of the speech in 15 cleft lip and palate children with late hard palate repair. *Scandinavian Journal of Plastic and Reconstructive Surgery and Hand Surgery*, 29, 21–31.

Lohmander-Agerskov, A., Söderpalm, E., Friede, H. and Lilja, J. (1998) A comparison of babbling and speech at pre-speech level, 3, and 5 years of age in children with cleft lip and palate treated with delayed hard palate closure. *Folia Phoniatrica et Logopaedica*, 50, 243–250.

Mars, M. and Houston, W.J. (1990) A preliminary study of facial growth and morphology in unoperated male unilateral cleft lip and palate subjects over 13 years of age. *Cleft Palate Journal*, 27, 7–10.

Myklebust, O. and Åbyholm, F.E. (1989) Speech results in CLP patients operated on with a von Langenbeck palatal closure. *Scandinavian Journal of Plastic and Reconstructive Surgery*, 23, 71–74.

Nyberg, J., Raud-Westberg, L., Neovius, E. *et al.* (2010) Speech results after one-stage palatoplasty with or without muscle reconstruction for isolated cleft palate. *Cleft Palate-Craniofacial Journal*, 47, 92–103.

O'Gara, M., Logemann, J. and Rademaker, A. (1994) Phonetic features by babies with unilateral cleft lip and palate. *Cleft Palate-Craniofacial Journal*, 31, 446–451.

Ortiz-Monasterio, F., Rebeil, A.S., Valderrama, M. and Cruz, R. (1959) Cephalometric measurements on adult patients with nonoperated cleft palates. *Plastic and Reconstructive Surgery*, 4, 53–61.

Park, S., Yasumi, S., Osamu, I. *et al.* (2000) The outcome of long-term follow-up after palatoplasty. *Plastic and Reconstructive Surgery*, 105, 12–17.

Persson, C., Elander, A., Lohmander-Agerskov, A. and Söderpalm, E. (2002) Speech outcomes in isolated cleft palate: impact of cleft extent and additional malformations. *Cleft Palate-Craniofacial Journal*, 39, 397–408.

Persson, C., Lohmander, A. and Elander, A. (2006) Speech in children born with an isolated cleft palate: a longitudinal perspective. *Cleft Palate-Craniofacial Journal*, 43, 295–309.

Peterson-Falzone, S.J. (1990) A cross-sectional analysis of speech results following palatal closure, in *Multidisciplinary Management of Cleft Lip and Palate* (eds J. Bardach and H.L. Morris), WB Saunders, Philadalphia, pp. 750–757.

Peterson-Falzone, S.J. (1996) The relationship between timing of cleft palate surgery and speech outcome: what have we learned, and where do we stand in the1990s? *Seminars in Orthodontics*, 2, 185–191.

Peterson-Falzone, S.J., Hardin-Jones, M.A. and Karnell, M.P. (2010) *Cleft Palate Speech*, 4th edn. Mosby, Philadelphia, pp. 149–160.

Pigott, R.W., Albery, E.H., Hathorn, I.S. *et al.* (2002) A comparison of three methods of repairing the hard palate. *Cleft Palate-Craniofacial Journal*, 39, 383–391.

Pradel, W., Senf, D., Mail, R. *et al.* (2009) One-stage palate repair improves speech outcome and early maxillary growth in patients with cleft lip and palate. *Journal of Physiology and Pharmacology*, **60**, 37–41.

Pulkkinen, J., Haapanen, M.L., Paaso, M. *et al.* (2001) Velopharyngeal function from the age of three to eight years in cleft palate patients. *Folia Phoniatrica et Logopedica*, **53**, 93–98.

Randal, P., LaRossa, D.D., Fakhraee, S.M. and Cohen, M.A. (1983) Cleft palate closure at 3 to 7 months of age: a preliminary report. *Plastic and Reconstructive Surgery*, **71**, 624–628.

Riski, J.E. and DeLong, E. (1984) Articulation development in children with cleft lip/palate. *Cleft Palate Journal*, **21**, 57–64.

Roberts, C.T., Semb, G. and Shaw, W.C. (1991) Strategies for the advancement of surgical methods in cleft lip and palate. *Cleft Palate-Craniofac Journal*, **28**, 141–149.

Rohrich, R.J., Love, E.J., Byrd, H.S. and Johns, D.F. (2000) Optimal timing of cleft palate closure. *Plastic and Reconstructive Surgery*, **106**, 413–421.

Ross, R.B. (1987) Treatment variavles affecting facial growth in complete unilateral cleft lip and palate. *Cleft Palate Journal*, **24**, 54–77.

Scherer, N.J., Williams, A.L. and Proctor-Williams, K. (2008) Early and later vocalization skills in children with and without cleft palate. *International Journal of Pediatric Otorhinolaryngology*, **72**, 827–840.

Sell, D. (2005) Issues in perceptual speech analysis in cleft palate and related disorders: a review. *International Journal of Language and Communication Disorders*, **40**, 103–121.

Sell, D., Grunwell, P., Mildinhall, S. *et al.* (2001) Cleft lip and palate care in the United Kingdom (UK) – The Clinical Standards Advisory Group (CSAG) study. Part 3 – Speech outcomes. *Cleft Palate-Craniofacial Journal*, **38**, 30–37.

Shaw, W.C., Semb, G., Nelson, P. et al. (2000) *The Eurocleft Project 1996–2000. Standards of Care for Cleft Lip and Palate in Europe. European Commission Biochemical and Health Research*, IOS Press, Amsterdam.

Sommerlad, B.C. (2008) Cleft palate repair, in *Comprehensice Cleft Care* (eds J.E. Losee and R.E. Kirschner), McGraw-Hill, pp. 413–429.

Spauwen, P.H.M., Goorhuis-Brouwer, S.M. and Schutte, H.K. (1992) Cleft palate rapeir: furlow versus von Langenbeck. *Journal of Cranio-Maxillofacial Surgery*, **20**, 18–20.

Timmons, M.J., Wyatt, R.A. and Murphy, T. (2001) Speech after repair of isolated cleft palate and cleft lip and palate. *British Journal of Plastic Surgery*, **54**, 377–384.

Van Demark, R.D., Gnoinski, W., Hotz, M.M. *et al.* (1989) Speech results of the Zürich approach in the treatment of unilateral cleft lip and palate. *Plastic and Reconstructive Surgery*, **83**, 605–613.

Van Lierde, K.M., Monstrey, S., Bonte, K. *et al.* (2004) The long-term speech outcome in Flemish young adults after two different types of palatoplasty. *International Journal of Pediatric Otorhinolaryngology*, **68**, 865–875.

Van Lierde, K.M., Luyten, A., Van Borsel, J. *et al.* (2010) Speech intelligibility of children with unilateral cleft lip and palate (Dutch cleft) following a one-stage Wardill-Kilner palatoplasty, as judged by their parents. *International Journal of Oral Maxillofacial Surgery*, **39**, 641–646.

WHO (World Health Organization) (2001) ICF: International Classification of Functioning, Disability and Health, WHO, Geneva, Switzerland.

Willadsen, E. and Albrechtsen, H. (2006) Phonetic description of babbling in Danish toddlers born with and without cleft lip and palate. *Cleft Palate-Craniofacial Journal*, **43**, 189–200.

Zansi, M., Cheroillod, J. and Hohlfeld, J. (2002) Phonetic and otological results after early palate closure in 18 consecutive children presenting with cleft lip and palate. *International Journal of Pediatric Otorhinolaryngology*, **66**, 131–137.

5

Secondary Management and Speech Outcome

John E. Riski

Children's Healthcare of Atlanta, Center for Craniofacial Disorders and Speech Pathology Laboratory, Atlanta, GA 30342-1654, USA

5.1   Introduction

Hypernasality, nasal air emission and compensatory articulation are the hallmarks of velopharyngeal incompetence (VPI). These speech symptoms mark the failed primary management of the patient with cleft palate. Despite best attempts, primary palatal management is successful in only 70–80% of individuals with cleft palate (Morris, 1973; Riski, 1979). Thus, there is a need for secondary surgical management. This chapter addresses common procedures for secondary surgical management, including the pharyngeal flap, muscle transposition to the posterior wall, velarplasty and posterior wall augmentation. Outcome in light of type of cleft, age at surgery and presence of a syndrome and other factors is reviewed. Finally, consideration is given to surgical revision and complications.

Reviewing and comparing results from studies of secondary surgery is difficult. Methods, pre-operative/post-operative analysis and patient populations vary widely in

Cleft Palate Speech: Assessment and Intervention, First Edition. Edited by Sara Howard, Anette Lohmander.
© 2011 John Wiley & Sons, Ltd. Published 2011 by John Wiley & Sons, Ltd.

reports. Methods for analysing velopharyngeal function vary from perceptual analysis only to multimodality assessment using perceptual judgments of resonance, objective instrumental measures, radiographic imaging and fibre-optic endoscopy. Judgments of improvement were based on perceptual ratings of 'improved resonance', 'improved speech' or 'elimination of nasal air escape'. In some studies improvement was based on observed velopharyngeal closure by nasendoscopy or videofluoroscopy, or by objective aerodynamic or nasometric measures. Definitions of success and failure varied from study to study. Many authors labelled patients with 'hyponasal' resonance as 'successes'. Others concluded that hyponasal resonance is another form of surgical failure.

5.2 Secondary Surgical Management of Velopharyngeal Incompetence

The concept of a secondary surgical procedure to manage VPI was first introduced by Passavant (1862). Passavant described a pharyngoplasty which surgically tethered the uvula to the posterior pharyngeal wall. Schoenborn (1876) described the elevation of a full-thickness, inferiorly based flap. The superiorly based flap was later described by Bardenheur (1892).

Augmentation of the posterior pharyngeal wall was first described by Wardill (1928). He created a permanent ridge of fibrous tissue on the posterior pharyngeal wall by making transverse incisions through the superior constrictor. The tissue was sutured vertically, creating a ridge for the elevated velum to contact. Hynes (1951, 1953), and later Orticochea (1968), described pharyngoplasties by muscle transposition. The procedure has undergone modification and refinement (Riski et al., 1984, 1992a). Others (Furlow et al., 1982) have injected material (Teflon) into the posterior pharyngeal wall to decrease the size of the nasopharynx.

5.3 Secondary Pharyngeal Flap

The pharyngeal flap has been completed with inferiorly and superiorly based flaps (Figure 5.1). The pharyngeal flap is a static obturator of the midportion of the nasopharynx. The lateral portals are closed by active mesial movement of the lateral pharyngeal walls (Shprintzen et al., 1979). Secondarily, circumferential scar contracture narrows the pharynx. Finally, contracture of the flap itself elevates the velum into the pharynx, diminishing the anterior–posterior dimension.

Crockett, Bumstead and Van Demark (1988) suggested that three variables should be controlled for successful pharyngeal flap surgery: flap width, flap height or level and lateral port size. Strategies have been developed to cope with these variables. The size of the lateral ports has been controlled (Hogan, 1973) and the width of the pharyngeal flaps has been tailored to the amount of wall motion (Shprintzen et al., 1979). Some researchers have suggested that little strategy, if any, is needed for small VPI. Randall (1972) observed that if the VPI is small, any method should have a good result.

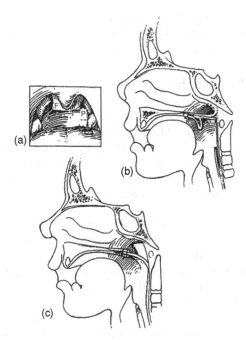

Figure 5.1 Pharyngeal flap pharyngoplasty. (a) An intra-oral view of the superiorly based, posterior pharyngeal flap demonstrating flap position (F) and lateral portals (P). (b) Lateral view of a superiorly based, posterior wall pharyngeal flap. The under surface of the pharyngeal wall flap is lined by a flap from the nasal surface of the velum. (c) Lateral view of an inferiorly based, posterior wall pharyngeal flap. The pharyngeal flap has been inset into a split made in the velum. (Reproduced with permission from J.E. Riski (2004), in K.R. Bzoch (Ed.) *Communicative Disorders Related to Cleft Lip and Palate*, 5th Edn (p. 198). Austin, TX: PRO-ED. Copyright 2004 by PRO-ED, Inc.).

5.3.1 Pharyngeal Flap Failure

Pharyngeal flaps fail because they are placed too low, they are to narrow or there is incomplete motion of the lateral pharyngeal walls to close the portals (Skolnick and McCall, 1972; Argamaso *et al.*, 1980). Crockett, Bumstead and Van Demark (1988) discussed failure in terms of three specific areas: method(s) of preoperative assessment, choice of operative procedure and mechanics of procedure, and uncontrolled wound healing and other host factors.

5.3.2 Pharyngeal Flap Revision

Failed pharyngeal flaps with large portals have been revised by further narrowing the portals with additional pharyngeal flaps sewn into the lateral margins of the original flap (Hirshowitz and Bar-David, 1976; Friedman *et al.*, 1992). Failed pharyngeal flaps have also been replaced completely by construction of new flaps (Barone *et al.*, 1994).

5.3.3 Improving Predictability of Port Size

Improving the predictability of port size has been attempted by lining the pharyngeal flaps (Owsley *et al.*, 1966) or by folding flaps, raw surface to raw surface (Isshiki and Morimoto, 1975; Johns *et al.*, 1994). Hogan (1973) constructed the lateral portals around catheters with a 4-mm diameter (area = 25 mm^2) to control the post-operative size. The rationale was based on several studies that demonstrated significant velopharyngeal incompetency when port size exceeded 20 mm^2 (Bjork, 1961; Isshiki, Honjow and Morimoto, 1968). Later, Hogan and Schwartz (1977) reported elimination of VPI in 93% of 150 patients operated on with this procedure. However, 4% remained hypernasal and 3% had port stenosis requiring a secondary procedure for correction.

Since lateral port control surgery was first proposed, the understanding of nasal and nasopharyngeal airway size has advanced considerably. Warren, Drake and Davis (1992) have documented minimal cross-sectional nasal areas for individuals with and without cleft. Nasal cross-sectional area increases with age and is generally smaller for individuals with cleft palate at any age. Nasal cross-sectional area increases to 20 mm^2 only after nine years of age in children with cleft palate and after six years of age for children without cleft palate. Thus, the possibility of obstructing the nasopharyngeal airway with port control surgery is great, especially in younger children.

5.3.4 Pharyngeal Flaps Tailored

General agreement exists that pharyngoplasties should be placed at the height of maximum velar or pharyngeal movement and that flaps should be of sufficient width to allow contact or closure by the excursion of the velum or lateral pharyngeal walls. The predictability of post-operative lateral wall movement is an important issue if flaps tailored to pre-operative movement are to be successful. However, there is some disagreement about the predictability of lateral wall movements post flap surgery. Lewis and Pashayan (1980) found no difference in amount of movement following flaps surgery. In contrast, Shprintzen, McCall and Skolnick (1980) reported that lateral wall movement remained the same in most patients but may also increase or decrease.

Shprintzen *et al.* (1979) achieved a 97% success rate when matching the width of the pharyngeal flap to the width of the nasopharyngeal gap. In contrast, success rate was only 62% when the pharyngeal flap with was not controlled for the size of the gap. Karling *et al.* (1999) compared outcomes in individuals receiving a wide pharyngeal flap because of limited wall movement to individuals receiving a narrow pharyngeal flap used in individuals with good wall movement. They found no difference in the results between the two groups. Armour *et al.* (2005) evaluated the outcome of pharyngeal flaps in 93 patients. Some had coronal pattern of closure and some had circular or sagittal closure patterns with mesial movement of the lateral pharyngeal walls. Post-operative Nasalance was better in the group with lateral wall motion (57%) than the coronal pattern group

(35%). In addition, hyponasality occurred 13% of the time in the coronal pattern group and only 7% of the time in the non-coronal pattern group.

5.4 Posterior Pharyngeal Wall Augmentation by Muscle Transposition

Hynes (1951, 1953) transposed muscle to create a muscular ridge on the posterior pharyngeal wall. He elevated superiorly based flaps from the salpingopharyngeus (1951) and later (1953) from the palatopharyngeus and the underlying superior constrictor. These flaps were inserted into a transverse incision in the posterior pharyngeal wall just below the eustachian tube orifices. He reported that adenoids prevented elevating the flaps to the necessary height. The initial results were 'dramatic improvement' in three of eight and 'less marked' improvement in five of eight (Hynes, 1951). He later reported 'perfect intelligibility' in 13 of 31 and no improvement in 4 of 41 (Hynes, 1953).

Orticochea (1968) advocated a pharyngoplasty that some (Riski *et al.*, 1984) believed was a modification of the Hynes pharyngoplasty. The surgery used superiorly based flaps from the posterior faucial pillar including the underlying palatopharyngeus. These flaps joined end to end in the midline of the posterior pharyngeal wall and then joined to an inferiorly based, posterior pharyngeal wall flap. The intent was to create an active diaphragm for velopharyngeal closure. The insertion site was in the oropharynx and well below the height of attempted velopharyngeal closure. Success was judged by intra-oral inspection of sphinctering of the orifice. Active sphinctering and success diminished with age (Orticochea, 1970). Overall velopharyngeal closure was observed in 45 of 73 (62%) patients. Sphinctering was reported in 36 of 43 (83.72%) patients under five years of age, but none of 14 patients over 16 years of age demonstrated closure.

Because of the poor results with the Orticochea technique surgeons began modifying the procedure. Jackson and Silverton (1977) substituted a superiorly based flap for the inferiorly based posterior wall flap in an attempt to raise the flap insertion and improve outcome. They reported improvement in 94.6% and resolution of hypernasality in 53% of patients. Others also reported improved results with this modification. Huskie and Jackson (1977) reported improvement in 23 of 26 (88%); two patients had residual, severe nasal air escape, six had moderate escape and eight had mild escape. Stratoudakis and Bambace (1984) eliminated hypernasality and nasal air escape in 10 of 16 patients. Roberts and Brown (1983), who tried to insert flaps as high as possible, reported improvement in 8 of 10 patients.

Riski *et al.* (1984) reviewed the results of 55 patients. Twenty six received the pharyngoplasty as reported by Orticochea and 29 underwent the procedure with the lateral flaps inserted into the posterior pharyngeal wall at the height of attempted velopharyngeal contact. The height of attempted velopharyngeal contact (relative to the first cervical vertebra (C1)) was identified by lateral phonation radiographs. Successful outcome was achieved in 16 of 26 (61%) patients using the technique as described by Orticochea and in 27 of 29 (93%) when using the modified insertion. These results were repeated in a larger series by Riski *et al.*, 1992a) and again in an even larger series by Losken *et al.* (2003)

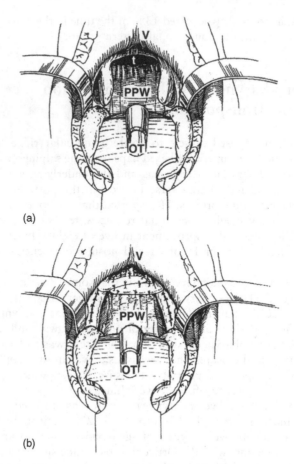

(a)

(b)

Figure 5.2   Intraoperative diagrams of sphincter pharyngoplasty. (a) The transverse incision (t) has been made in the posterior pharyngeal wall (PPW) and the lateral palatopharyngeus flaps elevated. The velum (V) has pulled out of the operative field. The orotracheal tube (OT) has been labelled. (b) The lateral flap is over the left and both have been sutured into the transverse incision. (Reproduced with permission from Riski *et al.* (1992a) *The Cleft Palate-Craniofacial Journal*, Allen Press Publishing Services.)

5.4.1   How Muscle Transposition Surgeries Function

Orticochea (1968) claimed the nasopharynx closed by active sphinctering of the palatopharyngeus flaps with the velum. This was determined by visual observation of sphinctering during the sound 'ah' (Orticochea, 1983). Even this observed sphinctering was found to diminish with age and was not observed in patients after 16 years of age.

The Hynes or sphincter pharyngoplasty is designed as a passive, muscular prominence that is contacted by the elevated velum (Hynes, 1953; Riski *et al.*, 1984; Riski *et al.*, 1992a) (Figure 5.2). Success of the procedure relies on placement at the level of active velar elevation (Riski *et al.*, 1984). Pigott (1993) suggested the procedure worked in any of three ways: by advancing the posterior wall, by reducing the lateral pharyngeal recess in a static manner, or as an active sphincter. The nature of the active sphinctering has been controversial. Ysunza *et al.* (1999), using electromyography, found that there is no activity of the palatopharyngeus muscle but there is activity of the superior constrictor and levator muscles. They concluded that the observed sphinctering seems to be caused by the contraction of the superior constrictor.

5.4.2   Why Transposition Pharyngoplasties Fail

Riski *et al.* (1992b) evaluated 30 patients with VPI following sphincter pharyngoplasty. Poor operative results were reported in 23 patients: low flap insertion (16), flap dehiscence (6) and flaps not approximated in midline (1). Poor patient selection appeared at fault in the remaining seven, including large velopharyngeal gap (4) and coexisting articulation disorders (3). Low flap insertion was also the primary reason for failure reported by Pryor *et al.* (2006). In contrast, Witt, Myckatyn and Marsh (1998) found the primary reason for failure was flap dehiscence. Failures related to dehiscence, low flap placement and end-to-end suturing of the flaps was also reported by Kasten *et al.* (1997).

5.4.3   Revisions of Transposition Failures

Riski *et al.* (1992a) reported on the revision of 13 failed sphincter pharyngoplasties. Eight of the failed pharyngoplasties were too low and five dehisced. Eleven had one revision and two had a second revision. Overall, 8 of 13 demonstrated resolved VPI; both who had a second revision remained hypernasal. Witt, Myckatyn and Marsh (1998) reported that 20 of 123 patients (16%) required surgical revision of a failed sphincter pharyngoplasty. Of these 20 patients, 17 were managed successfully. Losken *et al.* (2003) revised the sphincter pharyngoplasty in 32 of 250 patients. The revision was successful in 30 of 32 of the patients. Patients with velocardiofacial syndrome, more severe preoperative hypernasal resonance and larger velopharyngeal area were more likely to require pharyngoplasty revision.

5.4.4   Tailored Transposition Pharyngoplasties

The height of insertion for the sphincter pharyngoplasty on the posterior pharyngeal wall has been modified from the low insertion recommended by Orticochea (1968). Riski *et al.* (1984) offered a rationale for tailoring the height of flap insertion. The height of attempted velopharyngeal contact was identified relative to the anterior tubercle of the first cervical vertebra. The vertebra was identified by palpation at the time of surgery and the flaps were surgically inset at that predetermined height. Hypernasality was eliminated in only 61% when the flaps were placed as advocated by Orticochea. In contrast, hypernasality was eliminated in 93% of patients when the flaps were placed at the level of attempted velopharyngeal contact.

5.5   Studies Comparing Treatments of VPI

Few randomized studies of VPI treatment are available. This is presumed to relate to a clinician's hesitation to randomize a patient to a treatment that he or she believes may be inadequate or inappropriate. Marsh and Wray (1980) reported the results of managing 39 children with VPI, three to thirteen years of age. Each patient was randomized to management with a speech bulb or superiorly based pharyngeal flap. The speech bulb was successful in resolving VPI in 11 of 12 and the pharyngeal flap in 20 of 22. The authors observed that a prosthesis was only 40% the cost of surgery (in 1977 dollars). All patients randomized to surgery complied; however, the non-compliance for the prosthesis was 29%. In addition, 33% of patients randomized to the speech prosthesis later had a pharyngeal flap.

Pensler and Reich (1991) compared the outcome of 75 patients undergoing pharyngeal flap with only 10 patients with a sphincter pharyngoplasty. The authors reported a failure rate of 30% for each surgery. They concluded that either procedure could be used with equal effectiveness.

De Serres et al. (1999) evaluated the speech outcomes and complications of sphincter pharyngoplasty and pharyngeal flap. Patients with pharyngoplasty had a higher rate of resolution of VPI than those with pharyngeal flap (50% vs. 22.2%, respectively), although this was not statistically significant. However, only patients who underwent pharyngeal flap surgery had post-operative obstructive sleep apnoea (OSA). The authors concluded the sphincter pharyngoplasty may have a higher success rate with a lower risk of OSA.

Peat et al. (1994) selected one of four pharyngoplasties depending on the size and shape of the VPI determined endoscopically. Patients with poor palatal and lateral wall motion were treated with a Honig pharyngoplasty (superiorly based pharyngeal flap and a V–Y palatal push-back). Acceptable nasal resonance was achieved in 81% of 53 patients. Patients with good palatal elevation and poor lateral wall motion were treated with a modified Hynes pharyngoplasty. Acceptable nasal resonance was achieved in 81% of 63 patients. Eight patients with poor palatal movement and good lateral wall movement were treated with a superiorly based pharyngeal flap that was tailored to the width of the defect. Acceptable resonance was reported in 62.5%. Finally, eight patients with a small central defect were treated with a 'fish flap' that adds bulk to the nasal surface of the velum. Only 50% had acceptable resonance.

Abyholm et al. (2005) found better success for elimination of hypernasality at three months postoperatively in the pharyngeal flap group but no statistical difference between the pharyngeal flap and sphincter groups at 12 months.

Ysunza et al. (2002) randomly placed patients with VPI into one of two groups. One group received a pharyngeal flap and the other group received a sphincter pharyngoplasty. Each pharyngoplasty was then tailored based on imaging information. There was little difference in the outcome. The VPI was resolved in 89% of the patients receiving a pharyngeal flap and 85% of the patients receiving a sphincter pharyngoplasty. They concluded that tailoring the surgery based on imaging information was important.

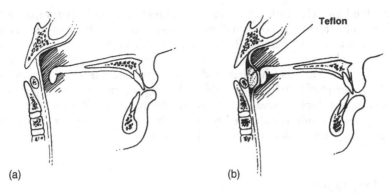

(a)   (b)

Figure 5.3 Teflon Injection. (a) Line drawing of lateral view demonstrating velopharyngeal incompetence. (b) Lateral view demonstrating position of Teflon injection into the posterior pharyngeal wall. The velum has elevated to contact the Teflon mass. (Reproduced with permission from J.E. Riski (2004), in K.R. Bzoch (Ed.) *Communicative Disorders Related to Cleft Lip and Palate*, 5th Edn (p. 216). Austin, TX: PRO-ED. Copyright 2004 by PRO-ED, Inc. [adapted from Furlow *et al.*, 1982].)

5.6 Posterior Pharyngeal Wall Augmentation by Implants and Injections

Autogenous or exogenous implants and injections have been used to augment the posterior pharyngeal wall. Despite the attractiveness of pharyngeal wall implants, especially for small VPIs, no material or procedure has proven safe or effective in the long term. The intent was to create a static bulge or pad on the posterior pharyngeal wall. The bulge would reduce the depth of the nasopharynx for easier obturation by velopharyngeal movement during speech. (Figure 5.3)

The first attempts included paraffin (Eckstein, 1904), cartilage (Hagerty and Hill, 1961), silicone (Blocksma, 1963) and proplast (Wolford, Oelschlaeger and Deal, 1989). Wolford, Oelschlaeger and Deal (1989) described the use of proplast in 26 patients. VPI was eliminated in 18 and minimal residual VPI remained in three. The implant was lost, secondary to infection, in four patients.

Teflon became a popular choice after it was used first to medialize a paralyzed vocal fold by Arnold (1961). A survey by Blocksma and Bralley (1969) found 47 surgeons performing retropharyngeal wall implants on 378 patients using 10 different materials. Results for all materials varied from 0% to 100% success. Teflon had a 0% failure rate. Bluestone *et al.* (1968) reported normal resonance in 5 of 12 patients. Sturim (1974) reported improvement in 22 of 23 patients, with 12 of 23 demonstrating good results. Smith and McCabe (1977) reported that 60% of 80 patients demonstrated good voice quality after Teflon injection and an additional 19% were improved but still hypernasal. Kuehn and Van Demark (1978) suggested that gaps greater than 2 mm should not be treated with Teflon injection. Furlow *et al.* (1982) reported a 74% success rate when used as a single procedure and 62% success rate when used to manage failed pharyngeal flaps.

Sipp, Ashland and Hartnick (2008) used injectable calcium hydroxyapatite in seven children with VPI stemming from small velopharyngeal gaps. Four of the patients had satisfactory result after 17 months. Three were considered failures and two underwent revision with a pharyngeal flap. Four of the children underwent magnetic resonance imaging within the postoperative area and there was no evidence of migration of the material. Leuchter *et al.* (2010) used a rhinopharyngeal autologous fat injection in 18 patients with mild velopharyngeal insufficiency. This required 28 total injections. There was a good overall result as measured by nasometry and only minor complications in two patients, one haematoma and one cervical pain.

5.7   Velarplasty

5.7.1   Island Flap Push-back

Palatal lengthening using an island flap push-back was first described by Millard (1963). Infrequently, it has been used to manage VPI with less satisfying results than other procedures. Lewin, Heller and Kojak (1975) reported 10 cases of VPI from submucous cleft palate and adenoidectomy. The Millard island flap repair eliminated hypernasality in 60%. Rintala and Rantala (1978) reported the results of an island flap push-back used as a secondary management of VPI in 57 patients. Closure was achieved in 'about' 50% and the degree of nasality diminished in 70%. Speech was rated as good in 50%, but speech was rarely normal. This surgery has been largely discarded.

5.7.2   Furlow Double-Opposing Z-Plasty as a Secondary Procedure

Furlow (1986) first described the double-opposing Z-plasty for primary repair of cleft palate (Figure 5.4). Twenty patients old enough for speech evaluation were studied. Eighteen had no velopharyngeal insufficiency and the remaining two had a mild insufficiency. Chen *et al.* (1994) documented velopharyngeal closure in 16 of 18 patients using the Furlow Z-plasty as a secondary procedure. Fifteen of the successful patients had velopharyngeal gaps less than 5 mm, whereas the two with residual VPI had gaps greater than 10 mm. Furlow (1994), in his review of the series, observed that retropositioning of the levator muscle sling seemed the chief benefit of the procedure.

D'Antonio *et al.* (2000) used radiographs and pressure flow assessment pre- and post-operatively to examine patients with submucous cleft palate who underwent the Furlow palatoplasty. They reported significant increases in velar length and thickness of the velum and both were associated with complete velopharyngeal closure postoperatively. In contrast, patients with incomplete closure tended to demonstrate relatively small percentage gains in both dimensions. They suggested that radiographic features (such as pharyngeal depth/velar length ratio) might be able to predict which patients may be most likely to benefit from Furlow Z-plasty. Patients with a nasopharyngeal depth/velar length ratio greater than expected did less well than those who had a favorable ratio.

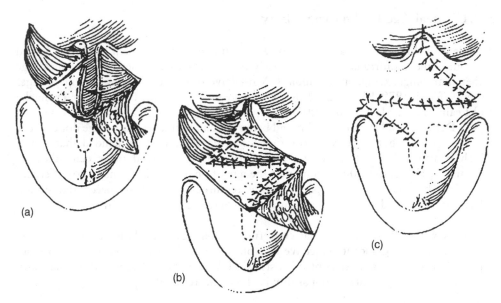

Figure 5.4 The Furlow double-opposing Z-plasty. (a) The oral surface flaps are elevated with the levator in the posterior flap (patient's left side) and only mucosa in the anterior flap (patient's right side). The nasal flaps are elevated with levator in the posterior flap (patient's right side) and only mucosa in the anterior flap (patient's left side). (b) The nasal side has been closed with right muscular flap posteriorly and the left mucosal flap anteriorly. (c) The oral side is then closed with the left muscular flap posteriorly and the right mucosal flap anteriorly. (Reproduced with permission from J.E. Riski (2004), in K.R. Bzoch (Ed.) *Communicative Disorders Related to Cleft Lip and Palate*, 5th Edn (p. 217). Austin, TX: PRO-ED. Copyright 2004 by PRO-ED, Inc. [adapted from Furlow, 1986].)

5.8 Other Considerations in Managing VPI

Consideration has been given to age of pharyngoplasty, type of cleft, presence of syndrome and the role of speech therapy. There is general agreement that patients with VPI make little or no progress in speech therapy until the VPI is managed (Riski, 1979; Riski and DeLong, 1984; Van Demark, 1974; Van Demark and Hardin, 1985). Exercises have not proved successful in increasing velopharyngeal function with the possible exception of continuous positive airway pressure (Kuehn *et al.*, 2002). When VPI is suspected or documented, speech therapy should be considered diagnostic and should be short term. Referral to a cleft palate–craniofacial team is appropriate after no more than several weeks of speech therapy.

The type of cleft may have a bearing on the need for pharyngoplasty. Van Demark and Hardin (1985) found the need for a pharyngoplasty increased with the severity of clefting. In contrast, Riski (1979) found the need for pharyngeal flaps was similar across cleft types in over the 300 patients.

5.8.1   Ideal Age for Pharyngoplasty

The ideal age for both primary and secondary cleft palate management has been debated for some time. Unfortunately and unwisely investigators have used chronological age rather than language age as a standard. Most have observed better results in younger patients (Riski, 1979; Riski *et al.*, 1984, 1992a; Leanderson *et al.*, 1974; Seyfer, Prohazka and Leahy, 1988; Meek *et al.*, 2003).

Van Demark and Hardin (1985) found better articulation when flaps were done before five years of age but there was no difference in nasality. They concluded that age at which pharyngeal flap surgery was performed was not critical in speech outcome. Similarly, Becker *et al.* (2004) found that the age of pharyngoplasty made no difference in the length of post-operative speech therapy required to normalize speech and did not affect the likelihood of subsequent surgical management for residual velopharyngeal incompetence.

Adults with VPI present special concerns for management. Younger and Dickson (1985) reported 'significant subjective and objective improvement' in eight adults but reported no data. In a more controlled study, Hall *et al.* (1991) reported normal resonance in 15 adult patients, hyponasality in three and residual hypernasality in two.

5.8.2   Presence of 22Q11.2 Deletion

Patients with velo-cardio-facial syndrome (VCFS) have vertebral and carotid arteries that are often shallow or displaced into the posterior pharyngeal wall. Further, there is frequent velar paralysis (Hultman *et al.*, 2000). Some have found poorer results when 22Q11.2 deletion is present. Losken *et al.* (2003) reported an 89% success rate with the sphincter pharyngoplasty in patients without syndromes. Later, Losken *et al.* (2006) reported only a 78% success rate in patients with 22Q11.2 deletion. Sie *et al.* (1998) reported that 15 of 24 patients (62.5%) had complete resolution of VPI; five of 24 (20.8%) had significant improvement; one of 24 (4.2%) had minimal to no change; and three of 24 (12.5%) were hyponasal. Following revision of failures they reported an overall success rate of 18 of 24 (75%). In contrast, Witt *et al.* (1999) reported that 18 of 19 patients were managed successfully with sphincter pharyngoplasty

Ysunza *et al.* (2009) reported better success (17 of 20, 85%) by using a tailored pharyngeal flap to manage VPI in children with VCFS. In contrast, success was only 66% (6 of 9) in patients who received a sphincter.

5.8.3   Primary versus Secondary Pharyngoplasty

A pharyngeal flap combined with palatoplasty is advocated when the palatal cleft is extremely wide (Tartan *et al.*, 1991). Both the pharyngeal flap and the sphincter pharyngoplasty have been used at the time of primary palatal. Reported results are higher than a palatoplasty alone. Dalston and Stuteville (1975) reported a success rate of 94% using a pharyngeal flap at the time of palatal plasty. Similarly, Riski *et al.* (1987) reported 100% success using the sphincter pharyngoplasty with primary palatoplasty. Controversy still exists about using any secondary procedure with primary palatoplasty because only

20% to 30% of patients will eventually require pharyngoplasty and because of the potential obstruction. The ability to predict which infants will eventually require a pharyngoplasty appears to be poor. Riski *et al.* (1987) found that only 50% of the children needed a pharyngoplasty. The remaining children achieved closure at the adenoids, well above the pharyngoplasty.

5.8.4   Hearing and Middle Ear Function

Primary repair of overt and submucous cleft palate often improves otologic and audiologic status (Pensler and Bauer, 1988). However, there has been little study and there is less agreement about the effect of pharyngoplasty on otologic status. Spauwen *et al.* (1988) evaluated 51 patients with inferiorly based pharyngeal flaps. 60% demonstrated a decrease in the frequency of otitis media. This was a more common in patients over than six years of age. The authors suggested that the pharyngeal flap corrects the vector of the force of the levator, which facilitates contraction of the dilator tubae muscle on the membraneous wall of the Eustachian tube. Also, oronasal reflux may be diminished, reducing irritation to eustachian tube orifice.

5.9   Complications Secondary to Pharyngoplasties

5.9.1   Airway Obstruction

Complications following a pharyngoplasty are not uncommon. The incidence of obstructive sleep apnoea (OSA) following pharyngeal flap ranges from 2.6% (Ysunza *et al.*, 1993) to 15% (Sirois *et al.*, 1994). Obstruction has been reported following the sphincter pharyngoplasty but appears to be less frequent (De Serres *et al.*, 1999; Sloan, 2000). Airway obstruction may be severe enough to warrant take-down of the flap (Caouette-Laberge *et al.*, 1992).

OSA is most common immediately following pharyngoplasty and resolves in the months following surgery (Orr, Levine and Buchanan, 1987). Shprintzen (1988) found that patients with narrow and wide flaps had the same incidence of OSA. The author postulated that the causes were obstruction of portals by large tonsils, contraction of the nasopharynx around the flap, post-operative nasopharyngeal oedema and a sudden change in breathing pattern.

Post-pharyngoplasty apnoea may be obstructive of central. Long-term apneas are usually central (Sirois *et al.*, 1994). Shortening the length of the flap to reduce pharyngeal contracture and use of nasopharyngeal tubes for nasal respiration until the patient is awake appears to reduce OSA (Shprintzen *et al.*, 1992).

5.10   Conclusions

Surgical management with pharyngeal flap, sphincter pharyngoplasty and Furlow double opposing Z-plasty, by themselves or in combination have rates of success in the range of 80–90%. The presence of a syndrome such as VCFS lowers the success rate by 10–15%. Tailoring surgery to the physiology and anatomy can improve the success of both pharyngeal flaps and sphincter pharyngoplasty. The Furlow double-opposing Z-plasty can be used successfully to treat 'small' velopharyngeal gaps. Posterior pharyngeal wall injections and implants are attractive options but have not had the success rate of surgical procedures.

Despite numerous modifications and refinements of secondary surgical procedures some the surgeries will fail. Two of the common causes of failure are inappropriate flap size (too small) and inappropriate flap height (too low). Both the pharyngeal flap and sphincter pharyngoplasty can be revised to improve outcome.

A pharyngoplasty is not without risk to the patient. The most common risk is airway obstruction. The recognition of obstructive sleep apnoea and its relationship to hyponasality has caused some clinicians to redefine VPI to include hyponasality.

A pharyngoplasty should have anatomic and physiologic bases. The clinician is challenged to incorporate available instrumentation into the evaluation process. The clinician may be guided by experience and by the *Parameters for Evaluation and Treatment of Patients with Cleft Lip/Palate or Other Craniofacial Anomalies* (American Cleft Palate–Craniofacial Association, 2009). This peer-reviewed document offers several recommendations for evaluation and treatment.

References

Abyholm, F., D'Antonio, L., Davidson Ward, S.L. *et al.* (2005) Pharyngeal flap and sphincterplasty for velopharyngeal insufficiency have equal outcome at 1 year postoperatively: results of a randomized trial. *Cleft Palate-Craniofacial Journal*, **42**, 501–511.

American Cleft Palate-Craniofacial Association Revised 2009). Parameters for evaluation and treatment of patients with cleft lip/palate or other craniofacial anomalies.

Argamaso, R.V., Shprintzen, R.J., Strauch, B. *et al.* (1980) The role of lateral pharyngeal wall movement in pharyngeal flap surgery. *Plastic and Reconstructive Surgery*, **66**, 214–219.

Armour, A., Fischbach, S., Klaiman, P. and Fisher, D.M. (2005) Does velopharyngeal closure pattern affect the success of pharyngeal flap pharyngoplasty? *Plastic and Reconstructive Surgery*, **115** (1), 45–52.

Arnold, G.E. (1961) Vocal rehabilitation of paralytic dysphonia VI. Further studies of intracordal injection of material. *Archives of Otolaryngology*, **73**, 290i–294i.

Bardenheur, D. (1892) Vorschlage zu plastischen operationen bei chirurgischen eingriffen in der mundhohle. *Archiv für Klinische Chirurgie*, **43**, 32.

Barone, C.M., Shprintzen, R.J., Strauch, B. *et al.* (1994) Pharyngeal flap revisions: flap elevation from a scarred posterior pharynx. *Plastic and Reconstructive Surgery*, **93**, 279–284.

Becker, D.B., Grames, L.M., Pilgram, T. *et al.* (2004) The effect of timing of surgery for velopharyngeal dysfunction on speech. *Journal of Craniofacial Surgery*, **15**, 804–809.

Bjork, L. (1961) Velopharyngeal function in connected speech. *Acta Radiologica Supplement*, **202**, 1–94.

Blocksma, R. (1963) Correction of velopharyngeal insufficiency by silastic pharyngeal implant. *Plastic and Reconstructive Surgery*, **31**, 268–274.

Blocksma, R. and Bralley, S. (1969) Present status of retropharyngeal implantation for velopharyngeal insufficiency. *Plastic and Reconstructive Surgery*, **43**, 242–247.

Bluestone, C.C., Musgrave, L.H., McWilliams, B.J. and Crozier, P.A. (1968) Teflon injection pharyngoplasty. *Cleft Palate Journal*, **5**, 19–22.

Caouette-Laberge, L., Egerszegi, E.P., de Remont, A.M. and Ottenseyer, I. (1992) Long-term follow-up after division of a pharyngeal flap for severe nasal obstruction. *Cleft Palate-Craniofacial Journal*, 29, 27–31.

Chen, P.K.-T., Wu, J.T.H., Chen, Y.R. and Noordhoff, S. (1994) Correction of secondary velopharyngeal insufficiency in cleft palate patients with the Furlow palatoplasty. *Plastic and Reconstructive Surgery*, 94, 933–941.

Crockett, D.M., Bumstead, R.M. and Van Demark, D.R. (1988) Experience with surgical management of velopharyngeal incompetence. *Otolaryngology – Head and Neck Surgery*, 99, 1–9.

Dalston, R.M. and Stuteville, O.H. (1975) A clinical investigation of the efficacy of primary nasopalatal pharyngoplasty. *Cleft Palate Journal*, 12, 177–192.

D'Antonio, L.L., Eichenberg, B.J., Zimmerman, G.J. *et al.* (2000) Radiographic and aerodynamic measures of velopharyngeal anatomy and function following Furlow Z-plasty. *Plastic and Reconstructive Surgery*, 106, 539–549.

De Serres, L.M., Deleyiannis, F.W., Eblen, L.E. *et al.* (1999) Results with sphincter pharyngoplasty and pharyngeal flap. *International Journal of Pediatric Otorhinolaryngology*, 48, 17–25.

Eckstein, H. (1904) Demonstration of paraffin prosthesis in defects of the face and palate (translation). *Dermatologica*, 11, 772–778.

Friedman, H.I., Hanes, P.C., Coston, G.N. *et al.* (1992) Augmentation of the failed pharyngeal flap. *Plastic and Reconstructive Surgery*, 90, 314–318.

Furlow, L.T. (1986) Cleft palate repair by double opposing Z-plasty. *Plastic and Reconstructive Surgery*, 78, 724–738.

Furlow, L.T. (1994) Discussion. Correction of velopharyngeal insufficiency in cleft palate patients with the Furlow palatoplasty. *Plastic and Reconstructive Surgery*, 94, 942–943.

Furlow, L.T., Williams, W.N., Eisenbach, C.R. and Bzoch, K.R. (1982) A long-term study on treating velopharyngeal insufficiency by Teflon injection. *Cleft Palate Journal*, 19, 47–56.

Hagerty, R.F. and Hill, M.J. (1961) Cartilage pharyngoplasty in cleft palate patients. *Surgery, Gynecology and Obstetrics*, 112, 350–356.

Hall, C.D., Golding-Kushner, K.J., Argamaso, R.V. and Strauch, B. (1991) Pharyngeal flap surgery in adults. *Cleft Palate Journal*, 28, 179–182.

Hirshowitz, B. and Bar-David, D. (1976) Repeated superiorly-based pharyngeal flap operation for persistent velopharyngeal incompetence. *Cleft Palate Journal*, 13, 45–53.

Hogan, V.M. (1973) Clarification of the surgical goals in cleft palate speech and the introduction of the lateral port control (LPC) pharyngeal flap. *Cleft Palate Journal*, 10, 337–345.

Hogan, V.M. and Schwartz, M.F. (1977) Velopharyngeal incompetence, *Reconstructive Plastic Surgery*, 4th edn (ed. J.M. Converse), Saunders, Philadelphia, pp. 2268–2283.

Hultman, C.S., Riski, J.E., Cohen, S.R. *et al.* (2000) Chiari malformation, cervical spine anomalies, and neurologic deficits in velocardiofacial syndrome. *Plastic and Reconstructive Surgery*, 106, 16–24.

Huskie, C.F. and Jackson, I.T. (1977) The sphincter pharyngoplasty-A new approach to the speech problem of velopharyngeal incompetence. *British Journal of Disorders of Communication*, 12, 31–35.

Hynes, W. (1951) Pharyngoplasty by muscle transposition. *British Journal of Plastic Surgery*, 3, 128–135.

Hynes, W. (1953) The results of pharyngoplasty by muscle transplantation in 'failed cleft palate' cases, with special reference to the influence of the pharynx on voice production. *Annals of the Royal College of Surgery England*, 13, 17–35.

Isshiki, N. and Morimoto, M. (1975) A new folded pharyngeal flap: preliminary report. *Plastic and Reconstructive Surgery*, 55, 461–465.

Isshiki, N., Honjow, I. and Morimoto, M. (1968) Effects of velopharyngeal competence on speech. *Cleft Palate Journal*, 5, 297–310.

Jackson, I.T. and Silverton, J.S. (1977) The sphincter pharyngoplasty as a secondary procedure in cleft palates. *Plastic and Reconstructive Surgery*, 59, 518–524.

Johns, D.F., Cannito, M.P., Rohrich, R.J. and Tebbetts, J.B. (1994) The self-lined superiorly based pull-through velopharyngoplasty: plastic-surgery-speech pathology interaction in the management of velopharyngeal insufficiency. *Plastic and Reconstructive Surgery*, 94, 436–445.

Karling, J., Henningsson, G., Larson, O. and Isberg, A. (1999) Comparison between two types of pharyngeal flap with regard to configuration at rest and function and speech outcome. *Cleft Palate-Craniofacial Journal*, 36, 154–165.

Kasten, S.J., Buchman, S.R., Stevenson, C. and Berger, M. (1997) Sphincter success rate: a retrospective analysis of revision sphincter pharyngoplasty. *Annals of Plastic Surgery*, 39, 583–589.

Kuehn, D.P. and Van Demark, D.R. (1978) Assessment of velopharyngeal competency following Teflon injection. *Cleft Palate Journal*, 15, 145–149.

Kuehn, D.P., Imrey, P.B., Tomes, L. *et al.* (2002) Efficacy of continuous positive airway pressure for treatment of hypernasality. *Cleft Palate Craniofacial Journal*, 39, 267–276.

Leanderson, R., Korlof, B., Nylen, B. and Eriksson, G. (1974) The age factor and reduction of open nasality following superiorly-based velopharyngeal flap operation in 124 cases. *Scandinavian Journal of Plastic and Reconstructive Surgery*, 8, 156–160.

Leuchter, I., Schweizer, V., Hohlfeld, J. and Pasche, P. (2010) Treatment of velopharyngeal insufficiency by autologous fat injection. *European Archives of Otorhinolaryngology*, 267, 977–983.

Lewin, M.L., Heller, J.C. and Kojak, D.J. (1975) Speech results after the Millard island flap repair in cleft palate and other velopharyngeal insufficiencies. *Cleft Palate Journal*, 12, 263–269.

Lewis, M.B. and Pashayan, H.M. (1980) The effects of pharyngeal flap surgery on lateral pharyngeal wall motion: a videoradiographic evaluation. *Cleft Palate Journal*, 17, 301–308.

Losken, A., Williams, J.K., Burstein, F.D. *et al.* (2003) An outcome evaluation of sphincter pharyngoplasty for the management of velopharyngeal insufficiency. *Plastic and Reconstructive Surgery*, 112, 1755–1761.

Losken, A., Williams, J.K., Burstein, F.D. *et al.* (2006) Surgical correction of velopharyngeal insufficiency in children with velocardiofacial syndrome. *Plastic and Reconstructive Surgery*, 117, 1493–1498.

Marsh, J.L. and Wray, R.C. (1980) Speech prosthesis versus pharyngeal flap: a randomized evaluation of the management of velopharyngeal incompetency. *Plastic and Reconstructive Surgery*, 65, 592–594.

Meek, M.F., Coert, J.H., Hofer, S.O. *et al.* (2003) Short-term and long-term results of speech improvement after surgery for velopharyngeal insufficiency with pharyngeal flaps in patients younger and older than 6 years old: 10-year experience. *Annals of Plastic Surgery*, 50, 13–17.

Millard, D.R. (1963) The island flap in cleft palate surgery. *Surgery, Gynecology and Obstetrics*, 116, 297.

Morris, H.L. (1973) Velopharyngeal competence and primary cleft palate surgery, 1960–1971: a critical review. *Cleft Palate Journal*, 10, 62–71.

Orr, W.C., Levine, N.S. and Buchanan, R.T. (1987) Effect of cleft palate repair and pharyngeal flap surgery on upper airway obstruction during sleep. *Plastic and Reconstructive Surgery*, 80, 226–232.

Orticochea, M. (1968) Construction of a dynamic muscle sphincter in cleft palates. *Plastic and Reconstructive Surgery*, 41, 323–327.

Orticochea, M. (1970) Results of the dynamic muscle sphincter operation in cleft palates. *British Journal of Plastic Surgery*, 23, 108–114.

Orticochea, M. (1983) A review of 236 cleft palate patients treated with dynamic muscle sphincter. *Plastic and Reconstructive Surgery*, 71, 180–188.

Owsley, J.Q., Lawson, L.I., Miller, E.R. and Blackfield, H.M. (1966) Experience with the high attached pharyngeal flap. *Plastic and Reconstructive Surgery*, 38, 232.

Passavant, G. (1862) Über die operation der angeborenen spalten des harten gaumens und der damit complicirten hasenscharten. *Archiv für Ohren- Nasen- und Kehlkopfheilkundearbeiten*, **3**, 193.

Peat, B.G., Albery, E.H., Jones, K. and Pigott, R.W. (1994) Tailoring velopharyngeal surgery: the influence of etiology and type of operation. *Plastic and Reconstructive Surgery*, **93**, 948–953.

Pensler, J.M. and Bauer, B.S. (1988) Levator repositioning and palatal lengthening for submucous clefts. *Plastic and Reconstructive Surgery*, **82**, 765–769.

Pensler, J.M. and Reich, D.S. (1991) A comparison of speech results after the pharyngeal flap and the dynamic sphincteroplasty procedures. *Annals of Plastic Surgery*, **26**, 441–443.

Pigott, R.W. (1993) The results of pharyngoplasty by muscle transplantation by Wilfred Hynes. *British Journal of Plastic Surgery*, **46**, 440–442.

Pryor, L.S., Lehman, J., Parker, M.G. *et al.* (2006) Outcomes in pharyngoplasty: a 10-year experience. *Cleft Palate-Craniofacial Journal*, **43**, 222–225.

Randall, P. (1972) Cleft palate, in *Plastic Surgery: A Concise Guide to Clinical Practice* (eds W.C. Grabb and J.W. Smith), Little, Brown, Boston, pp. 312–318.

Rintala, A.E. and Rantala, S.L. (1978) Secondary palatal repair by the island flap technique: a follow-up study. *Scandinavian Journal of Plastic and Reconstructive Surgery and Hand Surgery*, **12**, 257–260.

Riski, J.E. (1979) Articulation skills and oral-nasal resonance in children with pharyngeal flaps. *Cleft Palate Journal*, **16**, 421–428.Riski, J.E. (2004) Secondary Surgical Procedures to Correct Postoperative Velopharyngeal Incompetencies Found After Primary Palatoplasties, in *Communicative Disorders Related to Cleft Lip and Palate*, 5th edn (ed. K.R. Bzoch), PRO-ED, Austin, TX, p. 198.

Riski, J.E. and DeLong, E. (1984) Articulation development in children with cleft lip/palate. *Cleft Palate Journal*, **21**, 57–64.

Riski, J.E., Serafin, D., Riefkohl, R. *et al.* (1984) A rationale for modifying the site of insertion of the Orticochea pharyngoplasty. *Plastic and Reconstructive Surgery*, **73**, 882–894.

Riski, J.E., Georgiade, N.G., Serafin, D. *et al.* (1987) The Orticochea pharyngoplasty and primary palatoplasty. An evaluation. *Annals of Plastic Surgery*, **18**, 303–309.

Riski, J.E., Ruff, G.L., Georgiade, G.S. *et al.* (1992a) Evaluation of the sphincter pharyngoplasty. *Cleft Palate Journal*, **29**, 254–261.

Riski, J.E., Ruff, G.L., Georgiade, G.S. and Barwick, W.J. (1992b) Evaluation of failed sphincter pharyngoplasties. *Annals of Plastic Surgery*, **28**, 545–553.

Roberts, T.M.F. and Brown, B.S.J. (1983) Evaluation of a modified sphincter pharyngoplasty in the treatment of speech problems due to palatal insufficiency. *Annals of Plastic Surgery*, **10**, 209–213.

Schoenborn, D. (1876) Über eine neue methode der staphylorrlaphiei. *Archiv für Klinische Chirurgie*, **19**, 527.

Seyfer, A.E., Prohazka, D. and Leahy, E. (1988) The effectiveness of the superiorly-based pharyngeal flap in relation to the type of palatal defect and timing of the operation. *Plastic and Reconstructive Surgery*, **82**, 760–764.

Shprintzen, R.J. (1988) Pharyngeal flap surgery and the pediatric upper airway. *International Anesthesiology Clinics*, **26**, 79–88.

Shprintzen, R.J., Lewin, M.L., Croft, C.B. *et al.* (1979) A comprehensive study of pharyngeal flap surgery; Tailor-made flaps. *Cleft Palate Journal*, **16**, 46–55.

Shprintzen, R.J., McCall, G.N. and Skolnick, M.L. (1980) The effect of pharyngeal flap surgery on the movements of the lateral pharyngeal walls. *Plastic and Reconstructive Surgery*, **66**, 570–573.

Shprintzen, R.J., Singer, L., Sidoti, E.J. and Argamaso, R.V. (1992) Pharyngeal flap surgery: postoperative complications. *International Anesthesiology Clinics*, **30**, 115–124.

Sie, K.C., Tampakopoulou, D.A., de Serres, L.M. *et al.* (1998) Sphincter pharyngoplasty: speech outcome and complications. *Laryngoscope*, **108**, 1211–1217.

Sipp, J.A., Ashland, J. and Hartnick, C.J. (2008) Injection pharyngoplasty with calcium hydroxya-patite for treatment of velopalatal insufficiency. *Archives of Otolaryngology–Head and Neck Surgery*, **134**, 268–271.

Sirois, M., Caouette-Laberge, L., Spier, S. *et al.* (1994) Sleep apnea following pharyngeal flap. A feared complication. *Plastic and Reconstructive Surgery*, **93**, 943–947.

Skolnick, M.L. and McCall, G.N. (1972) Velopharyngeal competence and incompetence following pharyngeal flap surgery; Videofluoroscopic study in multiple projections. *Cleft Palate Journal*, **9**, 1–12.

Sloan, G.M. (2000) Posterior pharyngeal flap and sphincter pharyngoplasty: the state of the art. *Cleft Palate-Craniofacial Journal*, **37**, 112–122.

Smith, J.K. and McCabe, B.F. (1977) Teflon injection in the nasopharynx to improve velopharyn-geal closure. *Annals of Otology, Rhinology and Laryngology*, **86**, 559.

Spauwen, P.H., Ritsma, R.J., Huffstadt, B.J. *et al.* (1988) The inferiorly-based pharyngoplasty. Effects on chronic otitis media with effusion. *Cleft Palate Journal*, **25**, 26–32.

Stratoudakis, A.C. and Bambace, C. (1984) Sphincter pharyngoplasty for correction of velopha-ryngeal incompetence. *Annals of Plastic Surgery*, **12**, 243–248.

Sturim, H.S. (1974) Bleeding complications with pharyngeal flap construction in humans following Teflon pharyngoplasty. *Cleft Palate Journal*, **11**, 292–294.

Tartan, B.F., Sotereanos, G.C., Patterson, G.T. and Giuliani, M.J. (1991) Use of the pharyngeal flap with temporalis muscle for reconstruction of the unrepaired adult palatal cleft Report of two cases. *Journal of Oral and Maxillofacial Surgery*, **49**, 422–425.

Van Demark, D.R. (1974) A comparison of articulation abilities and velopharyngeal competence between Danish and Iowa children with cleft palate. *Cleft Palate Journal*, **11**, 463–470.

Van Demark, D.R. and Hardin, M.A. (1985) Longitudinal evaluation of articulation and velopha-ryngeal competence of patients with pharyngeal flaps. *Cleft Palate Journal*, **22**, 163–172.

Wardill, W.E.M. (1928) Results of operation for cleft palate. *British Journal of Surgery*, **16**, 127.

Warren, D.W., Drake, A.F. and Davis, J.U. (1992) Nasal airway in breathing and speech. *Cleft Palate-Craniofacial Journal*, **29**, 511–519.

Witt, P., Cohen, D., Grames, L.M. and Marsh, J. (1999) Sphincter pharyngoplasty for the surgical management of speech dysfunction associated with velocardiofacial syndrome. *British Journal of Plastic Surgery*, **52**, 613–618.

Witt, P.D., Myckatyn, T. and Marsh, J.L. (1998) Salvaging the failed pharyngoplasty: intervention outcome. *Cleft Palate-Craniofacial Journal*, **35**, 447–453.

Wolford, L.M., Oelschlaeger, M. and Deal, R. (1989) Proplast as a pharyngeal wall implant to correct velopharyngeal insufficiency. *Cleft Palate Journal*, **26**, 119–125.

Younger, R. and Dickson, R.I. (1985) Adult pharyngoplasty for velopharyngeal insufficiency. *Journal of Otolaryngology*, **14**, 158–162.

Ysunza, A., Garcia-Velasco, M., Garcia-Garcia, M. *et al.* (1993) Obstructive sleep apnea secondary to surgery for velopharyngeal insufficiency. *Cleft Palate-Craniofacial Journal*, **30**, 387–390.

Ysunza, A., Pamplona, M.C., Molina, F. *et al.* (1999) Velopharyngeal motion after sphincter pharyngoplasty: a videonasopharyngoscopic and electromyographic study. *Plastic and Reconstructive Surgery*, **104**, 905–910.

Ysunza, A., Pamplona, C., Ramírez, E. *et al.* (2002) Velopharyngeal surgery: a prospective rand-omized study of pharyngeal flaps and sphincter pharyngoplasties. *Plastic and Reconstructive Surgery*, **110**, 1401–1407.

Ysunza, A., Pamplona, M.C., Molina, F. and Hernández, A. (2009) Surgical planning for restoring velopharyngeal function in velocardiofacial syndrome. *International Journal of Pediatric Otorhinolaryngology*, **73**, 1572–1575.

6

Cleft Palate Speech in the Majority World: Models of Intervention and Speech Outcomes in Diverse Cultural and Language Contexts

Debbie Sell[1], Roopa Nagarajan[2] and Mary Wickenden[3]

[1] Great Ormond Street Hospital NHS Trust, North Thames Regional Cleft Service, London, WC1N 3JH, UK
[2] Sri Ramachandra Medical College and Research Institute, Department of Speech, Language and Hearing Sciences, Chennai, India
[3] University College London, Centre for International Health and Development, London, WC1N 1EH, UK

6.1 Introduction

It is salutary to reflect that almost a quarter of a million new babies with cleft lip and/or palate (CL+/–P) are born every year, of which 93% are in low income countries collectively described as the majority world[1] (Mars, Sell and Habel, 2008). Furthermore, this birth rate is occurring on a cumulative yearly basis, resulting in many millions of

[1] Varying terminology is used to describe regions of the world with contrasting levels of economic development, including 'high, middle and low income countries', 'developed vs developing', 'non-industrial countries', 'north vs south', 'first vs third world' and 'majority vs minority countries'. In this chapter the terms majority and minority world are used.

Cleft Palate Speech: Assessment and Intervention, First Edition. Edited by Sara Howard, Anette Lohmander.

under-treated and untreated individuals many of whom have major concerns about their severe speech disorders (Reeve *et al.*, 2004). In India alone, over a million individuals are yet to be reached, at least in part because cleft lip and palate (CL+/–P) is not a life threatening condition. However, life quality with an unoperated cleft lip and/or palate is severely affected (Reeve *et al.*, 2004; Bradbury and Habel, 2008), often exacerbated by an environment in which war, poverty, poor and minimal health care availability, life threatening diseases, no or limited access to surgical resources, socio-cultural influences and low life expectancy are all characteristic (Hodges, Wilson and Hodges, 2009).

For more than fifty years, surgical teams from the West have visited the majority world in order to perform surgery on patients with unoperated CL+/–P (Sell and Grunwell, 1994; Yeow *et al.*, 2002; Reeve *et al.*, 2004). More recently, project groups and non-government organizations (NGOs) have emerged, including the Smile Train, Operation Cleft, Transforming Faces Worldwide, Operation Smile, Rotoplast and Interplast. These organizations have developed different approaches to service delivery, depending on their particular philosophy, the availability of expertise and an understanding of local needs.

With regard to speech and language therapy, Hartley and Wirz (2002) reported low coverage of any services for communication disorders in the majority world, with those specialist services which do exist tending to replicate those in the minority world. Although only 5% of the global population has access to specialist rehabilitation services, the immense importance of communication is recognized. In relation to the majority world, it has been recognized as a 'basic human need' and follows closely behind food, shelter and safety.

Initially, there was minimal involvement of speech and language therapists (SLTs) in overseas surgical teams (Yeow *et al.*, 2002). Recently, the concept of developing sustainable local multidisciplinary teams has been more widely recognized (Mars, Sell and Habel, 2008; Ruiz-Razura, Cronin and Navarro, 2000; Yeow *et al.*, 2002). The inclusion of SLTs as members of the visiting team is much more commonplace (D'Antonio, 1990; Sell and Grunwell, 1990), although not routine (Aziz, Rhee and Redai, 2009). Sell (2008a) has reviewed the many reasons why SLTs should be included.

This chapter is in three parts. It begins with a review of existing knowledge about speech outcomes in a majority world context, detailing appropriate methodological approaches required for outcome studies. It explores ways in which speech services have and are being delivered, identifying the advantages and disadvantages of different models. There then follows a discussion of attitudes, cultural and language issues for both service providers and users in order to maximize the effectiveness of working within the majority world.

6.2   Speech Outcomes in a Majority World Context

Knowledge of speech outcomes in this environment is vital to ensure the best use of local resources and visiting medical teams and to counsel patients regarding realistic expectations of surgery with regards to speech (Bradbury and Habel, 2008). Reeve *et al.* (2004) found improvement in speech was the single most important anticipated outcome for patients and their families, with the assumption often made that surgery would make an immediate and dramatic positive difference. Sell (2008a) provides evidence that this is not always the case (see below). Sell (2008a) further argues that there is a need to report on more than just the impairment level[2], the consequences of the speech disorder on activity and participation must also be addressed (World Health Organization, 2001).

In 2008, the Smile Train convened an expert committee to advise on its speech strategy (D'Antonio et al., 2008). A review of speech initiatives in the majority world indicated there had been about 45 projects undertaken in 31 countries. Only four were outcome studies, three of which were data based (Sell and Grunwell, 1990; Jobe, D'Mello and Kumar, 2007; Murthy, Sendhilnathan and Hussain, 2010).

Sell and Grunwell (1994) undertook a critical review of studies of patients who had established their speech in the presence of an unoperated cleft palate. They concluded that many of the early studies were characterized by flawed methodologies with regard to contemporary expectations, conflicting findings and with usually no SLT involvement. Unfortunately, even contemporary studies, with the notable exception of Murthy et al. (2010), do not always meet rigorous scientific standards, such as controlling for bias, providing reliability data and ensuring an appropriate design for an intervention study, including a control group (Jobe, D'Mello and Kumar, 2007; Saboye et al., 2004). This can have worrying implications as multidisciplinary colleagues, desperate to improve speech, may be unaware of these limitations and pursue unproven treatments.

Speech studies under the auspices of the Sri Lankan Cleft Lip and Palate Project (SLCLPP) addressed some of the previous methodological flaws, and these principles should be considered and adhered to in outcome studies in a majority world context wherever possible. Of primary importance is the need for SLTs to lead in the design of the speech research. Independent variables need to be controlled, such as age and cleft type, and inclusion and exclusion criteria should be made explicit. Attention should be paid to an appropriate speech sample based on a study of the sound system of the local language (Sell, 1992; http://clispi.org.; Henningsson et al., 2008). If possible, a standardized approach to recording should be adopted. Judgements based on live recordings are unacceptable for outcome studies as reliability cannot be investigated and reported (Sell, 2005). As Kummer (2008) comments, often in this type of context there is minimal time for a detailed speech assessment and rating scales may be a very appropriate approach to analysis (Sell, Grunwell and Mars, 1994). In the SLCLPP, nasendoscopy and lateral cephalograms of patients at rest and phonating 'ee' were used to provide information on velopharyngeal function, and this may be a possibility in some environments. Small lightweight nasendoscopy equipment is now available (Figure 6.1). For all procedures, inter- and intra-rater reliability of observations should be addressed. Using such principles and methods, longitudinal studies on the pre-operative, post-operative and post-therapy speech and velopharyngeal function in adults and adolescents, and speech outcome studies in children, have been reported (Sell, 1992; Sell and Grunwell, 1990, 1993; Nayak, 1996; Birkett, 1999; Sell, 2008a; Murthy et al., 2010).

---

[2]The term 'Impairment' is commonly used as a shorthand for the 'body structure and function' aspect of disablement as described in the International Classification of Functioning, Disability and Health (ICF) (World Health Organization, 2001).

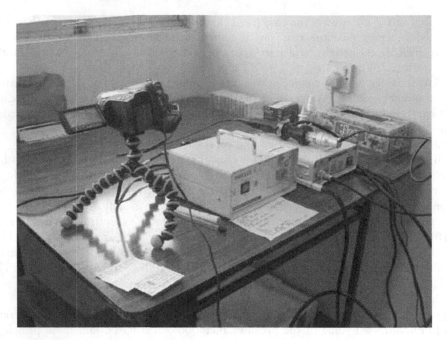

Figure 6.1 Lightweight nasendoscopy equipment.

6.2.1   Speech Outcomes

The nature of the pre-operative speech pattern, age at surgery, cleft type and years of school attendance have all been associated with speech outcome (Landis and Cuc, 1975; Sell, 1992).

Based on the Sri Lankan cohort and the studies by Ortiz-Monasterio and colleagues (Ortiz-Monasterio *et al.*, 1966, 1974) palate repair in adulthood (without pharyngoplasty) appears to be of little benefit to speech, no doubt in part due to the many technical difficulties described by Ortiz-Monasterio *et al.* (1966), Ward and James (1990) and Aziz, Rhee and Redai (2009). Sell (1992) reported a high incidence of velopharyngeal insufficiency of more than 80% in the adult and adolescent cohorts with complete CL+/–P, together with a high occurrence of fistulae in the adults and persistent and prevalent glottal errors. Murthy *et al.* (2010), in contrast, in their study of 131 patients over the age of ten years at surgery, with a mean age of 15.8 years, reported improvement in all speech parameters, although 'residual speech problems persist in most patients'. Indeed, all the patients remained hypernasal. Each speech parameter was statistically significantly different post-operatively; clinically this represented minimal to moderate improvement. The authors concluded that these 'marginally better' findings than previous studies may reflect the universal improvement in surgical techniques. In addition, there may be other important culturally related outcomes of palate repair in the adult which are unknown to overseas visitors. As Reeve *et al.* (2004, p. 174) state 'patients exist in a socio-cultural matrix in which the meaning of the condition they

Table 6.1 Speech Results of Sinhalese-speaking children in the SLCLPP.

Study	Number	Age at palatal surgery (years)	Cleft type	Surgery	Resonance: oral tone (%)	Articulation
Nayak (1996)	Group 1 = 15	1.04– 3.02	UCL+/–P	Von Langenbeck	73	60% normal or near normal
	Group 2 = 11	5.01– 7.02	UCL+/–P	Von Langenbeck	36	18% normal or near normal
Birkett (1999)	77	<8	UCL+/–P	Von Langenbeck	44	50% glottal

have and their futures are determined by a host of factors, including cultural, such as beliefs and practices …'. For example, it is possible that repair of the palate carries some status within the patient's local community, perhaps improving employment opportunities and conferring a status of healed or redeemed (Bradbury and Habel, 2008). Alternatively, palate repair may serve to encourage others to seek treatment, particularly children. It is important to be sensitive to local cultures when using the evidence base. Murthy *et al.* (2010) anecdotally reported improvement in eating following surgery.

Palate repair in childhood is strongly recommended (Sell, 1992; Sell 2008a), in contrast to the results of the adults and adolescents (Table 6.1). Furthermore, one third of patients greater than 24 months of age at palate repair achieved normal or near normal speech despite no speech and language therapy, audiological management or secondary velopharyngeal surgery. With regard to the latter, there is considerable controversy as to the safety of pharyngoplasty in a majority world environment, and this needs to be carefully considered within the context of the local facilities (Sell, 2008a). Furthermore, there is often a need for post-operative speech therapy for disordered articulation to maximize the benefits of such surgery and the difficulties of accessing such treatment are now explored.

6.3   Different Models of Provision

In the minority world, service delivery has been dictated predominantly by the impairment based model, not least because CL+/–P has its roots in medical management. The speech disorder is conceptualized as a deficit and the emphasis is on eliminating this. There is a current groundswell to move away from these purely curative approaches. Such models rely heavily on professional expertise. An example of this in the majority world is one where assessment and surgery are provided as an outreach programme. Here the tertiary based team travels to a place (often with minimal infrastructure) to provide services. Arguably most NGO projects come under this category, usually targeting the impairment focussed activities of a team.

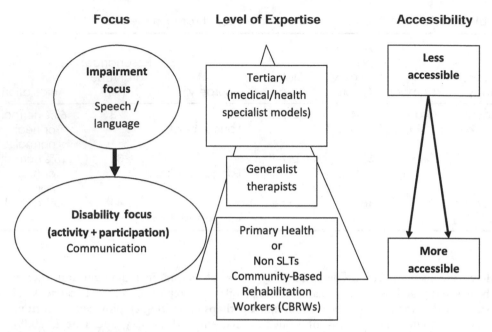

Figure 6.2 The relationship between impairment (specialist) and disability (community) models of services for communication impairments.

However, with the change in focus precipitated by the new conceptualization of disability suggested by the WHO ICF model (Part One, this volume), services and intervention can be provided at different levels; that is at the level of the impairment which may necessitate specialist services, or more broadly at the levels of activity and or participation (World Health Organization, 2001; Wickenden, 2008). The latter approach aims for acceptance of differences in communicative skills and facilitates inclusion in the community. Clearly this may be the more appropriate strategy for adults and many adolescents with very poor speech outcomes at the impairment level.

Figure 6.2 illustrates how the specialist impairment and broader disability models contrast with reference to their focus, level of expertise and the number of individuals who can be reached. The more 'expert' the service provided, the more likely it is to be both primarily impairment focussed and accessible to a relatively small proportion of the total population.

Of course this approach paints a very dichotomized picture of how models of service differ. There are some examples of specialist services providing very effective disability focussed work alongside impairment work, and below is an example of a non-specialist community based project undertaking impairment work together with a disability focussed intervention. D'Antonio (2002) usefully pointed out how the development of speech services requires a different commitment and time frame than surgical care. In many countries in Asia, Africa and South America the profession of speech and language therapy is non-existent even if basic surgery is possible. Even where there is a therapist, the number of SLTs with expertise in cleft care is often few, for example in India, Sri Lanka and Brazil. A lack of knowledge of the language, cultural and social factors, and very different work practices in the local health system may make it difficult for an SLT from another country/region to work effectively, as discussed below.

D'Antonio (2002) suggested that alternative models of service delivery need to be explored in the majority world, in particular harnessing existing community based approaches (D'Antonio, 1990; Prathanee, Dechongkit and Manochiopinig, 2006; D'Antonio and Nagarajan, 2003; Nagarajan, 2006). Models and approaches to speech intervention in the majority world are shown in Table 6.2, which is, of course, not exhaustive.

Although the structure and manner in which these models have been implemented has been described (Sell, 2008b; Wirt et al., 1990; D'Antonio and Nagarajan, 2003; Prathanee, Dechongkit and Manochiopinig, 2006; Pamplona et al., 2005; Barker et al., 2009) there is a need for many of these approaches to be validated through research. Determining the best approach to evaluation regardless of whether they have impairment and/or disability outcomes also needs careful consideration. In addition, there are other important issues to take into account when adopting a particular model, such as infrastructure and financing, partner institutions or highly motivated local individuals, and the availability of a multidisciplinary team to address problems which arise (Lamabadusuriya and Mars, 2008).

A detailed example of a community based project (in Thiruvannamalai, a rural district in South India) working in partnership with a tertiary centre (in Chennai) is provided here. Importantly, the drive for the project was the local district rehabilitation officer, who recognized that individuals with CL+/–P were frequently excluded from society and speech services might be helpful in addressing this. In stage one, 105 community based rehabilitation workers (CBRWs), all of whom were special educators, teachers or rehabilitation NGO workers, were trained about CL+/–P and screening for communication disorders. They then identified and referred more than 196 individuals with CL+/–P to screening camps held throughout the district. Each child was screened for communication disorders by the volunteer CBRW and two specialist SLTs from the tertiary centre. The screening included a rating of articulation (correct/incorrect), resonance (normal/abnormal) and intelligibility on a four point anchored scale. Agreement between the SLT and CBRW was variable: affricates 60%, nasals 82%, resonance 76% and intelligibility 56%. The poorer agreement for intelligibility was in part caused by differing screening methods of the CBRWs and SLTs (Nagarajan, D'Antonio and Chandran, 2006).

In stage two, a needs assessment was undertaken. The speech of 129 children over the age of three years was fully assessed by the specialist SLTs, together with the collection of socio-economic and demographic data. 39% of children did not demonstrate specific communication disorders, 43% showed impairments in both articulation and resonance, 12% showed only articulation errors while 3% had only resonance impairments. Those in need of further investigation for VPI, surgery of unrepaired palates and/or fistulae were referred to the tertiary centre. Those requiring therapy were identified. This needs assessment was very helpful in understanding the challenges faced by the families in accessing services. It also provided 'unmet need' data for the tertiary centre and gave an understanding of the range of disorders that existed within this community (Nagarajan, Subramaniyan and Savitha, 2009).

In stage three, the nine CBRWs were trained in the recognition and correction of articulation errors including glottal stops. Nineteen individuals (aged 10–20 years) with repaired CL+/–P and no associated conditions, with errors in the production of /k/ /g/

Table 6.2 Models and approaches to speech intervention in the majority world.

Model of intervention	Main features	Underlying principles	Strengths/Advantages	Challenges/Disadvantages	Example organization, Place
Community based rehabilitation (CBR)	Involves non-SLTs in intervention Community settings, e.g. teachers, community health workers, parents	Appropriate skills can be passed on A community based health care/rehabilitation network exists	Matched to local culture and existing services and structures Cheap Accessible to many communities, e.g. poor/rural May address non-health disability issues well, e.g. inclusion/attitudes/poverty	Lack of specialist knowledge and backup Very prescriptive if working on impairment Narrow range of impairments only can be addressed May lack credibility/status	Thiruvanamallai, India (Transforming Faces Worldwide) Thailand
Specialist fly in, fly out or 'Parachute' projects	Specialists from another country or region make short visits	Short term interventions can be effective Main focus is on impairment Demonstrates need	Can pass on skills to local staff Can act as resource at a distance Can act as catalyst for policy/service development	Sustainability Expensive and potentially culturally not well matched to context May not address disability issues	Operation Smile Rotaplast
SLT Students fly in, fly out	SLT students from another country make short visits	As above	As above	Sustainability and quality issues Students lack of clinical experience and of training others	City Cambodia Project (Supported by National CLAPA, UK) Vietnam (McAllister Australia) Dalhousie University

Reverse fly in, fly out	Professionals from majority world visit developed services in minority world	Visiting professionals can learn from observing specialists in a tertiary multidisciplinary context	Knowledge gained about specialist models Inspires visitors to be ambitious about what is possible High status for visitors on return home May lead to establishment of a one-off elite/model service on return May lead to the development of locally appropriate SLT services	Expensive May be difficult to implement on return home because of different structures, language and culture May only provide service to urban elite	Clinical internships SLCLP Project Fulbright style scholarships Ethiopia Project (Holmefjord and Kvinnsland, 2010)
Transfer of skills	Specialists run courses for local trainees who may be specialists, or non-specialists including parents Visits vary in length from few weeks or few years	Knowledge sharing Basic principles can be translated and adapted to local context with local input	Longer term than 2 or 3 above and with specific training remit Can potentially reach more people and spread services to rural and poorest areas Visitors have training skills	Trainers need to understand local context and adapt approach Trainees may expand their role beyond the remit of the training Follow up sustainability and no multidisciplinary team (MDT)	Earthspeak Smile Train (D'Antonio, 2003) Nepal, Bangladesh

(Continued)

Table 6.2 (Continued)

Model of intervention	Main features	Underlying principles	Strengths/Advantages	Challenges/Disadvantages	Example organization, Place
Camp model	Specialists and students/volunteers provide intensive intervention programmes & residential programmes	Intensive five days a week 4–5 hours a day of one-on-one and group work	Allows for supervised intervention even when provided by non-specialists. Can meet needs in under-served regions. Can support CBR approaches	Usually restricted to school holidays. Expensive. Follow up, sustainability and no local MDT	Mexico, Nepal, Sri Lanka, Earthspeak
Generalist SLTs but no specialist service	Local SLTS seeing cleft cases as part of general caseloads in diverse settings	Generalist SLTs can do cleft work	Local SLTS know the language and context well, and can address other communication disabilities, linked to local services and systems	Quality issues. Lack of time. No specialist knowledge of CL+/-P speech work. Lack of specialist support and MDT working. Enormous caseloads leading to 'low dose' effects	
Tertiary level specialist SLT service	Expert model	Effective intervention needs specialist knowledge	Links to primary and secondary services. Acts as a resource for generalists and others	Expensive and scarce. Accessible only to urban/rich. High status	North America, Europe, Australia and selected sites in Asia, Africa and Latin America

/d/ /t/ were included in the programme. Each CBRW was paired with one individual. The programme was delivered for eight weeks (30 minute sessions twice weekly) at either the school or home. The specialist SLT monitored the program through weekly field visits. Nine of the 19 individuals completed the eight week course. Inclement weather, logistics and ill health prevented the remaining 10 from completing the programme. Post-programme analysis revealed that all nine individuals met the criteria of correct production of target at word level. Three had generalized correct production to sentence and conversational levels. This continuing unique project needs careful evaluation, as it may be that this model could be replicated elsewhere (Subramaniyan *et al.*, 2009). The challenges of such a model have been many. The pace and reach of the activities are completely dictated by local conditions including the skills and capacities of the volunteer CBRWs.

There are different ways in which such projects can be evaluated. For example, by the number of patients referred who otherwise were not being seen by a tertiary team, the number who receive direct speech services, or the number with significant speech improvement. However, perhaps of more significance is the value to individuals and the local community. As the activities of the project have spread at grass roots level, user involvement, recently popularized in the minority world, has been effectively mobilized. Parents, the beneficiaries and the local community have become involved in the organization, planning and ownership of home/school based speech correction services.

6.4   Attitudes/Cultural Aspects

It is well recognized in the field of disability that across cultures there is a wide variety of attitudes, beliefs and practices in relation to people who are perceived as different. Thus, although the clinical features of impairments and, to a large extent, incidence rates are very similar globally, the way societies respond to disabled people varies greatly (Scheer and Groce, 1988). Cleft features and their consequences may or may not be seen as disabling depending on the cultural context. Thus, unusual facial appearance or unclear speech may be socially significant or may be disregarded. People with clefts, who have cosmetically successful repairs and intelligible speech, may not be viewed as either impaired or disabled. However, there are many in poor, rural and remote regions of the majority world who do not have these benefits, and are as socially excluded as those with other types of impairment. Thus much of the literature on poverty and discrimination of disabled people may be relevant to those with unrepaired clefts or poor surgical and speech outcomes (Barron and Amerena, 2007).

In many regions of the majority world, and indeed very poor parts of the minority world, accurate factual information about the causes and consequences of different impairments is scarce, and so people depend on local knowledge and beliefs to inform how they behave towards someone who is different. Where specialist services are sparse, health information is often unavailable, and when most people live rurally, traditional folk beliefs prevail. Many poor regions do have basic community health facilities, using modern medicine to deal mainly with acute illness. However, community workers are unlikely to have specialist knowledge about the causes and types of CL+/–P, still less about practicalities such as managing feeding or improving unclear speech. These workers themselves may have a mix of traditional and modern beliefs or attitudes.

Families' attitudes to intervention will be heavily influenced by their immediate community. They may have tried local traditional remedies or healers, as well as perhaps, if they are lucky, made long and expensive journeys to specialist facilities in the cities. Dagher and Ross (2004) have shown that traditional healers play an important role in the lives of South African families. One of the skills of the specialist (whether surgeon, dentist or SLT) is in not alienating people who come with a range of beliefs about what has caused the cleft, what 'cure' might be possible and the kind of life the individual can expect in the future. This requires an acknowledgement of a different set of beliefs and an ability to mesh the options that modern medicine can offer onto these, in acceptable ways for the family.

Some styles of service provision which are seen as optimal in the minority world may be seen as alien elsewhere. For example, a multidisciplinary team where members negotiate the treatment plan together, may be seen as odd in hierarchical societies, where the status of health professionals is very high and the senior person's opinion usually prevails. Similarly, the now common practice of asking the patient and family for their views may be perceived as incompetence. It may be seen as especially inappropriate to ask either women or children for their views. Even though most countries are signatories to the two United Nations conventions (the Rights of the Child (UN, 1989) and the Rights of Disabled Persons (UN, 2006)), these two traditionally powerless groups' opinions are still often overlooked. It is important to find out who should and can be involved in decisions. For example, failing to include grandparents or uncles can be very insulting. Equally it may be difficult to gain the views of 'low status' members of a household, such as child carers or servants, who may be responsible for childcare and potentially are significant in intervention.

Concepts of confidentiality and privacy vary greatly, and it can be quite normal for a consultation to take place in front of a large crowd of curious onlookers. Observers may perceive the professional closing the clinic door as defensive or the family selfish.

Attitudes to education in many majority countries are often formal and disciplined, and parents may take this kind of approach to therapy tasks too. Parents may insist on the child sitting on an adult chair and reciting on demand, and may be uncomfortable with a more informal style such as the professional sitting on the floor and 'following the child's lead' in play or conversation. Play based practice as a vehicle for therapy may also be unfamiliar. When encouraging home or school practice, parents and teachers need to be persuaded to change styles and to use praise. This may be an unfamiliar practice, perhaps regarded as indulgent and unnecessary. Accepting the child's best efforts as good enough, even if not yet 'perfect', may also be alien.

Attitudes to child rearing and learning vary greatly globally. It is important that any programme which plans to introduce intervention approaches to help with cleft speech matches the local beliefs and practices as closely as possible. While in some communities literacy rates may be low, there is often a heavy emphasis on children acquiring literacy. Thus, therapy activities using toys and pictures rather than written materials may be seen as of low value or dubious effectiveness. Materials should ideally be locally sourced or produced to give parents the confidence that they can replicate activities at home and not feel under pressure to use or buy unfamiliar, expensive or culturally inappropriate items.

The concept that pre-school or nursery attendance may facilitate communication skills and increased confidence may be unfamiliar. Difficulties may occur in trying to secure a school place for a child with poor speech. In countries where attendance rates are low or class sizes huge, it is often difficult for children with additional difficulties to gain admission. Conversely, often older children drop out of school because of bullying about speech (Bradbury and Habel, 2008). The introduction of gesture, signing and picture communication systems for a child with very unintelligible speech may also be met with opposition. In some very remote or poor regions, children with cleft speech or other impairments may not be identified until school age and beyond (Murthy *et al.*, 2010). Thus it may be that intervention (surgery or therapy) may begin late and should be linked to school, thereby encouraging attendance.

As in the minority world, understanding about what constitutes 'progress' may be different and families can be disappointed when dramatic changes in speech do not occur quickly. Thus an explanation of the gradual process of change is needed, using locally appropriate analogies (e.g. a plant growing), in order to motivate everyone to continue with the intervention. As professionals' skills are highly regarded, families may lack confidence in doing home based 'practice'. Parents who are used to 'expert models' of health care may find 'transplant' or 'empowerment' models (i.e. parents as partners in therapy) demanding and difficult to adapt to, because they conflict with their expectations (Appleton and Minchom, 1991). Recruiting an older sibling, cousin, grandparent or the local CBR or community worker to do 'therapy' may work better.

It is important to be aware that the urban rich elite will access specialist services much more easily than the rural poor. They will understand the approaches used in modern medicine and child-centred education, and so will more easily make use of advice and information. However, for the vast majority, it is important that agencies developing cleft services find approaches to serve disadvantaged populations in ways that take their economic, social and cultural circumstances into account. Otherwise, specialist services which mimic too closely those of the minority world can inadvertently exacerbate existing inequalities.

It is important to use the WHO ICF (World Health Organization, 2001) model to consider input at the impairment, activity and participation levels. Community workers should be trained to provide the following: information about clefts and hearing and access to specialist centres for assessment and surgery, community awareness, advocacy for education and social inclusion, human and legal rights, access to work, marriage, family and financial support. They work very broadly to improve inclusion and acceptance of all within a local community.

6.4.1 Working Across Languages

Many of the models of service provision outlined above involve specialists visiting regions outside their own. Working across languages or contexts adds complexity to the task, but can be successful if sensitively planned and executed. Being bilingual or multilingual is more common than being monolingual globally, and often the elite in majority countries do speak high status international languages such as English, French, Spanish or Arabic. So, a visitor may find that there is no communication gap with professional colleagues. However, it cannot be assumed that local people (either patients or trainee 'therapists') will speak anything but their local (perhaps several) and regional languages. Thus the people who are to receive services or be trained may be multilingual but not in the languages of the visiting 'experts'. It is important that the power and status issues around language are carefully considered and that intervention is provided in the appropriate language, without reinforcing any negative attitudes toward particular languages, by assessing, treating or teaching only in higher status ones.

Research on bilingual intervention shows that assessment and intervention should generally be provided in the mother tongue of the family, at least initially (Duncan, 1989). Children initially learn the local language of the home, and then are exposed to the regional or national language at school. Thus they are often 'successively' rather than 'simultaneously' bilingual. With regards to cleft speech it is important to consider age of palatal surgery in relation to the child's learning of languages. They may show a different pattern of speech characteristics in their first and second languages, for example if they have learnt the second language after palate repair. The cleft speech pattern has become habitual in the first language pre-surgery, but post-surgery the child integrates consonants as it acquires the second language (Borud et al., 2000). Changing the speech pattern in the first language is important but likely more challenging.

It is usually inappropriate to transfer assessments or treatment programmes from one language and culture to another, at least not without substantial adaptation and careful thought. There will be lack of transferability both of the technical aspects of the languages (e.g. vocabulary, phonological, grammatical and pragmatic rules) and cultural aspects, such as acceptability and recognizability of pictures and types of tasks. There is often very little data about developmental norms for speech or language acquisition in many local languages, although linguistic studies by local or foreign academics may be available. It is always better to use non-standardized but locally appropriate assessments than inappropriate standardized ones which don't match the language or context.

Preparation before working in an unfamiliar language environment is essential. Visiting SLTs must recruit the assistance of local speakers as interpreters, as well as to help design and carry out appropriate assessment and interventions. Teachers, linguists and parents can provide excellent information about how the language works, including its phonotactic rules. They can make reliable judgements about whether an individual's speech is 'normal' if they are asked the right questions or trained to listen out for particular aspects; for example:

- Does the child sound different from other children of similar age?

- Can the child pronounce all the consonants of the sound system?

- Which sounds are missing or incorrect? In what way?

- Does the way the child says the sounds cause confusion about the meaning of the words? (e.g. loss of contrast in a minimal pair)

- In a bilingual individual, is speech better in one language than the other?

Activities given to community workers or parents to practice should be demonstrated by a local speaker not a foreigner.

When using any of the intervention models (Table 6.2) it is crucial that those who do *not* speak the local languages are skilled and flexible in the way they work with local interpreters (Wallin and Ahlstrom, 2006). The challenging aspect of this is that the 'interpreter' may not be trained either in the interpreting or training role, in health care and still less in the specifics of a speciality such as SLT or cleft work.

6.5 Conclusion

This brief chapter describes a structure for understanding the way in which speech services may be conceptualized and in so doing evaluates the strengths and weaknesses of different models. Addressing activity and participation aspects is particularly important given the frequently severe speech disorders that present in contexts where timely multidisciplinary cleft services and impairment based SLT provision are scarce. Although there will always be a need for specialist speech services focussing on impairment, these need to be developed in parallel and in collaboration with community services. A broader social model approach which promotes positive attitudes and human rights is essential to ensure that the disabling effects of the impairment are minimized and social inclusion is maximized.

References

Appleton, P.L. and Minchom, P.E. (1991) Models of parent partnership and child development centres. *Child: Care, Health and Development*, **17**, 27–38.

Aziz, S.R., Rhee, S.T. and Redai, I. (2009) Cleft surgery in rural Bangladesh: reflections and experiences. *Journal of Oral and Maxillofacial Surgery*, **67**, 1581–1588.

Barker, C., Bergin, F., Williams, C. *et al.* (2009) Taking speech and language therapy to Cambodia. *Bulletin of the Royal College of Speech and Language Therapists*, **682**, 18–19.

Barron, T. and Amerena, P. (eds) (2007) Disability and Inclusive Development, Leonard Cheshire International, London.

Birkett, L. (1999) A study of speech results and timing of surgery in a Sri Lankan UCLP population. MSc project, University of London.

Borud, L.J., Ceradini, D., Eng, N. and Court, C.C. (2000) Second language acquisition following pharyngeal flap surgery in non-English-speaking immigrants. *Plastic and Reconstructive Surgery*, **106**, 640–644.

Bradbury, E. and Habel, A. (2008) Psychological and Social Aspects of CL/P in the Developing World, in *Management of Cleft Lip and Palate in the Developing World* (eds M. Mars, D. Sell and A. Habel), John Wiley & Sons Ltd, Chichester, pp. 159–170.

Dagher, D. and Ross, E. (2004) Approaches of South African traditional healers regarding the treatment of cleft lip and palate. *Cleft Palate-Craniofacial Journal*, **41** (5), 461–469.

D'Antonio, L.L. (1990) Commentary to Ward & James. *Cleft Palate Journal*, **27**, 15–17.

D'Antonio, L.L. (2002) The interdisciplinary approach to cleft care and beyond. Keynote address: symposium and workshop on 'Speech disorders in individuals with CLP: assessment, therapy and surgical management'. Sri Ramachandra University, Chennai, India.

D'Antonio, L.L. (2003) Speech training symposium, China. The Smile Train.

D'Antonio, L.L. and Nagarajan, R. (2003) Use of a consensus building approach to plan speech services for children with cleft palate in India. *Folia Phoniatrica et Logopaedica*, **55**, 306–314.

D'Antonio, L.L., Louw, B., Nagarajan, R. *et al.* (2008) Strategies for increasing speech services in underserved regions of the world: report of the Smile Train ad hoc speech advisory group. The Smile Train Medical Advisory Board Meeting (June 2008), New York.

Duncan, D. (ed.) (1989) *Working with Bilingual Language Disability*, Chapman & Hall, London.

Hartley, S. and Wirz, S. (2002) Development of a communication disability model and its implication on service delivery in low-income countries. *Social Science & Medicine*, 10, 1543–1547.

Henningsson, G., Kuehn, D.P., Sell, D. *et al.* (2008) Universal parameters for reporting speech outcomes in individuals with cleft palate. *Cleft Palate-Craniofacial Journal*, 45, 1–17.

Hodges, S., Wilson, J. and Hodges, A. (2009) Plastic and reconstructive surgery in Uganda – 10 years experience. *Pediatric Anesthesia*, 19, 12–18.

Holmefjord, A. and Kvinnsland, B. (2010) Speech therapy in Ethiopia. Poster presentation at the 13th meeting of international clinical linguistics and phonetics association, Oslo.

Jobe, A.L., D'Mello, J. and Kumar, S. (2007) Speech understandability of repaired cleft palate patients pre and post caregiver training. *Indian Journal of Plastic Surgery*, 20, 122–128.

Kummer, A. (2008) Cleft lip/palate missions to developing countries, in *Cleft Palate and Craniofacial Anomalies: Effects on Speech and Resonance*, 2nd edn (ed. A. Kummer), Thompson Delmar Learning, New York, pp. 609–625.

Lamabadusuriya, S.P. and Mars, M. (2008) The Sri Lankan cleft lip and palate project (2008), in *Management of Cleft Lip and Palate in the Developing World* (eds M. Mars, D. Sell and A. Habel), John Wiley & Sons Ltd, Chichester, pp. 95–111.

Landis, P. and Cuc, T. (1975) Articulation patterns and speech intelligibility of 54 Vietnamese children with unoperated oral clefts: clinical observations and impressions. *Cleft Palate Journal*, 12, 234–243.

Mars, M., Sell, D. and Habel, A. (2008) Introduction, in *Management of Cleft Lip and Palate in the Developing World* (eds M. Mars, D. Sell and A. Habel), John Wiley & Sons Ltd, Chichester, pp. 1–4.

Murthy, J., Sendhilnathan, S. and Hussain, S.A. (2010) Speech outcome following late primary repair. *Cleft Palate-Craniofacial Journal*, 47, 156–161.

Nagarajan, R. (2006) Development of community based speech services for individuals with CLP in India: lessons for around the world. Presentation at an international video conference on the treatment of speech disorders in individuals with cleft lip and palate. Loma Linda University, California, USA, and Sri Ramachandra Medical College, Chennai, India.

Nagarajan, R. D'Antonio, L.L. and Chandran, K. (2006) When speech pathologists are not available: Training community workers. American Cleft Palate Association convention, Vancouver, Canada (April 2006).

Nagarajan, R., Subramaniyan, B. and Savitha, V.H. (2009) Designing community based resource worker delivered speech correction program: strengths and barriers. Presentation at the 11th international congress on cleft lip and palate and related Craniofacial Anomalies, Fortaleza, Brazil (September, 2009).

Nayak, J. (1996) A systematic study correlating speech results of Sri Lankan UCLP participants with timing of surgery. MSc project, University of London.

Ortiz-Monasterio, F., Serrano, R.A., Barrera, G.P. *et al.* (1966) A study of untreated adult cleft palate patients. *Plastic and Reconstructive Surgery*, 38, 36–41.

Ortiz-Monasterio, F., Olmeda, A., Trigos, I. *et al.* (1974) Final results from the delayed treatment of patients with clefts of the lip and palate. *Scandinavian Journal of Plastic Surgery*, 8, 109–115.

Pamplona, C., Ysunza, A., Patino, C. *et al.* (2005) Speech summer camp for treating articulation disorders in cleft palate patients. *International Journal of Pediatic Otorhinolaryngology*, 69, 351–359.

Prathanee, B., Dechongkit, S. and Manochiopinig, S. (2006) Development of community-based speech therapy model: for children with cleft lip/palate in Northeast Thailand. *Journal of the Medical Association of Thailand*, 89, 500–507.

Reeve, M., Groce, N., Persing, J. and Magge, S. (2004) An international surgical exchange program for children with cleft lip/cleft palate in Manaus, Brazil: patient and family expectations of outcome. *Journal of Craniofacial Surgery*, **15**, 170–174.

Ruiz-Razura, A., Cronin, E. and Navarro, C. (2000) Creating long-term benefits in CLP volunteer missions. *Plastic and Reconstructive Surgery*, **105**, 195–201.

Saboye, J., Chancholle, A.-R., Tournier, J.-J. and Maurette, I. (2004) Palatopharyngoplasty an 'all in one surgery'. Our experience in Phillipines. *Annales de Chirugie Plastique Esthétique*, **49**, 261–264.

Scheer, J. and Groce, N.E. (1988) Impairment as a human constant: cross-cultural and historical perspectives on variation. *Journal of Social Issues*, **44**, 23–37.

Sell, D. (1992) Speech in Sri Lankan cleft palate subjects with delayed palatoplasty. PhD thesis, De Montfort University, Leicester, UK (formerly Leicester Polytechnic, UK).

Sell, D. (2005) Issues in perceptual speech analysis in cleft palate and related disorders: a review. *International Journal of Language and Communication Disorders*, **40**, 103–121.

Sell, D. (2008a) Speech in the unoperated or late operated patient, in *Management of Cleft Lip and Palate in the Developing World* (eds M. Mars, D. Sell and A. Habel), John Wiley & Sons Ltd, Chichester, pp. 177–192.

Sell, D. (2008b) Speech therapy and CLP in the developing world context, in *Management of Cleft Lip and Palate in the Developing World* (eds M. Mars, D. Sell and A. Habel), John Wiley & Sons Ltd, Chichester, pp. 193–202.

Sell, D. and Grunwell, P. (1990) Preliminary speech results in a subgroup of unoperated Sri Lankan adolescents following late palatal surgery. *Cleft Palate Journal*, **27**, 162–168.

Sell, D. and Grunwell, P. (1993) Speech in late operated cleft palate subjects, in *Analysing Cleft Palate Speech* (ed. P. Grunwell), Whurr, London, pp. 112–141.

Sell, D. and Grunwell, P. (1994) Speech studies and the unoperated cleft palate subject. *European Journal of Disorders of Communication*, **9**, 151–164.

Sell, D., Grunwell, P. and Mars, M. (1994) A methodology for the evaluation of severely disordered cleft palate speech. *Clinical Linguistics & Phonetics*, **8**, 219–233.

Subramaniyan, B., Nagarajan, R., Vijay Kumar, K.V. and Savitha, V.H. (2009) Correction of stop consonants errors by community based resource workers: an efficacy study. 11th international congress on cleft lip and palate and related Craniofacial Anomalies, Fortaleza, Brazil (September, 2009).

UN (1989) Convention on the Rights of the Child, http://www2.ohchr.org/english/law/pdf/crc.pdf (accessed 16 March 2011).

UN (2006) Convention on the Rights of Persons with Disabilities, http://www.un.org/esa/socdev/enable/rights/convtexte.htm (accessed 16 March 2011).

Wallin, A.-M. and Ahlstrom, G. (2006) Cross-cultural interview studies using interpreters: systematic literature review. *Journal of Advanced Nursing*, **55**, 723–735.

Ward, C.M. and James, I. (1990) Surgery of 346 patients with unoperated CLP in Sri Lanka. *Cleft Palate Journal*, **27**, 11–14.

Wickenden, M. (2008) Disability, culture and CLP, in *Management of Cleft Lip and Palate in the Developing World* (eds M. Mars, D. Sell and A. Habel), John Wiley & Sons Ltd, Chichester, pp. 145–158.

Wirt, A., Wyatt, R., Sell, D. *et al.* (1990) Training counterparts in cleft palate speech therapy in the developing world: an extended report. *European Journal of Disorders of Communication*, **25**, 355–367.

World Health Organization (2001) *International Classification of Functioning Disability and Health (ICF)*, WHO, Geneva.

Yeow, V., Lee-Seng-Teik, T., Lambrecht, T.J. *et al.* (2002) International task force on volunteer cleft missions. *Journal of Craniofacial Surgery*, **13**, 18–25.

Part Two

Speech Assessment and Intervention

Anette Lohmander[1] and Sara Howard[2]

[1] Karolinska Institutet, Department of Clinical Science, Intervention and Technique, Division of Speech and Language Pathology, SE 141 86, Stockholm, Sweden

[2] University of Sheffield, Department of Human Communication Sciences, Sheffield, S10 2TA, UK

Assessment and evaluation of speech and language in individuals born with cleft lip and palate (CLP) is a main objective in CLP treatment and research. Speech is a major outcome after surgical intervention and the basis for decisions about the need for further treatment.

Thus, methodologies for assessment must be valid and reliable. A critical review of studies on speech outcome after CLP treatment during a 20-year-period (1980–1999) revealed major flaws and lack of information in many of the articles (Lohmander and Olsson, 2004). It was obvious that standardized procedures for data collection and analysis had not been the practice in many studies (Chapter 4). To be able to use clinical data for audit and research it is necessary to develop and use standardized procedures. Sell (2005) summarizes the related requirements very well. Her experiences, together with those of her colleagues, are based on the development of procedures for data collection and analysis in the United Kingdom. They have successfully developed and used standardized procedures in research, for national audits and for education and training (Sell et al., 2001; John et al., 2006; Sell et al., 2009). The methodology developed for the Scandcleft project is another good example with a standardized procedure for data collection (Lohmander, Willadsen *et al.*, 2009) and analysis, based on the framework by Hutters and Henningsson (2004). Further information is available on the website 'Cleft palate international speech issues' (www.CLISPI.org), originally developed in the Eurocran project (www.eurocran.org). Similarly, 'universal parameters' have also been suggested for reporting speech outcome (Henningsson *et al.*, 2008).

Perceptual analysis of cleft palate speech includes transcription and/or scale rating of deviances or skills. The second part of this book contains a comprehensive chapter on transcription, and use of ratings scales is addressed in other chapters. In the chapter on cross-linguistic issues, the specific problems comparing speech in different languages are described.

A description of resonance characteristics is usually included in the assessment of speakers with cleft palate and usually a rating procedure is used for evaluation (Lohmander and Olsson, 2004). This sounds reasonable, since the decision as to whether a speaker is hypernasal is the subjective decision of an observer, based on perceptual judgement. The problem, however, is that such ratings are still not presented with convincing reliability (Kuehn and Moller, 2000). This could be attributed to variable internal standards acquired by different individuals and also to the fact that the internal standards could be unstable over time, independent of the experience level of the observer (Kreiman *et al.*, 1993; Keuning, Wieneke and Dejonckere, 1999). It is easier to agree on a normal outcome of a variable than on a pathological one (Kreiman *et al.*, 1993), and problems other than hypernasality may interfere with judgement and even masque the impression of hypernasality (Fletcher and Bishop, 1970; Kent, 1996). The same experiences have been found regarding the assessment of voice quality (Chapter 10). Both descriptive category judgments and rating of severity will continue to be useful in describing changes in voice or resonance after surgical or behavioural intervention. Continuing effort to increase the level of agreement is, therefore, highly needed and figures on reliability shall be reported. In the chapters on nasality (Chapter 11) and intelligibility (Chapter 16) more information on different methods for rating are discussed.

Instrumental analysis is often used as a complement to perceptual analysis in order to understand and verify the subjective opinion. One chapter here describes instrumental assessment of articulation, and two further chapters describe various instrumental methods for assessment of velopharyngeal function and speech symptoms associated with velopharyngeal impairment (VPI). One reliable correlate may be an overall variable for perceptual assessment of velopharyngeal function, such as has sometimes has been used for evaluation of velopharyngeal function during speech (McWilliams, Morris and Shelton, 1990). Such an overarching variable has been found to be representative of the observers' overall impression of degree of impairment (Dotevall *et al.*, 2002). Overall variables or composite scores have recently been used in addition to the assessment of speech errors related to cleft palate (John *et al.*, 2006)

Assessment and intervention of the early communication of infants and children with cleft palate, including both articulation and phonology, followed by phonological approaches to intervention for speech difficulties in cleft palate are covered in two chapters and psycholinguistic aspects in a further one.

Issues of activity and participation are dealt with in two chapters and, finally, the importance of current evidence regarding intervention in the area of speech and language pathology is presented in the final chapter in the book. Many research questions can be raised from this information and it is hoped that the reader will be inspired to help increasing the level of evidence within the area of cleft palate.

References

Dotevall, H., Lohmander, A., Ejnell, H. and Bake, B. (2002) Perceptual evaluation of speech and velopharyngeal function in children with and without cleft palate and the relationship to nasal airflow patterns. *Cleft Palate-Craniofacial Journal*, **39**, 409–424.Fletcher, S.G. and Bishop, M.E. (1970) Measurement of nasality with TONAR. *Cleft Palate Journal*, **7**, 610–621.

Henningsson, G., Kuehn, D.P., Sell, D. *et al.* (Speech Parameters Group) (2008).Universal parameters for reporting speech outcomes in individuals with cleft palate. *Cleft Palate-Craniofacial Journal*, **45**, 1–17.

Hutters, B. and Henningsson, G. (2004) Speech outcome following treatment in crosslinguistic cleft palate studies: methodological implications. *Cleft Palate-Craniofacial Journal*, **41**, 544–549.

John, A., Sell, D., Sweeney, T. *et al.* (2006) The cleft audit protocol for speech–augmented: a validated and reliable measure for auditing cleft speech. *Cleft Palate-Craniofacial Journal*, **43**, 272–288.

Kent, R.D. (1996) Hearing and believing: some limits to the auditory-perceptual assessment of speech and voice disorders. *American Journal of Speech and Language Pathology*, **5**, 7–23.

Keuning, K.H.D., Wieneke, G.H. and Dejonckere, P.H. (1999) The intrajudge reliability of the perceptual rating of cleft palate speech before and after pharyngeal flap surgery: the effect of judges and speech samples. *Cleft Palate-Craniofacial Journal*, **36**, 328–333.

Kreiman, J., Gerratt, B.R., Kempster, G.B. *et al.* (1993) Perceptual evaluation of voice quality: review, tutorial, and a framework for future research. *Journal of Speech and Hearing Research*, **36**, 21–40.

Kuehn, D. and Moller, K. (2000) Speech and language issues in the cleft palate population: the state of the art. *Cleft Palate-Craniofacial Journal*, **37**, 1–35.

Lohmander, A. and Olsson, M. (2004) Perceptual assessment of speech in patients with cleft palate: a critical review. *Cleft Palate-Craniofacial Journal*, **41**, 64–70.Lohmander, A., Willadsen, E., Persson, C. *et al.* (2009) Methodology for speech assessment in the Scandcleft project. *Cleft Palate-Craniofacial Journal*, **46** (4), 347–362.

McWilliams, B.J., Morris, L.M. and Shelton, R.L. (1990) Cleft Palate Speech, BC Decker, Philadelphia.

Sell, D. (2005) Issues in perceptual speech analysis in cleft palate and related disorders: a review. *International Journal of Language and Communication Disorders*, **40**, 103–121.

Sell, D.A., Grunwell, P., Mildenhall, S. *et al.* (2001) Cleft lip and palate care in the United Kingdom–the clinical standards advisory group (CSAG) study. Part 3: speech outcomes. *Cleft Palate-Craniofacial Journal*, **38**, 30–37.

Sell, D., John, A., Harding-Bell, A. *et al.* (2009) Cleft audit protocol for speech (CAPS-A): a comprehensive training package for speech analysis. *International Journal of Language and Communication Disorders*, **44**, 529–548.

7

Phonetic Transcription for Speech Related to Cleft Palate

Sara Howard

University of Sheffield, Department of Human Communication Sciences, Sheffield, S10 2TA, UK

7.1 Introduction

A central question in the analysis of speech production associated with cleft palate is why a particular speaker sounds the way they do. To begin to answer this question it is necessary, at minimum, to make a phonetic analysis of the speaker's speech production. This may consist of perceptual analysis or instrumental analysis, or a combination of the two. In terms of instrumental analysis, the speech output of individuals with a cleft lip and/or palate has been effectively investigated using a wide range of instrumental and imaging techniques, including spectrography, electropalatography, nasometry, nasal airflow measures, videofluoroscopy and nasendoscopy (Chapters 8, 11 and 12). However, despite the undoubtedly valuable information provided by such analyses, researchers continue to remind us that the 'gold standard' for clinical assessment of speech related to cleft palate remains that of perceptual analysis using narrow phonetic transcription (Sell, 2005; Peterson-Falzone et al., 2006). This chapter explores the use of phonetic transcription in the assessment of speech production associated with cleft palate,

Cleft Palate Speech: Assessment and Intervention, First Edition. Edited by Sara Howard, Anette Lohmander.
© 2011 John Wiley & Sons, Ltd. Published 2011 by John Wiley & Sons, Ltd.

considering the aims and objectives of perceptual analysis, the various symbol systems available for clinical transcription, potential benefits and pitfalls, and the specific challenges to transcription presented by the speech production of individuals with a cleft palate.

7.2   What is Phonetic Transcription?

Phonetic transcription is one approach to the perceptual analysis of speech production. It can be contrasted with the use of perceptual ratings scales which estimate degree or severity of specific speech characteristics (e.g. nasality, intelligibility), the latter being a popular approach in the analysis of speech associated with cleft palate, but one which is, like transcription, not without its difficulties and drawbacks (Flipsen, 2006; Whitehill, 2002). Lohmander and Olsson (2004) have provided a detailed review of different perceptual methodologies in speech analysis related to cleft palate, and chapters in this volume by (Chapters 11 and 16) discuss the use of perceptual rating scales in the analysis of speech production in individuals with a cleft palate. Phonetic transcription can be thought of as a method of translating fleeting auditory and visual impressions of speech production into a permanent record comprising a string of written symbols (typically in the first instance using pencil and paper). As such, it is at best an incomplete record, and clearly the linear string of symbols does not have a totally transparent relationship with the subtle and constantly changing movements of the vocal organs and the resulting acoustic signal.

It is important to consider what is being implied by the use of a particular phonetic symbol. Describing phonetic transcription as a form of *perceptual* analysis suggests that the transcription is a record of what is heard (and seen) when the speech was produced. Often it is felt possible to assume a close relationship between that percept and a set of underlying articulatory, phonatory and resonatory behaviours. This assumption forms the basis of the International Phonetic Alphabet (IPA, 1999), such that use of the symbol [t] implies that a voiceless alveolar plosive, entailing a specific configuration of abducted vocal folds, tongue tip elevation to the alveolar ridge, velopharyngeal closure, and so on, has been heard. However, because of the well-known phenomenon of motor equivalence (whereby speakers may be able to produce the same auditory percept using different articulatory movements (Perkell, 1997)), it cannot always be assumed that each auditory percept has a simple one-to-one relationship to a specific set of articulatory behaviours. As Howard and Heselwood (2002a, p. 388) observe, 'in the absence of instrumental evidence ... what [t] in a transcription can only mean is that there was a sound that sounded as if it was made [with the articulatory movements described above]'. Comparisons of perceptual and instrumental analysis of atypical speech production of various kinds, including that associated with cleft palate, have often revealed surprising relationships between what the listener has experienced and what the vocal organs can be seen to have done for a particular sound or word (Gibbon, 1990; Howard, 1994; Heselwood, 2009); this important issue is returned to below.

A phonetic transcription will reflect both the transcriber's skills (and limitations) in perceptual analysis, as well as their specific aims and objectives in embarking on a transcription in the first place, but they can be confident that the process of making a transcription will provide valuable information and insights into a speaker's abilities and difficulties (Howard and Heselwood, 2002a, Shriberg, Hinke and Trost-Steffen, 1987). Crucially, a good phonetic transcription can capture the auditory effect of atypical speech production upon a listener; in other words it can help to explain why a speaker sounds the way they do, as a clinical precursor to considering what might be done about it.

7.3   Why Transcribe?

Before embarking on any transcription, it is imperative to consider the purposes of our analysis and to ask ourselves why we are spending time and effort on this activity. What aspect or aspects of the speech production do we want to capture, for what reason? It may be, for example, that we are specifically interested in identifying the contextual distribution of audible nasal emission or nasal turbulence in the individual's speech. We may just want to distinguish between the speaker's realizations of /s/ and /ʃ/, or perhaps to examine the production of those consonants usually produced by the tip of the tongue, rather than evaluating the production of all consonants and vowels. We might have the ambitious aim of uncovering the phonetic parameters of speaker intelligibility in spontaneous speech production, which would entail transcription not only of individual sound segments, but also of voice quality and prosodic features such as stress, pitch, rate, loudness and pauses. Alternatively, our phonetic analysis might aim to form the basis of a phonological analysis, which will help in the task of differential diagnosis, by for example permitting us to distinguish between typical developmental phonological processes and unusual cleft-related speech behaviours (Harding and Grunwell, 1996; Chapter 15), or to explore the possible impact of a hearing impairment or motor speech problem on the speech output. We may aim to transcribe a very specific set of words or phrases from a formal assessment, for the purposes of clinical audit or to share with other clinicians or researchers, or so that we can compare pre- and post-intervention speech production. We may, in turn, be interested in comparing perceptual and instrumental data for a particular sound segment or class of sounds. The purpose of our transcription will determine both the kind and the amount of material we elicit, the level of detail of our transcription and its comprehensiveness. As Crystal (1987, p. 16) remarks 'If we have made a transcription *at the right level for our purposes*, it should be unnecessary to have to refer back to the tape' [author's italics].

More generally, a fundamental motivation for spending valuable clinical time making a phonetic transcription of atypical speech is that the information it can provide may reveal hitherto unnoticed speech behaviours or patterns which are nevertheless clinically significant. Furthermore, it may serve to undo some of our possible preconceptions about the speaker's likely productions. Howard (1993), for example, describes a young girl with a cleft palate who had been described, on the basis of a broad phonemic transcription, as having severe phonological problems, including amongst other things the lack of a contrast between /f/ and /v/ in her sound system. Detailed transcription, however, revealed the presence of a consistent contrast, realised by unusual means, whereby the voiceless fricative /f/ was produced as a weakly articulated voiceless labiodental fricative [f̨], whereas its voiced counterpart was produced either as a strongly articulated voiceless labiodental fricative [f̟] or as a voiced labiodental approximant [ʋ]. Thus, although this child was not able to combine vocal fold vibration with a fricative stricture, to produce the required voiced turbulence, she was able to signal a consistent if unusual contrast which familiar listeners tuned in to over time. Having an open mind in making our transcriptions is probably particularly important where we are dealing with speakers with complex speech difficulties and high levels of unintelligibility. As Kelly and Local (1989, p. 26) remark 'it is not possible to have too much phonetic detail … at the beginning of work on language material we can't, in any interesting sense, know before-hand what it going to be important'. There are two responses one might have to this observation: one would be to feel daunted by the demands of detailed analysis; the other, which is arguably preferable, is to feel excited about the fascinating task which lies ahead.

7.4 What to Transcribe and How to Transcribe It

Making good quality sound recordings (which currently will typically be in the form of digital videos) will be vital in supporting the transcription process (John *et al.*, 2006). Although live observation of an individual's speech production is undeniably helpful for clinical analysis, it has long been established that atypical speech production is too complex to transcribe accurately *in situ* (Amorosa *et al.*, 1985), which may have a det-rimental effect on transcription reliability (Lohmander and Olsson, 2004), so recourse to recordings is inevitable if we wish to make transcriptions which will be clinically valuable.

Establishing clear aims and objectives for our transcription, as discussed above, will help us to determine the type of speech sample we collect. Traditional speech assessments have generally consisted of the elicitation of a list of single words by picture naming, with pictures selected to capture the consonant phonemes of the language in question in different word and syllable contexts. More recently, however, there has been greater acknowledgement of the importance of gathering information on sound production in larger linguistic constructions (e.g. the phonetically-balanced phrases used in the GOS. SP.ASS and the Scandcleft Project (Sell, Harding and Grunwell, 1999; Lohmander *et al.*, 2009)) and in spontaneous connected speech (Sell *et al.*, 2001; Howard, 2007; Howard, Wells and Local, 2008; Peterson-Falzone, Hardin-Jones and Karnell, 2010). Ideally a sample of each of these types of data should be collected and analysed. Certainly where there are issues with a speaker's overall intelligibility, analysis of both the articulatory and prosodic aspects of their connected speech production may be vital in order to understand why listeners have difficulties understanding them (Howard, 2007). On the other hand, analysis of single sounds, and sounds in single words, can give us informa-tion about the speaker's articulatory abilities in less demanding contexts, and a com-parison of single word production in picture naming, word repetition and nonsense word production will provide a fuller picture of the individual's overall speech processing abilities and difficulties (Chapter 13).

The focus of phonetic and phonological analysis for speech related to cleft palate, as for other types of impaired speech production, is generally on the production of conso-nants, with vowels being often somewhat neglected. However, although technically and perceptually challenging, it may be illuminating in some cases to spend some time on the careful transcription of vowels, (Howard and Heselwood, 2002b). Not only is it clear that different vowels will be susceptible to a greater or lesser degree to hypernasality

(Lewis, Watterson and Quint, 2000), and that sometimes speakers with a cleft palate may substitute nasal consonants for vowels within single syllables (Michi *et al.*, 1986), or over whole utterances (Howard, 2004), but also the close interrelationship of consonants and vowels within the syllable frame means that vowels may affect consonant production, and vice versa, in unusual ways in atypical speech production (Bates, Watson and Scobbie, 2002).

Transcribing the speech of individuals with a cleft palate requires the use of a broad range of symbols and diacritics, many of which we will not have encountered in the transcription of normal speech production (Ball *et al.*, 2009). Currently the most widely used symbols for the transcription of speech related to cleft palate are those contained in the IPA and ExtIPA (The Extensions to the IPA for the transcription of atypical speech (IPA, 1999; Duckworth *et al.*, 1990)), although other symbols exist, including those, for example, developed by Trost (1981), which are widely used in the USA (Peterson-Falzone *et al.*, 2006). Work is continuing to solve some of the particular challenges to transcription offered by speech production in cleft palate, and to reach an international consensus, such that all the symbols and notational devices necessary for transcription can eventually be integrated into ExtIPA (Trost-Cardamone *et al.*, 2010; Howard, McLeod and Ball, in preparation). The IPA and ExtIPA combined provide us with an extensive range of notational devices for the transcription of speech associated with cleft palate (Appendices 7.A and 7.B). ExtIPA includes symbols to designate unusual places of articulations, unusual resonance and airflow, and unusual phonatory behaviours, as well as notations to capture a range of prosodic features, arranged on a chart which mirrors the organization of the IPA chart. To signal aspects of voice quality which extend over domains longer than the segment, we can use the notations offered by the VoQS system (Ball, Esling and Dickson, 1995, based on Laver, 1980) (Appendix 7.C). Some of these resources are now explored in relation to the speech production of individuals with a cleft lip and/or palate.

7.5 Features of Cleft Speech Production

In the following section, we look at some of the most commonly attested features of speech associated with a cleft lip and/or palate, and consider how these might be transcribed phonetically. The examples below are not meant to be exhaustive, but to give a flavour of how the symbols in the IPA and ExtIPA can help us to get our auditory and visual perceptions of speech production down on paper. More comprehensive accounts of ExtIPA are available elsewhere (Duckworth *et al.*, 1990; Howard, McLeod and Ball, in preparation).

7.5.1 Atypical Place of Articulation

As discussed in Chapters 1 and 3, the unusual dentition and occlusion frequently encountered in individuals with a cleft lip and/or palate sometimes lead to unusual relationships between active and passive articulators in the production of target sound segments. Thus, for example, a speaker with the protruded mandible characteristic of a Class 3 occlusion may realize bilabial and labiodentals consonants (/p, b, m, f, v/) using a dentolabial (reverse labiodental) place of articulation. For such a speaker, the phrase FIVE MORE PEARS would be produced as [faɪʋ m̪ɔ p̪eəz]. Conversely, where a Class 2 occlusion results in a retracted mandible, bilabials may be realised as labiodentals (thus MORE PEAS AND BEANS would be realised as ['m̪ɔ piz əm̪ 'b̪inz]. A marked Class 2 occlusion could even result in bilabials having a labioalveolar articulation, such that MORE PEAS AND BEANS could be realised as ['m̺ɔ piz əm̺ 'b̺inz]. A feature which is perceptually identifiable in individuals with a cleft palate, and which has also been identified using instrumental analysis (Howard, 2001) is the sliding articulation, whereby the place of articulation of a segment perceptibly changes during its production. This may be most easily perceptually identified on fricative articulations, for example where a speaker's tongue dorsum slides forward from a velar place of articulation to the hard palate during the realization of /s/ as [xc] in SOAP [xcəup].

Whereas some unusual places of articulation will result from unusual structural relationships in the oral cavity (specifically malocclusions), other instances of atypical place of articulation seem to stem from compensatory behaviours related to the reduction of hypernasality and nasal air emission (Hutters and Brondsted, 1987). Different types of retracted realizations of alveolar and postalveolar sounds fall within this category, and commonly reported features associated with a cleft palate include palatal, velar, uvular, pharyngeal and glottal realizations of such targets. Most of these places of articulation are well provided for for the purposes of transcription on the IPA chart, although as noted by Peterson-Falzone *et al.* (2006) and Trost-Cardamone *et al.* (2010), there are relatively few symbols available for the transcription of pharyngeal and epiglottal articulations. It may be, in future, that further symbols could be introduced to the ExtIPA chart to capture the range of pharyngeal and epiglottal articulations encountered in speech production related to cleft.

7.5.2   Atypical Resonance and Airstream

A key area where a combination of IPA and ExtIPA symbols helps to capture aspects of atypical speech production commonly associated with cleft palate is that of resonance and oral/nasal airflow. The IPA allows us to make a useful distinction between nasal, nasalized and oral sounds, by the use of nasal and oral symbols and the nasal tilde: thus [m] is a voiced, bilabial nasal stop; [b] is a voiced bilabial oral stop (plosive) and [ɑ̃] is a nasalized low back unrounded vowel. A common use of the nasal tilde in the transcription of speech related to cleft palate is in combination with an oral symbol, to denote a nasalized oral consonant (e.g. [b̃] or [z̃]), which sounds somewhere between fully oral and fully nasal. Although there is an interesting discussion to be had about the way in which an oral stop (plosive), such as the /b/ in A BEAR realised as [ɜ̃ 'b̃ɛ̃ə], could actually be realised with audible nasal resonance (the implication being that air is resonating audibly in the nasal cavity during the hold phase of the stop) and how much our perception is actually of the surrounding context of nasalized vowels (Grunwell and Harding, 1996; Ball, 2010), this is a widely used and useful notation.

The IPA, of course, was designed for the purpose of transcribing typical speech production and we have to look to ExtIPA for further symbols to capture many of the atypical features of resonance and airflow evident in many individuals with a cleft palate.

Thus, for example, ExtIPA offers a diacritic (the denasal tilde) to indicate denasalization of nasal consonants, although the degree of denasalization is not further elaborated on and in practice the use of the diacritic appears to vary; thus, for example, some transcribers transcribe A MAN as [ə ˈbæd] if it is felt that the nasal consonant targets were produced with no perceptible nasal resonance whatsoever, or as [ə ˈm̃æñ] if it is felt that the consonants were somewhat but not totally denasalized. Others would use the second transcription for both realizations. Once again, it is an interesting phonetic question to ask whether we can have such a thing as a partially denasalized nasal, and what that might imply in speech production terms. Duckworth *et al.* (1990, p. 276) suggest that the denasal tilde 'describes the absence of expected nasal resonance', which of course implies that a perceptual judgement is being made relative to a listener's expectations for a typical production of a lexical item or utterance. (We will return to the question of the listener's knowledge of the intended target below, but for further discussion see also Ball, 2008). Where an oral consonant is realised but we can perceive air escaping nasally simultaneously (audible nasal escape), we can also look to ExtIPA for our transcription (thus, SAFE as [s̃eɪf̃]). Where the nasal airstream is particularly noisy, we can use a different diacritic to denote the presence of nasal turbulence simultaneous with an oral articulation (e.g. SAFE as [s̰eɪf̰]; TOP as [s̰eɪf̰]). A velopharyngeal fricative produced without simultaneous oral articulatory activity would be transcribed with the symbol [fŋ]: thus SAFE as [fŋeɪfŋ], although this is generally felt to occur only rarely in speech related to cleft palate, as usually the friction is simultaneous with an attempt by the speaker to produce an oral target. ExtIPA includes symbols for 'nareal fricatives' [n̥, m̥, ŋ̊], but once again these do not appear to have been adopted in either the clinical or research contexts and Harding and Grunwell (1996) argue specifically against their use.

7.5.3 Atypical Phonation

Atypical voice qualities, such as breathiness and hoarseness, have frequently been in speakers with a cleft palate (Chapter 10). In such cases, as we have noted earlier, the notations offered by VoQS can help us to capture different voice qualities. Thus, the phrase THE MAN IN THE MOON spoken with a breathy, creaky and harsh voice respectively can be captured the following transcriptions [{Vʰ ðə ˈmæn ɪn ðə ˈmun Vʰ}]; [{V! ðə ˈmæn ɪn ðə ˈmun V!}]; [{V! ðə ˈmæn ɪn ðə ˈmun V!}], where the brace notation indicates that the particular voice quality persisted throughout the portion of the utterance included within the braces.

Unusual vocal fold behaviour confined to individual sound segments is less common in speech related to a cleft palate: speakers typically don't have major problems signalling voiced–voiceless contrasts (although see Howard, 1993). Where such features do occur, however, they can be transcribed using notations from ExtIPA. For example, features such as pre- and post-voicing of voiceless segments, which signal a lack of coordination in timing between the movements of the articulators and the action of the vocal folds, can be signalled with ExtIPA diacritics (e.g. the realization of the word DOG with a pre-voiced /g/ and post-voiced /g/ would be transcribed [ˌvdɒgˌv]), and there are also diacritics to indicate partial voicing of target voiceless consonants (FISH as [f̬ɪʃ̬]) or partial or total devoicing of target voiced consonants (ABOUT as [əˈb̥aut]; ZOO as [ˌ̥zu]).

7.5.4   Atypical Airstreams

A number of studies have attested to the use of atypical airstream by individuals with a cleft palate (see, e.g. Howard, 1993, for implosives; Howard, 1993, and Gibbon *et al.*, 2008, for clicks, Al Awaji, 2008, for ejectives, Harding-Bell (personal communication) for ingressive fricatives). Most of these can be transcribed using the symbols for non-pulmonic consonants provided by the IPA; an ingressive airstream can be indicated, using the ExtIPA symbol [↓], thus FACE as [feɪs↓] indicating that the speaker switched from an egressive to an ingressive airstream mechanism for the final consonant of the word.

7.5.5   Indeterminate Sounds

Sometimes it can be difficult, particularly with very unintelligible speech production, to decide on the appropriate symbol to capture a particular sound segment, even though we may be able to identify with certainty some of its phonetic characteristics. A useful feature of ExtIPA is that it allows for this kind of uncertainly and provides a way of recording the maximum amount of information in our transcription, using its range of notations for indeterminate sounds. Thus a segment which is very clearly a voiced nasal, but whose place of articulation in not clear, is transcribed (N̠) (v̄) and an alveolar plosive with indeterminate voicing as (Pl.) (Alv). We can even note the presence of a segment where we do not feel confident about accurately identifying any of its component phonetic features, as (¯). This may seem an odd thing to do, but if we are interested in the speaker's ability to signal the phonotactic structures of words, then the presence or absence of consonants and vowels at particular points in syllable structure is relevant and useful information.

One of the fascinating (and challenging) things about speech related to cleft palate, is that it can be atypical in so many different ways: all or any of the subsystems of speech production may be affected (airstream; articulation; phonation; resonance) and each speaker will present with an individual set of speech behaviours which combine to produce a unique perceptual signature. Judicious combination of the notations provided in the IPA, ExtIPA and VoQS permit us to capture a great deal, even if not all, of this variation.

7.6   Pitfalls of Transcription

7.6.1   Reliability and the Relationship between Perceptual and Instrumental Analysis

One of the biggest criticisms of phonetic transcription, and one which has appeared frequently over many years in the literature on speech analysis, is that it is subjective and unreliable (a useful review is provided by Shriberg and Lof, 1991). Critics point out that when agreement between transcribers is assessed, any increase in the number of transcribers being compared results in a corresponding decrease in levels of agreement. Furthermore, as the degree of narrowness of transcription increases, this also brings with it a decrease in transcriber agreement: clearly a problem for clinical transcription, where we are often aiming to make our transcriptions as detailed as possible. However, as Cucchiarini (1996) points out, we should be careful not to take these observations at face value without further exploring the ways in which agreement has been calculated. Cucchiarini makes the important point that many studies calculate symbol-to-symbol agreement, rather than attempting the more complex task of assessing the closeness of actual listener perceptions. Thus, if we compare three transcriptions for a single realization of the word BED: [p⁼ɛt], [b̥ɛd̥] and [ˌbɛdˌ], we can see that none of the consonant symbols or diacritics for the first two transcriptions match, despite the fact that the two transcribers have attempted to capture a very similar percept in terms of voice onset time, as compared to the second and third transcriptions, where the close match of the consonant symbols belies the very different percepts in terms of voicing which are implied by the transcriptions. Shriberg, Kwiatkowski and Hoffman (1984), meanwhile, provide valuable guidelines on making consensus transcriptions, where a final agreed version is reached by discussion and the application of a set of clear operational procedures. A number of studies stress the importance of transcription training and consensus listening to develop skills and improve reliability (Gooch et al., 2001; Hayden and Klimacka, 2000; John et al., 2006).

A further criticism of perceptual analyses is that they lack the rigour and objectivity (and therefore, the argument goes, also lack the value) of instrumental analyses. But to rush too hastily to condemn transcription because of the ways in which it differs from instrumental analysis would be a mistake. A transcription claims to be nothing other than the record of a listener's perceptions – it attempts to capture the listener's perspective in the communicative event. Instrumental analyses are undoubtedly very effective in objectively identifying and quantifying aspects and details of speech behaviour which are not identifiable or quantifiable by human eyes and ears, but no instrumental analysis can tell us what a speaker sounded like to a listener. The two methods of analysis should be seen as valuable complementary resources, not set in competition with each other. A phonetic transcription takes a listener-orientated perspective to an utterance; an instrumental analysis focuses on the utterance from the perspective of the speaker's intentions, regardless of whether or not these are discerned by the listener (Hewlett, 1985). Howard and Heselwood (2002a) and Heselwood (2009) provide further discussion of this important question. Certainly, humans cannot identify to the millisecond a particular durational event in speech, nor can they provide quantitative analyses of the relative contribution of oral and nasal resonance to an utterance: instruments can and do provide these kinds of useful data. Humans, in fact, can't see and hear everything that the vocal organs do during speech production, a source of consternation for some transcribers. But of course, if humans were attentive at all times to all of the detailed features of speech production, we wouldn't be very good communicators, because we would simply have far too much information to process, which would certainly slow down the rate of conversational interaction, if not bring it to a complete halt. Typical human speech perception relies on a variety of well-attested strategies and processes to maximize the efficiency of spoken interaction. Ironically it is the very existence of these processes which may impede the process of phonetic transcription, so it is worth taking a little time to explore them, and to consider whether and to what degree they might be overcome.

7.6.2   Listener Expectations

A particular dilemma for the transcription of atypical speech is that, in most cases, we know in advance the identity of the words the speaker has produced, often by virtue of the fact that they are the product of picture naming or word and phrase repetition. The very obvious justification for this state of affairs is that clinical phonetic and phonological analysis is dependent on comparing a speaker's production to a notional target production, so knowledge of the target is inherent in the overall process. Furthermore, of course, where a speaker is markedly unintelligible there is also a need for some degree of control over our knowledge of what they are saying at the lexical level, when this may be far from apparent from their actual speech. However, this knowledge comes at a price – as soon as we know the target, our perception of the speech produced is likely to be influenced by our expectations, based on the segmental and prosodic properties of a typical realization of the target. As Oller and Eilers (1975) remark, we may not only hear things which are not actually present in the speech signal, but we may also fail to hear things which are. This tendency may be exacerbated in longer utterances where the phonemic restoration effect (first demonstrated by Warren, 1970) leads us as listeners to 'hear' sounds which are not present on the basis of the overall meaning of a multiword utterance. Lexical and linguistic content, then, may have a profound effect on what we think we hear. But this is not the only set of pre-conceptions we bring to the task of clinical transcription. A particular label or diagnosis may predispose us to expect certain speech production features (which may not necessarily be present in the data) and potentially to ignore other features which are less predictable from the label, but are nevertheless relevant and significant features of the individual's phonetic and phonological behaviour (Amorosa et al., 1985), although this issue is not clear-cut where speech associated with a cleft palate is involved (Ramig, 1982). Being aware of these human tendencies helps us guard against their effects on transcription.

7.6.3   Linearity

We have previously noted that one of the challenges for phonetic transcription is that of using a linear string of symbols (from a finite set) to reflect the highly complex and constantly changing speech signal. Whilst freely admitting that the amount of detail we can aim for in our transcriptions will in no way match the complexity of the acoustic information to be derived from a spectrogram, we can, nevertheless, with judicious use of a combination of symbols and diacritics, capture at least some aspects of coarticulation and the ways in which activity across different subsystems of speech production (phonation, resonance, articulation, airstream) are coordinated. Howard and Heselwood (2002a) give the example of the word PEN, realised as [ᵥbɛ̃nᵥ], where the use of the nasal tilde and the pre- and post-voicing diacritics suggest not only the typical pattern of nasalization of a vowel preceding a nasal consonant, but also the atypical discoordination between activity of the articulators and the vocal folds across the utterance.

7.6.4 Categorical Perception and Phonemic False Evaluation

A further challenge for perceptual analysis stems from the speech processing phenomenon known as categorical perception (Liberman *et al.*, 1967). Thus, it has been widely demonstrated that as listeners we are greatly affected by the phonemic categories we have become attuned to over the course of speech development in our native language. As a native speaker of English, for example, if I am presented with a set of plosive articulations with a wide variety of voice onset times, regardless of this variation I will tend to place them all automatically into one of two categories, voiced or voiceless, as reflected in the phonological system of English. A native speaker of Thai, presented with exactly the same stimuli, is likely to use three categories which reflect the three-way voicing distinction in their language (voiceless aspirated; voiceless unaspirated; voiced). Equally, and clearly relevant to cleft palate, a native speaker of a language such a French, which has both oral and nasalized vowels, will be predisposed to use these two categories and may find it more difficult to make scalar judgements about the degree to which a vowel is nasalized.

Categorical perception leads, with atypical speech data, to a further potential pitfall for transcribers, known as phonemic false evaluation (Buckingham and Yule, 1987), where we may misidentify a sound by forcing it to fit into the categories of our native language. A telling example of this phenomenon from speech production associated with cleft palate relates to the common realization of alveolar and/or velar targets as palatal articulations (sometimes also referred to as middorsum palatal stops, Trost, 1981). Thus TEACUP may be produced as ['cicʌp] and CARD as [cɑɟ]. If these realizations were forced through the perceptual filter of the English sound system, which only has two lingual places of articulation for plosives, alveolar and velar, we would be likely to identify the misarticulations of /t/ and /d/ as [k] and [g] and that of /k/ as [t], on the misguided assumption that an alveolar realization which didn't sound alveolar must be velar, and vice versa. Santelman, Sussman and Chapman (1999) explored this precise issue in a study looking at listeners' abilities to identify and discriminate between alveolar, palatal and velar realizations in speech related to cleft palate, concluding encouragingly that with sufficient training listeners were able to step outside the perceptual categories of their own native language to deal with unusual sounds. It is important to note that training in the sound distinctions was an important part of the process, and this reflects the observation of Gooch *et al.* (2001) that rigorous training in phonetic transcription is vital in order to make useful perceptual analyses of speech production related to a cleft palate (Howard and Heselwood, 2002a).

7.6.5 Visual Influences on Speech Perception and Transcription

We noted earlier that for the purposes of phonetic transcription it is important to have high quality sound recordings, which will typically be in digital video format, so that we have access to visual as well as auditory information about the speech production. In general, combining the visual and auditory data will lead to richer transcriptions (Lohmander and Olsson, 2004), but we should be aware that in some circumstances the visual and auditory signals may conflict with each other and that this could have a detrimental effect on our transcriptions. McGurk and McDonald (1976) demonstrated in experimental conditions that confronting a listener with such conflicting signals (e.g. by presenting them with an audio-taped [g] simultaneous with a silent video of a speaker producing [b], would lead to misperception, in this case the identification of the mystery segment as [d]). Nelson and Hodge (2000) explored the implications of the McGurk effect for atypical speech production in a child with bilateral facial paralysis, showing how listeners misperceived the child's productions of bilabial segments because of conflicting auditory and visual cues. Furthermore, the overall perceptual and/or socio-phonetic salience of a specific misarticulation may influence our transcription. Shriberg, Kwiatkowski and Hoffman (1984, p. 457), for example, distinguish between dentalized realizations of alveolar fricatives, which they refer to as 'socially relevant articulation errors', and dentalized realizations of their plosive and nasal cognates, which may be less noticeable to a listener.

Further discussion of these issues in the context of phonetic transcription for clinical purposes is given elsewhere (Howard and Heselwood, 2002a; Heselwood and Howard (2008).

7.7 Conclusion

Narrow phonetic transcription of the speech production of individuals with a cleft palate is both challenging and rewarding. This account has attempted to explore both the challenges and the rewards, with the aim of convincing the reader of the value of spending time and effort honing and refining transcription skills and using them to enhance phonetic analyses of cleft speech. Being convinced of the value of transcription is perhaps the most important factor in the whole process. Shriberg, Hinke and Trost-Steffen (1987, p. 171) note, tellingly, that narrow phonetic transcription requires 'technical knowledge, auditory perceptual skills and *a positive attitude*' [author's italics]. Equipped with all three it is likely that the transcriber will be able to make observations and records which will make a significant contribution to assessment and intervention, reflecting transcriptions position as the 'gold standard' (Sell, 2005) in cleft speech analysis.

Appendices

7.A The IPA chart. Procedures to Correct Postoperative Velopharyngeal Incompetencies Found after Primary Palatoplasties, by J.E. Riski, 2004, Communicative Disorders Related to Cleft Lip and Palate.

THE INTERNATIONAL PHONETIC ALPHABET (revised to 2005)

CONSONANTS (PULMONIC)

© 2005 IPA

	Bilabial	Labiodental	Dental	Alveolar	Postalveolar	Retroflex	Palatal	Velar	Uvular	Pharyngeal	Glottal
Plosive	p b			t d		ʈ ɖ	c ɟ	k ɡ	q ɢ		ʔ
Nasal	m	ɱ		n		ɳ	ɲ	ŋ	ɴ		
Trill	ʙ			r					ʀ		
Tap or Flap		ⱱ		ɾ		ɽ					
Fricative	ɸ β	f v	θ ð	s z	ʃ ʒ	ʂ ʐ	ç ʝ	x ɣ	χ ʁ	ħ ʕ	h ɦ
Lateral fricative				ɬ ɮ							
Approximant		ʋ		ɹ		ɻ	j	ɰ			
Lateral approximant				l		ɭ	ʎ	ʟ			

Where symbols appear in pairs, the one to the right represents a voiced consonant. Shaded areas denote articulations judged impossible.

CONSONANTS (NON-PULMONIC)

Clicks		Voiced implosives		Ejectives	
ʘ	Bilabial	ɓ	Bilabial	ʼ	Examples:
ǀ	Dental	ɗ	Dental/alveolar	pʼ	Bilabial
ǃ	(Post)alveolar	ʄ	Palatal	tʼ	Dental/alveolar
ǂ	Palatoalveolar	ɠ	Velar	kʼ	Velar
ǁ	Alveolar lateral	ʛ	Uvular	sʼ	Alveolar fricative

OTHER SYMBOLS

ʍ	Voiceless labial-velar fricative	ɕ ʑ	Alveolo-palatal fricatives
w	Voiced labial-velar approximant	ɺ	Voiced alveolar lateral flap
ɥ	Voiced labial-palatal approximant	ɧ	Simultaneous ʃ and x
ʜ	Voiceless epiglottal fricative		
ʢ	Voiced epiglottal fricative		Affricates and double articulations can be represented by two symbols joined by a tie bar if necessary. k͡p t͡s
ʡ	Epiglottal plosive		

VOWELS

	Front		Central		Back
Close	i • y	— ɨ • ʉ —		ɯ • u	
	ɪ ʏ			ʊ	
Close-mid	e • ø —	ɘ • ɵ —	ɤ • o		
		ə			
Open-mid	ɛ • œ — ɜ • ɞ — ʌ • ɔ				
	æ	ɐ			
Open	a • ɶ —	ɑ • ɒ			

Where symbols appear in pairs, the one to the right represents a rounded vowel.

SUPRASEGMENTALS

ˈ	Primary stress
ˌ	Secondary stress ˌfoʊnəˈtɪʃən
ː	Long eː
ˑ	Half-long eˑ
˘	Extra-short ĕ
ǀ	Minor (foot) group
ǁ	Major (intonation) group
.	Syllable break ɹi.ækt
‿	Linking (absence of a break)

TONES AND WORD ACCENTS

LEVEL				CONTOUR		
e̋ or	˥	Extra high	ě or	˩˥		Rising
é	˦	High	ê	˥˩		Falling
ē	˧	Mid	e᷄	˧˥		High rising
è	˨	Low	e᷅	˩˧		Low rising
ȅ	˩	Extra low	e᷈	˧˩˧		Rising-falling
↓	Downstep		↗	Global rise		
↑	Upstep		↘	Global fall		

DIACRITICS

Diacritics may be placed above a symbol with a descender, e.g. ŋ̊

̥	Voiceless	n̥ d̥	̤	Breathy voiced	b̤ a̤	̪	Dental t̪ d̪
̬	Voiced	s̬ t̬	̰	Creaky voiced	b̰ a̰	̺	Apical t̺ d̺
ʰ	Aspirated	tʰ dʰ	̼	Linguolabial	t̼ d̼	̻	Laminal t̻ d̻
̹	More rounded	ɔ̹	ʷ	Labialized	tʷ dʷ	̃	Nasalized ẽ
̜	Less rounded	ɔ̜	ʲ	Palatalized	tʲ dʲ	ⁿ	Nasal release dⁿ
̟	Advanced	u̟	ˠ	Velarized	tˠ dˠ	ˡ	Lateral release dˡ
̠	Retracted	e̠	ˤ	Pharyngealized	tˤ dˤ	̚	No audible release d̚
̈	Centralized	ë	̴	Velarized or pharyngealized	ɫ		
̽	Mid-centralized	e̽	̝	Raised	e̝	(ɹ̝ = voiced alveolar fricative)	
̩	Syllabic	n̩	̞	Lowered	e̞	(β̞ = voiced bilabial approximant)	
̯	Non-syllabic	e̯	̘	Advanced Tongue Root	e̘		
˞	Rhoticity	ɚ a˞	̙	Retracted Tongue Root	e̙		

7.B The ExtIPA chart. Procedures to Correct Postoperative Velopharyngeal Incompetencies Found after Primary Palatoplasties, by J.E. Riski, 2004, Communicative Disorders Related to Cleft Lip and Palate.

extIPA SYMBOLS FOR DISORDERED SPEECH

(Revised to 2002)

CONSONANTS (other than on the IPA Chart)

	bilabial	labiodental	dentolabial	labioalv.	linguolabial	interdental	bidental	alveolar	velar	velophar.
Plosive		p̪ b̪	p͆ b͆	p̪͇ b̪͇	t̼ d̼	t̪͆ d̪͆				
Nasal			m͆	m̪͇	n̼	n̪͆				
Trill					r̼	r̪͆				
Fricative median			f͆ v͆	f̪͇ v̪͇	θ̼ ð̼	θ̪͆ ð̪͆	h̪͆ ɦ̪͆			ʩ
Fricative lateral+median								ʪ ʫ		
Fricative nareal	m̾							n̾	ŋ̾	
Percussive	ʬ						ʭ			
Approximant lateral					l̼	l̪͆				

Where symbols appear in pairs, the one to the right represents a voiced consonant. Shaded areas denote articulations judged impossible.

DIACRITICS

͍	labial spreading	s͍	͈	strong articulation	f͈	͊	denasal	m͊
͆	dentolabial	v͆	͉	weak articulation	v͉	͋	nasal escape	v͋
͆ ̪	interdental/bidental	n̪͆	\	reiterated articulation	p\p\p	͌	velopharyngeal friction	s͌
͇	alveolar	t͇	͎	whistled articulation	s͎	↓	ingressive airflow	p↓
̼	linguolabial	d̼	͢	sliding articulation	θ͢s	↑	egressive airflow	!↑

CONNECTED SPEECH

(.)	short pause
(..)	medium pause
(...)	long pause
f	loud speech [{$_f$ laʊd $_f$}]
ff	louder speech [{$_{ff}$ laʊdɚ $_{ff}$}]
p	quiet speech [{$_p$ kwaɪət $_p$}]
pp	quieter speech [{$_{pp}$ kwaɪətɚ $_{pp}$}]
allegro	fast speech [{$_{allegro}$ fɑst $_{allegro}$}]
lento	slow speech [{$_{lento}$ sloʊ $_{lento}$}]
crescendo, ralentando, etc. may also be used	

VOICING

ˬ	pre-voicing	ˬz
ˬ	post-voicing	zˬ
₍̥₎	partial devoicing	₍z̥₎
₍̥	initial partial devoicing	₍z̥
̥₎	final partial devoicing	z̥₎
₍̬₎	partial voicing	₍s̬₎
₍̬	initial partial voicing	₍s̬
̬₎	final partial voicing	s̬₎
=	unaspirated	p=
h	pre-aspiration	ʰp

OTHERS

◯, (C̲)	indeterminate sound, consonant	(( ))	extraneous noise	((2 sylls))
(V̲), (P̲l̲.v̲l̲s̲)	indeterminate vowel, voiceless plosive, etc.	¡	sublaminal lower alveolar percussive click	
(N̲), (v̲)	indeterminate nasal, probably [v], etc.	!¡	alveolar and sublaminal clicks (cluck-click)	
( )	silent articulation (ʃ), (m)	*	sound with no available symbol	

7.C The VoQS chart. Reproduced with permission from Ball *et al.* (1995); © 1994 Martin J. Ball, John Esling, Craig Dickson.

VoQS: Voice Quality Symbols

Airstream Types

Œ	œsophageal speech	И	electrolarynx speech
Ю	tracheo-œsophageal speech	↓	pulmonic ingressive speech

Phonation types

V	modal voice	F	falsetto
W	whisper	C	creak
V̤	whispery voice (murmur)	V̰	creaky voice
Vʰ	breathy voice	C̣	whispery creak
V!	harsh voice	V!!	ventricular phonation
V̬!!	diplophonia	V̤!!	whispery ventricular phonation
V̟	anterior or pressed phonation	W̠	posterior whisper

Supralaryngeal Settings

L̝	raised larynx	L̞	lowered larynx
Vᶣ	labialized voice (open round)	Vʷ	labialized voice (close round)
V͍	spread-lip voice	Vᶹ	labio-dentalized voice
V̺	linguo-apicalized voice	V̻	linguo-laminalized voice
V˞	retroflex voice	V̪	dentalized voice
V̳	alveolarized voice	V̳ʲ	palatoalveolarized voice
Vʲ	palatalized voice	Vˠ	velarized voice
Vʶ	uvularized voice	Vˤ	pharyngealized voice
V̝ˤ	laryngo-pharyngealized voice	Vᴴ	faucalized voice
Ṽ	nasalized voice	V͊	denasalized voice
J̞	open jaw voice	J̝	close jaw voice
J͔	right offset jaw voice	J͕	left offset jaw voice
J̟	protruded jaw voice	Θ	protruded tongue voice

USE OF LABELED BRACES & NUMERALS TO MARK STRETCHES OF SPEECH AND DEGREES AND COMBINATIONS OF VOICE QUALITY:

[ˈðɪs ɪz ˈnɔɹməl ˈvɔɪs {3V! ˈðɪs ɪz ˈveɹi ˈhɑɹʃ ˈvɔɪs 3V} ˈðɪs ɪz ˈnɔɹməl ˈvɔɪs wʌns ˈmɔɹ {L̞ 1V! ˈðɪs ɪz ˈlɛs ˈhɑɹʃ ˈvɔɪs wɪð ˈloʊə˞d ˈlæɹɪŋks 1V!L̞}]

References

Al Awaji, N. (2008) Speech characteristics of Saudi children with cleft palate. MSc dissertation, University of Sheffield, UK.

Amorosa, H., von Benda, U., Wagner, E. and Keck, A. (1985) Transcribing detail in the speech of unintelligible children: a comparison of procedures. *British Journal of Disorders of Communication*, 20, 281–287.

Ball, M.J. (2008) Transcribing disordered speech: by target or by production? *Clinical Linguistics & Phonetics*, 22 (10–11), 864–870.

Ball, M.J. (2010) The IPA and ExtIPA: Resources for cleft palate speech. Presentation at the 13th Conference of the International Clinical Phonetics & Linguistics Association, Oslo, Norway (June 2010).

Ball, M.J., Esling, J. and Dickson, G. (1995) The VoQS system for the transcription of voice quality. *Clinical Linguistics & Phonetics*, 25, 61–70.

Ball, M.J., Müller, N., Rutter, B. and Klopfenstein, M. (2009) My client is using non-English sounds! A tutorial in advanced phonetic transcription. *Contemporary Issues in Communication Sciences*, 36, 133–141.

Bates, S.A.R., Watson, J.M.M. and Scobbie, J.M. (2002) Context conditioned error patterns in disordered systems, in *Vowel Disorders* (eds M.J. Ball and F.E. Gibbon), Butterworth-Heinemann, London, pp. 145–185.

Buckingham, H. and Yule, G. (1987) Phonemic false evaluation: theoretical and clinical aspects. *Clinical Linguistics & Phonetics*, 1, 113–125.

Crystal, D. (1987) *Clinical Linguistics*, Arnold, London.

Cucchiarini, C. (1996) Assessing transcription agreement: methodological aspects. *Clinical Linguistics & Phonetics*, 10, 131–156.

Duckworth, M., Allen, G., Hardcastle, W.J. and Ball, M.J. (1990) Extensions to the International Phonetic Alphabet for the transcription of atypical speech. *Clinical Linguistics & Phonetics*, 4, 273–280.

Flipsen, P. (2006) Measuring the intelligibility of conversational speech in children. *Clinical Linguistics & Phonetics*, 20, 303–312.

Gibbon, F.E. (1990) Lingual activity in two speech disordered children's attempts to produce velar and alveolar stop consonants: evidence from electropalatographic (EPG) data. *British Journal of Disorders of Communication*, 25, 329–340.

Gibbon, F.E., Lee, A., Yuen, I. and Crampin, L. (2008) Clicks produced as compensatory articulations in two adults with velocardiofacial syndrome. *Cleft Palate-Craniofacial Journal*, 45, 381–392.

Gooch, J.L., Hardin-Jones, M., Chapman, K. *et al.* (2001) Reliability of listener judgments of compensatory articulations. *Cleft Palate-Craniofacial Journal*, 38, 59–67.

Grunwell, P. and Harding, A. (1996) A note on: describing types of nasality. *Clinical Linguistics & Phonetics*, 10, 157–161.

Harding, A. and Grunwell, P. (1996) Characteristics of cleft palate speech. *European Journal of Disorders of Communication*, 31, 331–358.

Hayden, C. and Klimacka, L. (2000) Inter-rater reliability in cleft palate speech assessment. *Journal of Clinical Excellence*, 2, 169–173.

Heselwood, B.C. (2009) A phenomenalist defence of narrow phonetic transcription as a clinical and research tool. *Linguistics: The Challenge of Clinical Application (Proceedings of the 2nd International Conference on Clinical Linguistics)* (eds V. Marrero and I. Pineda), Euphonia Ediciones, Madrid.

Heselwood, B. and Howard, S.J. (2008) Clinical phonetic transcription, in *The Handbook of Clinical Linguistics* (eds M.J. Ball, M.R. Perkins, N. Müller and S.J. Howard), John Wiley & Sons Ltd, Chichester, pp. 381–399.

Hewlett, N. (1985) Phonological versus phonetic disorders: some suggested modifications to the current use of the distinction. *British Journal of Disorders of Communication*, **20**, 155–164.

Howard, S.J. (1993) Articulatory constraints on a phonological system: a case study of cleft palate speech. *Clinical Linguistics & Phonetics*, **7**, 299–317.

Howard, S.J. (1994) Spontaneous phonetic reorganization following articulation therapy: an electropalatographic study, in *Proceedings of the 3rd Congress of the International Clinical Phonetics and Linguistics Association* (eds R. Aulanko and A.-M. Korpijaakko-Huuhka), University of Helsinki Press, Helsinki, pp. 67–74.

Howard, S.J. (2001) The realization of affricates in a group of individuals with atypical speech production: a perceptual and instrumental study. *Clinical Linguistics & Phonetics*, **15**, 133–138.

Howard, S.J. (2004) Connected speech processes in developmental speech impairment: observations from an electropalatographic perspective. *Clinical Linguistics & Phonetics*, **18**, 405–417.

Howard, S.J. (2007) The interplay between articulation and prosody in children with impaired speech: observations from electropalatographic and perceptual analysis. *The International Journal of Speech-Language Pathology*, **9**, 20–35.

Howard, S.J. and Heselwood, B.C. (2002a) Learning and Teaching Phonetic Transcription for Clinical Purposes. *Clinical Linguistics and Phonetics*, **16**, 371–401.

Howard, S.J. and Heselwood, B.C. (2002b) The contribution of phonetics to the study of vowel development and disorders, in *Vowel Disorders* (eds M. Ball and F.E. Gibbon), Butterworth-Heinemann, Boston, pp. 37–82.

Howard, S.J., McLeod, S. and Ball, M.J. The Handbook of ExtIPA, in preparation.

Howard, S.J., Wells, B. and Local, J. (2008) Connected speech, in *The Handbook of Clinical Linguistics* (eds M.J. Ball, M.R. Perkins, N. Müller and S.J. Howard), John Wiley & Sons Ltd, Chichester, pp. 583–602.

Hutters, B. and Brønsted, K. (1987) Strategies in cleft palate speech – with special reference to Danish. *Cleft Palate-Craniofacial Journal*, **24** (2), 126–136.

IPA (1999) *Handbook of the International Phonetic Association*, Cambridge University Press, Cambridge.

John, A., Sell, D., Sweeney, T. *et al.* (2006) The cleft audit protocol for speech – Augmented: a validated and reliable measure for auditing cleft speech. *Cleft Palate-Craniofacial Journal*, **43**, 272–289.

Kelly, J. and Local, J. (1989) *Doing Phonology,* Manchester University Press, Manchester.

Laver, J. (1980) *The Phonetic Description of Voice Quality*, Cambridge University Press, Cambridge.

Lewis, K.E., Watterson, T.L. and Quint, T. (2000) The effect of vowels on nasalance scores. *Cleft Palate-Craniofacial Journal*, **37**, 584–589.

Liberman, A.M., Cooper, F.S., Shankweiler, D.P. and Studdert-Kennedy, M. (1967) Perception of the speech code. *Psychological Review*, **74**, 431–461.

Lohmander, A. and Olsson, M. (2004) Methodology for perceptual assessment of speech in patients with cleft palate: a critical review of the literature. *Cleft Palate-Craniofacial Journal*, **41**, 64–70.

Lohmander, A., Willadsen, E., Persson, C. *et al.* (2009) Methodology for speech assessment in the Scandcleft Project – An international randomized clinical trial on palatal surgery: experiences from the pilot study. *Cleft Palate-Craniofacial Journal*, **46**, 347–362.

McGurk, H. and McDonald, J. (1976) Hearing lips and seeing voices. *Nature*, **264**, 746–748.

Michi, K.-I., Suzuki, N., Yamashita, Y. and Imai, S. (1986) Visual training and correction of articulation disorders by use of dynamic palatography: serial observation in a case of cleft palate. *Journal of Speech and Hearing Disorders*, **51**, 226–238.

Nelson, M.A. and Hodge, M.M. (2000) Effects of facial paralysis and audiovisual information on stop place identification. *Journal of Speech, Language, and Hearing Research*, **43**, 158–171.

Oller, D.K. and Eilers, R.E. (1975) Phonetic expectation and listener validity. *Phonetica*, **31** (3–4), 288–304.

Perkell, J.S. (1997) Articulatory processes, in *The Handbook of Phonetic Sciences* (eds J. Laver and W.J. Hardcastle), Blackwell, Oxford, pp. 333–370.

Peterson-Falzone, S., Trost-Cardamone, J., Karnell, M. and Hardin-Jones, M. (2006) *The Clinician's Guide to Treating Cleft Palate Speech*, Mosby, St Louis.

Peterson-Falzone, S., Hardin-Jones, M. and Karnell, M. (2010) *Cleft Palate Speech*, 4th edn. Mosby, St Louis.

Ramig, L. (1982) Effects of visibility of a prepalatal cleft on the evaluation of speech. *The Cleft Palate Journal*, **19**, 270–274.

Santelman, L., Sussman, J. and Chapman, K. (1999) Perception of middorsum palatal stops. *The Cleft Palate-Craniofacial Journal*, **36**, 233–242.

Sell, D. (2005) Issues in perceptual speech analysis in cleft palate and related disorders: a review. *International Journal of Language and Communication Disorders*, **40**, 103–121.

Sell, D., Harding, A. and Grunwell, P. (1999) GOS.SP.ASS'98: an assessment for speech disorders associated with cleft palate and/or velopharyngeal dysfunction (revised). *International Journal of Language and Communication Disorders*, **40**, 103–121.

Sell, D., Grunwell, P., Mildinhall, S. *et al.* (2001) Cleft lip and palate care in the United Kingdom – the Clinical Standards Advisory Group (CSAG) study. Part 3: speech outcomes. *Cleft Palate – Craniofacial Journal*, **38**, 30–37.

Shriberg, L.D. and Lof, G. (1991) Reliability studies in broad and narrow phonetic transcription. *Clinical Linguistics & Phonetics*, **5**, 225–279.

Shriberg, L.D., Kwiatkowski, J. and Hoffman, K. (1984) A procedure for phonetic transcription by consensus. *Journal of Speech and Hearing Research*, **27**, 456–465.

Shriberg, L.D., Hinke, R. and Trost-Steffen, C. (1987) A procedure to select and train persons for narrow phonetic transcription. *Clinical Linguistics & Phonetics*, **1**, 171–189.

Trost, J. (1981) Articulatory additions to the classical description of the speech of persons with cleft palate. *Cleft Palate Journal*, **18** (3), 193–203.

Trost-Cardamone, J., Howard, S., Ball, M. *et al.* (2010) The transcription of cleft speech. Panel presentation at the 13th Conference of the International Clinical Phonetics & Linguistics Association, Oslo, Norway (June 2010).

Warren, R.M. (1970) Perceptual restoration of missing speech sounds. *Science*, **167**, 392–393.

Whitehill, T.L. (2002) Assessing intelligibility in speakers with cleft palate: a critical review of the literature. *Cleft Palate-Craniofacial Journal*, **39**, 50–58.

8

Instrumentation in the Analysis of the Structure and Function of the Velopharyngeal Mechanism

Debbie Sell and Valerie Pereira

Great Ormond Street Hospital NHS Trust, North Thames Regional Cleft Service, London, WC1N 3JH, UK

Correlation of visual perception of closure of the isthmus with the sound of closure permits the surgeon to disentangle it from the mass of other faults of cleft palate speech, which can otherwise confuse the concept of escape. Thus the surgeon may find himself in a very strong position in discussion with a speech therapist.... . ...! (Pigott, 1977)

8.1   Introduction

This chapter provides an overview of the instrumentation used in the direct visualization of the velopharyngeal mechanism and documents current thinking. In so doing, it challenges some longstanding principles and highlights variability in practice, and finally indicates the direction in which diagnostics are moving, in particular the use of MRI. It provides a synopsis of the relevant aspects of craniofacial growth and maturational

Cleft Palate Speech: Assessment and Intervention, First Edition. Edited by Sara Howard, Anette Lohmander.
© 2011 John Wiley & Sons, Ltd. Published 2011 by John Wiley & Sons, Ltd.

changes affecting velopharyngeal dysfunction (VPD). Multiview videofluoroscopy and nasendoscopy, the gold standard investigations, are described with particular regard to quantitative and qualitative measurement for outcome studies.

VPD is present when a speech impairment results from incomplete closure of the velopharyngeal sphincter, sometimes described as inappropriate coupling of the oral and nasal cavities. It has its origins in cleft palate management, yet is associated with other aetiologies (Loney and Bloem, 1987). Velopharyngeal dysfunction is often used as a generic term before investigations, and the diagnosis has been made. Trost-Cardamone (1989) suggested that velopharyngeal insufficiency (VPI) should be used for structural deficits where there is a lack of sufficient tissue, such as following cleft palate repair, post tumour resection, post adenoidectomy and over roomy or capacious velopharynx. Velopharyngeal incompetency is applied to neurologically based disorders, such as dyspraxia or dysarthria. Velopharyngeal mislearning refers to learnt maladaptive articulation in which there is habitual use of incorrect direction of the oral air stream, for example active nasal fricatives, or hypernasality associated with severe hearing impairment as a result of incorrect timing of velopharyngeal closure. It is possible for there to be coexisting aetiologies. Based on a survey of the UK Regional Cleft Centres, the noncleft VPD workload consists of more than a thousand referrals annually. Regardless of aetiology, the consequences of impaired velopharyngeal function on speech varies from only minor symptoms to a major impact on speech intelligibility limiting quality of life such as activity and participation (Barr et al., 2007).

It may be helpful to briefly reflect on relevant aspects of craniofacial growth and maturational changes, an area often not considered, but very relevant when undertaking investigations of velopharyngeal function. It is increasingly apparent that patients with borderline VPD or minor symptoms in speech in childhood need to be monitored beyond puberty. With regard to adenoids their growth is rapid and is reported to fill the nasopharyngeal cavity by age four, peaking around age twelve (Mason and Warren, 1980; Chapter 1). Involution of the adenoids is reported to occur between the ages of six and sixteen (Finkelstein et al., 1996). As a result, in infancy and childhood, closure can be described as 'velo-adenoidal' and after adenoid involution and indeed craniofacial growth have occurred as 'velopharyngeal'.

Changes occur to the pharynx during the pre-pubertal and pubertal growth spurt. In the infant, the soft palate lies parallel to the roof of the pharynx, and moves partly in a superior–inferior direction to achieve closure. Over time, not only does the soft palate develop a 90 degree bend of the knee (Skolnick and Cohn, 1989), but with craniofacial growth there is a gradual rotational shift of the nasopharynx, resulting in the pharynx becoming increasingly vertical in the adult (Finkelstein et al., 1996). Velopharyngeal closure now occurs in an anterior–posterior direction against the posterior pharyngeal wall (PPW), where the point of contact would normally be just above the atlas promontory or the first cervical vertebra. In addition, at puberty the maxilla and, therefore, the soft palate move forward and downward. There is also an increase in the length and thickness of the soft palate and velar stretch as 'an increase in the intrinsic length of the soft palate during function' (Simpson and Austin, 1972, p. 2). Velopharyngeal closure, however, is usually maintained through this period of change, and yet, in patients with a history of cleft palate, VPI may result particularly if only touch velopharyngeal closure was achieved in the pre-pubertal stage. Interestingly, maxillary retrusion may offset a deterioration in velopharyngeal function.

8.2 Visualization of the Velopharyngeal Mechanism

Direct observation of the velopharyngeal mechanism during speech was popularised with the parallel developments of multiview videofluoroscopy in the USA (Skolnick, 1970) and nasopharyngosocopy in the United Kingdom (Pigott, Benson and White, 1969). Forty years on, these techniques remain the mainstay of evaluation. They provide information about structure, movement and extent of closure, and some indication of timing. They are used to determine the nature of management, most usually the need for and type of surgery, but also the other interventions of speech therapy or speech prostheses. They are helpful in counselling families and in predicting the success of an intervention. They are used for visual biofeedback therapy (Brunner *et al.*, 2005) to accurately fit speech prostheses (Karnell, Rosenstein and Fine, 1987; Sell, Mars and Worrell, 2006), in the evaluation of excessive nasal airflow during the playing of wind/brass instruments (Malick, Moon and Canady, 2007) and, importantly, to document both the successful and failed outcomes of intervention (Witt and D'Antonio, 1993; Sommerlad, 2005), which is essential in order for teams and surgeons to have information on their surgical protocols.

8.3 Multiview Videofluoroscopy

Multiview videofluoroscopy, including equipment, operation of a fluoroscopic system, interpretation and analysis of images recorded, have been extensively described by Skolnick and Cohn (1989). The utility of videofluoroscopy for both clinical and research purposes continues to be reported (Sommerlad *et al.*, 2002; Havstam *et al.*, 2005; Dudas *et al.*, 2006) and measurement systems described (Golding-Kushner *et al.*, 1990; Birch, Sommerlad and Bhatt, 1994; Birch *et al.*, 1999). There is great variation in practice and some of the reasons for this are discussed below.

8.3.1 Procedure

Skolnick (1970) described four multiview videofluoroscopy views: lateral, frontal, Towne's and base, although since then there has been extensive discussion in the literature with regards to whether all these views are necessary. A radiopaque material such as barium sulfate has to be used for all views other than the lateral view. This is applied in a liquid form using a syringe through one nasal passage, thinly coating the mucosal surfaces of the palate and pharyngeal walls. The field of radiation should be as narrow as possible to minimize exposure to the patient. As the absorbed dose is proportional to the exposure time (Isberg *et al.*, 1989), it is recommended that total radiation time is kept to a maximum of two minutes (Golding-Kushner *et al.*, 1990). Practitioners should be vigilant over the length of an X-ray exposure and follow the ALARA (As Low As Reasonably Acceptable) principle, thereby achieving the required diagnostic information with the minimum possible radiation dose. Sommerlad (2005) advocated a 30-second well collimated lateral videofluoroscopy which produces the equivalent of two dental bitewings of exposure.

Usually the minimum speech sample is counting from one to ten, repeating consonant-vowels such as [pa pa pa, pi pi pi, ta ta ta, ti ti ti, sa sa sa, si si si, ma ma ma, mi mi mi], vowels [a] and [i], and two sentences, one containing plosives, for example 'Bob is a baby boy', and the second containing fricatives, for example 'I saw Sam sitting on a bus'. If the movement pattern is consistent then this should suffice. Sometimes the speech and language therapist (SLT) may wish to include particular probes based on perceptual assessment in order to see variability related to the phonetic content or errors heard, to confirm place of articulation for particular targets, and less often to evaluate the movement pattern associated with nasal consonants.

8.3.2   Multivideofluoroscopy Views

Base View The patient is positioned in a sphinx-like position with back arched and head hyperextended backwards providing an 'en face' view of the velopharyngeal sphincter. However, this can be a difficult position to maintain. Additional factors that may confound the validity of the view include large adenoids, overlaying structures and posterior movements of the tongue towards the pharynx (Stringer and Witzel, 1989).

Frontal View The frontal view is used for observing the extent, length, symmetry and horizontal movements of the lateral pharyngeal walls (LPWs) during speech. The aim is also to determine the relationship of the soft palate or pharyngeal flap to the maximum horizontal movements of the LPWs. The patient is in either a supine or standing position with the image intensifier suitably positioned.

Towne's View The Towne's view requires the same positioning as for a frontal view with the additional hyperflexion of the head towards the neck. This can be a difficult position for young children to maintain. Skolnick and Cohn (1989) stated that this head position may reduce the volume of the nasopharynx, resulting in possible false negatives of velopharyngeal insufficiency, particularly in those with borderline velopharyngeal closure. However, Stringer and Witzel (1989) found that the information obtained from the Towne's view compared well with nasendoscopy.

Lateral View The patient is positioned between the table and the fluoroscopic screen with the head in neutral position. Sommerlad, Rowland and Harland (1994) described the use of a children's 3D View-Master device (Figure 8.1) which is attached to the X-ray table. This functions as a head fixation device ensuring correct head position and no movements and strict collimation of the radiation field (Isberg *et al.*, 1989). It can be adjusted for height and has a lead protective attachment to shield the eyes from irradiation. Importantly, the device incorporates a circular test object set in the mid-sagittal plane so that velar measurements can be made.

It is important to ensure that the rami of the mandible are superimposed on each other to prevent a double contour indicating that the patient's head is slightly tilted or rotated. The lateral view shows the anatomy of the soft palate and the PPW in mid-sagittal plane, in the rest or breathing position and their movements during speech. The clinician makes the following observations:

• Length and configuration of the soft palate, for example thickness in relation to the spatial configuration and depth of the pharynx.

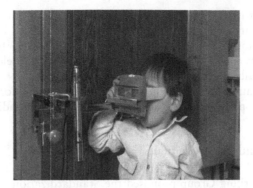

Figure 8.1 Figure showing the 3D View-Master. Note head fixation, alignment and circular test object.

- Presence, size and position of the adenoids and tonsils; involvement in velopharyngeal closure. Note whether low lying tonsils will be significant in any surgical solution.

- Movement of the PPW and its part in velopharyngeal closure.

- Presence of Passavant's Ridge and any role in velopharyngeal closure.

- Plane of (attempted) velopharyngeal closure against the PPW.

- Position of the levator veli palatini muscles, degree of levator eminence or 'knee' and soft palate movement.

- Position of pharyngoplasty or pharyngeal flap, and any tethering of the soft palate.

- Shape of the pharynx.

- 'Firmness' of velopharyngeal closure, that is the extent of contact of the soft palate with the PPW starting from the high point of the 'knee' continuing downwards (probably reflecting contraction of musculus uvulae).

Important observations can also be made of the tongue, the articulation pattern and its interaction with the soft palate and velopharyngeal closure or attempted closure. It is important to ensure palate movement is true movement and not the result of tongue humping, which gives a false impression of velopharyngeal closure. Sometimes the favoured pattern of velar consonants, or more subtle double articulations involving the velar position, may be a clue to this possibility. In contrast, tongue humping may not be detected perceptually. Nevertheless, this is not true velopharyngeal closure and should be managed accordingly. Another observation may be the tongue articulating against the PPW, transcribed as pharyngeal consonants, a pattern usually associated with VPD.

Unrelated to this, but useful to observe, is the use of the mid dorsum of the tongue to produce palatal type articulations.

Several velar function parameters can be evaluated objectively from this view, using a computerized measurement system; they are described further below. However, timing can only be superficially noted from lateral videofluoroscopy.

Finally, this view can be useful for the identification of source of nasal regurgitation, be it through the nasopharynx and/or oronasal fistula, using a radiopaque drink.

8.3.3 Analyses and Measurement

The International Working Group proposed the Standardization method for reporting multiview videofluorosocopy and nasopharyngoscopy (Golding-Kushner *et al.*, 1990). This involves both qualitative and quantitative or ratiometric measurements. For example, in the lateral view, velar movement towards the PPW is rated using a ratio-metric scoring system from 0.0 to 1.0, where 1.0 indicates complete closure. Parameters such as palatal length, pharyngeal depth and estimation of gap size are excluded as the authors stated that these are not standardized and could not be assessed. However, the reliability of quantitative measurements of videofluoroscopy remains a continuing issue. Several authors reported applying the Golding-Kushner scale (Armour *et al.*, 2005; Lam *et al.*, 2006; Sie and Chen, 2007), a 'ratio' method (Ysunza, Pamplona and Toledo, 1992), a 'percentage closure' method (Dudas *et al.*, 2006), or a five-point proportional scale (Henningsson and Isberg, 1991) to analyse videofluoroscopic data, but have failed to report any inter-rater reliability measures. Using subjective rating scales, Liedman-Boshko *et al.* (2005) reported a mean exact inter-observer agreement of 65% when assessing closure activity from the frontal view, whilst Pereira *et al.* (2008) reported only a fair to moderate inter-rater reliability (Kappa 0.3–0.5) when assessing degree of velo-pharyngeal closure from lateral view.

A measurement system that enables absolute and relative measures of velopharyngeal function using specialized software has been described with very high inter-rater agree-ment (Birch, Sommerlad and Bhatt, 1994; Birch *et al.*, 1999). Sommerlad *et al.* (1994) stated 'lateral videofluoroscopy provides the most accurate method of measuring velar movement' and that the use of a computerized method of measurement provides 'a reproducible objective means of quantifying such movement' (p. 409).

Image Pro (Media Cybernetics, Bethesda, MD) is an image processing, enhancing and analysis software that allows for the manual measurements of angles as well as point-to-point linear distances for 2D and 3D images. The methodology, described by Birch *et al.* (Birch, Sommerlad and Bhatt, 1994; Birch *et al.*, 1999), involves the editing of the speech sample to isolate the soft palate at maximum closure on production of /i/ and the soft palate at rest, and the consecutive digitization of the videofluoroscopic frames into a container format known as Audio Video Interleave (AVI). For absolute measure-ments, spatial calibration of the videofluoroscopic images during live capture is essential, accomplished with the use of a circular test object (Figure 8.1) which is attached to the head fixation alignment device. It is located in the same midsagittal plane as the patient's head and screened at the same magnification. When removed, the patient's midsagittal head position can then be aligned with the calibrated measurement plane. Measurement uncertainties relating to factors such as the nonlinearity in the imaging

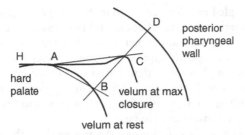

Figure 8.2 Anatomical landmarks used in the computerized analyses of velar function. Velar extensibility = AC/AB, Closure ratio = BC/BD, Velocity = BC/Time. (Reproduced with permission from Sommerlad *et al.*, 2002; *The Cleft Palate-Craniofacial Journal*, Allen Press Publishing Services.)

system were found to be less than 2% (Birch *et al.*, 1999). This system allows for the measurement of the extension of the soft palate at maximum closure, angular lift, soft palate velocity and gap size (Figure 8.2).

The clinical and research utility of this measurement technique has been demonstrated in several studies (Sommerlad *et al.*, 1994; Sommerlad *et al.*, 2002).

8.4 Nasendoscopy Procedure

Nasopharyngoscopy or, more commonly, nasendoscopy is a minimally invasive procedure that allows visual observation and analysis of the velopharyngeal mechanism during speech (Pigott, Benson and White, 1969; Pigott, 1977). Sell *et al.* (2008) detailed the procedure in the position paper of the UK Royal College of Speech and Language Therapists (RCSLT). The reader is also referred to other sources (Karnell, 1994; Shprintzen, 1995; Kummer, 2008a). Topical anaesthesia, such as Lidocaine Hydrochloride 5% and Phenylephrine Hydrochloride 0.5%, is usually applied to one nostril only, based on the sniff test. Local anaesthesia can be delivered via a catheter method or, more commonly, a spray. Mostly, children require a local anaesthetic in order to ensure compliance (Sell, 2007), whereas older patients may not (Leder *et al.*, 1997; Evans, 2007). Structural characteristics of the nasal passage also determine the need for local anaesthesia, particularly in patients with a deviated nasal septum typically associated with cleft lip and palate. With children, the environment should be child friendly, low key and de-medicalized with both patient and the endoscopist sitting on small chairs. Usually, a second adult needs to steady the child's head, and younger children may need to be positioned on the parent's lap facing forward with their back and head supported against the parent's chest. Distraction techniques are often employed, especially if children are anxious.

Initially rigid or end viewing endoscopes were used but latterly flexible endoscopes are greatly preferred, as they are both more easily passed into the nasopharynx and tolerated. The fibre-optic nasendoscope is passed, optimally through the middle meatus but otherwise the inferior meatus, to the nasopharynx, where the soft palate, lateral and PPWs and surrounding structures can be viewed. Ideally the moveable tip of the endoscope should be angled and rotated so that the velopharynx is in full view at rest. In the cleft palate population, structural abnormalities may restrict such optimum positioning. Velopharyngeal structure and function are assessed at rest, during speech and non-speech tasks, using the speech sample previously described for videofluoroscopy and, in a similar way, tailored to the patient based on the perceptual speech assessment. It may be important to try and stress the mechanism by encouraging speaking at speed and/or counting from 60 to 70. It is essential that the procedure is recorded (e.g. DVD) and the data archived for subsequent viewing.

By moving the scope up and down through the mechanism, the anatomical structures in the naso- and oropharynx can be observed, and the three-dimensional nature of activity is appreciated. Sell *et al.* (2008) outlined the possible features that should be evaluated, although the focus of the evaluation will depend on the surgical philosophy of the team. Anatomical features include observation of the nasal surface of the soft palate. A v-shaped notch is suggestive of the incorrect insertion of the levator palatini muscles into the back of the hard palate, commonly associated with the spectrum of submucous cleft palate (SMCP) or a poorly repaired cleft palate. A flat nasal surface might suggest an absence or hypoplasia of musculus uvulae, also associated with SMCP. Visualization of adenoids is useful, and in particular their presentation, be they projecting, irregular or indented (Sell *et al.*, 2008), together with some impression of size. On rare occasions, tonsils can be seen within the velopharynx at the level of (attempted) closure but usually they are below this plane. It is important to visualize one-sided defects, such as those resulting from a structural asymmetry as seen in hemifacial microsomia, hypoplasia or palatal palsy. The abnormal position of the carotid arteries, abnormal growths or structures and scarring on the PPW should be noted. Following pharyngeal flap surgery, its position and width, and some impression of its level and any residual gaps either side of the flap during speech can be seen and documented.

Functional features include identifying the presence, relative size, location and configuration of the velopharyngeal gap(s), the relative movements of the soft palate, LPWs and PPW, and the resultant pattern of velopharyngeal closure, be it coronal, sagittal, circular, circular with Passavant's Ridge (Croft, Shprintzen and Rakoff, 1981). Consistency of movements across different speech sounds and levels of speech (i.e. consonant-vowel syllables, single words, sentence repetition, conversational speech) is important to evaluate. There may be variability across speech levels, which may be dependant too on the phonetic content.

There have been several reports of success of the procedure in young children (Sommerlad, 1981; D'Antonio *et al.*, 1988; Shprintzen and Golding-Kushner, 1989; Lotz *et al.*, 1993). Generally, success rates have increased as the scopes have become smaller in diameter and flexible, and as child friendly techniques and environment have been used. Lotz *et al.* (1993) stated that failure related more to examiners' methods and skills than to the child's tolerance of the instrumentation. Success depends on factors such as examiner experience, confidence and time commitment. Van der Ham and Sell (2000) reported a 95% success rate in a consecutive series of 127 patients with an age range of 3.06–25 years, a third of whom were syndromic. Seventy-six per cent of this latter group was successfully endoscoped. They suggested that this investigation should be kept low key as part of a series of speech assessments, regularly undertaken by examiners, with the use of distraction techniques and a simple straightforward honest explanation.

Recently there has been a move in the United Kingdom and Sweden towards SLTs undertaking nasendoscopy in the Regional Cleft Services. This has been endorsed by the Royal College of Speech and Language Therapists in the United Kingdom (Sell *et al.*, 2008) and is an appropriate practice of Consultant Allied Health Practitioners (Sell *et al.*, 2008).

8.4.1 Problems with Reliability and Validity

There have been many different approaches used for reporting endoscopic findings including the use of descriptive scales with no quantitative measures (Croft, Shprintzen and Rakoff, 1981; Siegel-Sadewitz and Shprintzen, 1986; Witzel and Posnick, 1989), equidistant rating scales (Ibuki, Karnell *et al.*, 1983; Karnell *et al.*, 1983; Henningsson and Isberg, 1986; D'Antonio *et al.*, 1989; Sell and Ma, 1996; Sie, Tampakopolou and de Serres, 1998) and direct tracings (Croft, Shprintzen and Rakoff, 1981; Isberg and Henningsson, 1987; Witzel and Posnick, 1989). In the main these approaches have not been evaluated for their reliability, and studies were reported as unreliable or reliable only 'under certain conditions'. Reliability and validity are affected by the user's training, background, experience, and visual and auditory perceptual strengths. D'Antonio *et al.* (1989) found that reliability improved using expert group consensus judgements.

The Standardization method for reporting multiview videofluorosocopy and nasopharyngoscopy (Golding-Kushner *et al.*, 1990) was proposed to address the need for a method to quantify velopharyngeal movements and describe qualitative aspects (Figure 8.3). Reliability of the method was not addressed within the proposal, as this was presented 'for consideration only'.

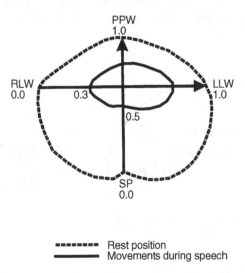

Figure 8.3 Diagram illustrating the standardization ratio measurement system. Note the medial position of the right lateral pharyngeal wall (RLW) to a rating of 0.3, and soft palate (SP) during speech to 0.5.

Using this approach Ysunza, Pamplona and Toledo (1992) reported 93% agreement in nasendoscopy between two examiners, but the variables measured were not specified. Others reported using the method, but did not report reliability data (Ysunza *et al.*, 1997; Witt *et al.*, 1999; Sie *et al.*, 2001; Vandevoort, Mercer and Albery, 2001). Yoon *et al.* (2006) undertook a study of inter- and intra-rater reliability within the same team of different professionals, based on interpretation of qualitative visual information. They reported the need to improve reliability but concluded the approach provided 'reasonably reliable findings' with some variability related to profession and experience. This same group then undertook a multicentre reliability study of 16 otolaryngologists (Sie *et al.*, 2008). They concluded good intra-rater but only fair inter-rater reliability overall. Both the latter studies advocated the need for training and reported poorer reliability on qualitative judgements such as gap size, pharyngeal pulsations and notching of the soft palate than might have been expected.

Henningsson *et al.* (1996) undertook an intra- and inter-reliability of the Standardization method following a period of joint training of three raters from both speech pathology and surgical backgrounds. Inter-rater reliability was unsatisfactory in the pilot study. Following further training and modifications to the original measuring system, many factors were identified as contributing to the persisting poor inter-rater reliability.

A fundamental premise of the Standardization method is the need to determine the medial position of the LPWs in speech in relation to the rest position. To do this the whole of the sphincter needs to be in view at rest, but this is often problematic, as it may not be possible to get the ideal distance of the scope from the velopharyngeal mechanism, and is sometimes further compounded by a poor angle of the scope. These are often induced and constrained by the anatomy. The mid-points of the component parts of the velopharyngeal mechanism at rest and at maximum movement during speech are then difficult to determine.

In the often found coronal pattern of movement, LPW movements are often obscured by soft palate movement. Figure 8.4 shows the rest position and maximum movement

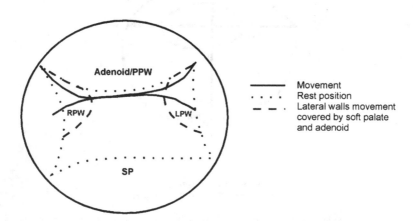

Figure 8.4   Diagram illustrating the obliteration of the LPWS by the soft palate during speech.

in speech, demonstrating the obliteration of the LPWs by the soft palate in association with large adenoid, thereby making measurements of LPW movements impossible.

In the eight patients with pharyngeal flaps there were problems in making measurements, as the assumption of LPW movement occurring against the midline flap was found to be too simplistic. Movements are sometimes in a 'vertical' direction, and thus cannot be measured according to the method. There is also an underlying assumption that all movements occur at the same level but evidence from videofluoroscopy illustrates that movements occur at different levels in the velopharynx (Shprintzen, 1995).

Therefore, in summary, there are several drawbacks to the Standardization method: mostly it has applicability when maximum movements occur in the midlines of the structures, at the same level and are symmetrical and consistent. Unfortunately, this is often not the case, which probably affects the reliability of the method and brings into question its validity.

However, most importantly, this ratiometric approach does not remove the intrinsic limitations of distortion and magnification in nasendoscopy (Pigott and Makepeace, 1982). Gap size is determined not only by actual size but also by the distance from the lens of the scope and its position within the field of view. The lens system produces a wide-angle effect with barrel distortions, which become progressively more pronounced as the distance from the centre increases (Ibuki, Karnell and Morris, 1983; Casper, Brewer and Colton, 1988; Hibi *et al.*, 1988). Gilleard (2008) in an investigation of the optical characteristics of two different flexible nasendoscopes confirmed large variability in the dimensions of the area related to the distance of the scope from the velopharyngeal sphincter, compounded by barrel distortion. He concluded that absolute quantifiable and ratiometric measurements of the velopharyngeal port is of little use unless the nasendoscopic images are calibrated, as 'even a single millimetre difference in object–lens distance and/or variation in object position ... will result in a change of visualized area that is too significant to be ignored'. This is only possible if patients undergo simultaneous videofluoroscopy using a split-screen technique, initially proposed by Pigott and Makepeace (1982) but not adopted in clinical practice. Gilleard (2008) casts doubt on the finding of Lam *et al.*'s study (2006) that nasendoscopy is an equally valid tool to multiview videofluoroscopy for assessing the relative size of the velopharyngeal port. Returning to the words of Pigott and Makepeace (1982), the originators of nasendoscopy, the endoscopic image is predominantly qualitative but within its limitations '*it portrays the real world of the isthmus*'.

An overview of the strengths and drawbacks of nasendoscopy and videofluoroscopy is given in Table 8.1. Our premise is that they both have an important role in the assessment of speech and velopharyngeal function.

8.5 Magnetic Resonance Imaging (MRI)

Several studies (Kuehn *et al.*, 2001; Ettema *et al.*, 2002; Kane *et al.*, 2002) have suggested that MRI is and will become a superior technique to both nasendoscopy and videofluoroscopy, offering much flexibility and capacity in assessing structures and their motion. It has many advantages: it is non-invasive, repeatable and reproducible, and no ionizing radiation is required. Images can be gathered in one plane and reconstructed with similar spatial resolution in any other plane and in multiple dimensions on repeated

Table 8.1 Strengths and drawbacks of nasendoscopy and videofluoroscopy.

	Strengths	Drawbacks
Videofluoroscopy	Easy to use Can be very quick Shorter speech sample Lateral view can be used in very young children Provides information about 'the entire vocal tract, most importantly the cephalaudal level of maximal closure of the palate, important in planning sphincter pharyngoplasty and pharyngeal flap surgery' (Lam et al., 2006) Information gained on the velar knee, the position of the levator muscles, the involvement of the tongue in assisting closure, involvement of adenoids, tonsils, Passavants Ridge and PPW Source of nasal regurgitation can be identified Valid relative and absolute velar measurements can be made Helps determine level of pharyngoplasty/pharyngeal flap Monitoring of outcome of treatment over time Helpful in determining place of articulation	Two-dimensional view only Overlapping shadows masque image Positional difficulties Radiation Expensive equipment Lack of availability in a Developing World context Asymmetry impossible to see in lateral view Cooperation problematic for multiviews in young children, related to barium insertion, movement and positioning Expertise required Cannot be undertaken by SLT alone Lateral view may underestimate degree of velopharyngeal closure and result in false positives and does not reveal residual gaps following pharyngeal flap. Limited information on timing

Nasendoscopy	Continuous non-time-limited visualization of the velopharynx	Two-dimensional view only
	Information about anatomy	Quantification not possible
	Able to see structures in detail	Cannot determine level of attempted closure or quantify movements
	Can see small openings not detectable on videofluoroscopy	Underestimation of LPW movement
	Scar tissue, tonsillar hypertrophy, adenoid guttering, pharyngeal pulsations.	Requires training and continuing regular practice
	Diagnostic, for example SMCP	Does not demonstrate position of velar muscles
	Symmetry of palatal movement	Lens distortion, distance and angle issues
	Some information on LPW movement	Gap size lacks validity
	Helps determine the width of the flap and its level	Invasive
	Monitoring of outcome treatment over time	Age and developmental level related constraints
	No radiation exposure	Anatomic constraints preventing ideal view
	Relatively inexpensive	Interaction with articulation characteristics
	SLT-led investigation	Does not show information on timing problems

occasions with excellent soft tissue contrast and high spatial resolution. It can visualize the underlying musculature, may identify muscle fibres from their origin to their point of insertion and, in particular, has the potential to provide unique detail about the levator palatini muscles. It may further inform how the musculus uvulae acts to increase the area of contact of the soft palate along the PPW. Indeed, Kuehn *et al.* (2001) describe it as a potential outcome tool to determine the effectiveness of primary palate repair, contributing to an understanding of why there is VPI and the likely need for secondary speech management. MRI also allows investigation of a wider oropharyngeal area. It can be used to visualize the entire velopharyngeal sphincter in the sagittal, coronal and axial planes, and does not require the repositioning of the patient for each view. This type of digital data can be passed to an off-line image analysis programme with no loss of contrast or spatial resolution.

There are, however, several disadvantages: high spatial resolution images are single slice static except in gated MRI (Kane *et al.*, 2002), the measurement of single sounds only and not connected speech requiring a relatively long data acquisition time, machine noise and claustrophobia, and the possible effects of gravity on VPD in the supine condition. Its costs and availability will limit it becoming a routine clinical tool in the foreseeable future, but it has very exciting potential to increase knowledge and understanding of velopharyngeal function.

Tian and Redett (2009) have developed a protocol for MRI scanning and have introduced new measurements, including velar stretch, levator muscle contraction, pharyngeal constriction and the effective velopharyngeal ratio. They criticized the typical use of the entire soft palate in the measurement of velar length and need ratio, advocating that only the section of the soft palate from its attachment to the posterior border of the hard palate and where the intravelar muscles are inserted should be measured to reflect the effective velopharyngeal ratio, as the part below this does not contribute to velopharyngeal closure.

8.6   Variability in Practice

In the early days of these investigations, teaching by authorities recommended a comprehensive series of investigations (Skolnick and McCall, 1972; Pigott, 1974; Henningsson and Isberg, 1991) involving the majority of the videofluoroscopy views and nasendoscopy in order to increase the success of intervention (Shprintzen *et al.*, 1979; Shprintzen and Golding-Kushner, 1989). Indeed, it was advocated that surgical intervention should not be considered until all this information had been gathered, often delaying surgery until at least four to five years of age and beyond (Witzel and Stringer, 1990).

By the 1990s, the Standardization Group modified this to a minimum of a frontal, lateral and either a basal view or nasendoscopy view (Golding-Kushner *et al.*, 1990), subsequently supported by Kuehn and Moller (2000). However, practice has not always reflected these recommendations. In 1984, a survey in the United States showed that only 3% of respondents were using multiview videofluoroscopy (Pannbacker *et al.*, 1984). D'Antonio, Achauer and Vander (1993) reported that 90% of teams had access to nasendoscopy. More recently, Kummer (2008a) reported that only 21% of 123 respondents use videofluoroscopy in contrast to 50% using nasendoscopy. Shprintzen and Marrinan (2009) stated that few centres employ both techniques, preferring to rely on nasopharyngoscopy alone. In contrast, Sell's survey of the 16 United Kingdom cleft centres revealed that 100% of centres use lateral videofluoroscopy and 70% use nasendoscopy, suggesting considerable variability in international practice. Choice of investigation is frequently determined by availability, examiner preference, experience and training. Rowe and D'Antonio (2005) stated that in the United States nasendoscopy has often been chosen as the investigation of choice, because of the need for barium insertion, radiation and the difficulties of interpreting multiview videofluoroscopy. Skolnick and Cohn (1989) estimated a radiation absorbed dose (rad) of between 0.5 and 0.025, which is comparable to a single lateral cephalometric X-ray at 0.25 rad (Kummer, 2008a), in contrast to Sommerlad's recommendation described above. Newer systems such as the Artis Zee use advanced dose reduction technology, minimizing radiation dosage (http://www.medical.siemens.com).

There is also controversy about the processes, timing and order of investigations, and personnel involved. For example, some centres always use barium for videofluoroscopy; others undertake lateral videofluoroscopy without it. With regard to personnel, in the United States, VPD management is often undertaken by paediatric otolaryngology (Willging, 2003; Rowe and D'Antonio, 2005; Rudnick and Sie, 2008) but in the United Kingdom this is firmly located within the remit of the Cleft Teams. In Scandinavia, nasendoscopy is undertaken by phoniatricians. In some United Kingdom centres, videofluoroscopy has become an SLT–radiographer led clinical practice. Sell's survey showed that only one-third of the centres have a radiologist present. Approximately half of the centres reported this as a joint SLT–consultant cleft surgeon investigation. Given that nasendoscopy is now within the practice of SLTs this is a relatively inexpensive and easily accessed investigation (Sell *et al.*, 2008). An SLT is able to integrate both the visual and auditory information based on the perceptual assessment, and can use these skills to adapt the speech sample during the investigation and probe stimulability. Indeed, it may well be that the simultaneous use of visual and auditory analysis of speech not only enriches the SLT's perceptual assessment, but maybe enhances the reliability of judgements. But what matters most is not which profession undertakes the investigations, but that they are undertaken by experienced clinicians followed always by joint interpretation and decision making by the surgeon/SLT and other team members.

Recently there has been a trend to suggest one investigation is better than the other. Kummer (2008b) stated that nasendoscopy, although complementary to radiographic studies, is in most cases superior to videofluoroscopy. Many authorities have, however, concluded that multiview videofluoroscopy and nasendoscopy each provide unique and overlapping information and that neither approach is better than the other. Practice varies widely. Some centres always use nasendoscopy (Rudnick and Sie, 2008), others lateral videofluoroscopy (Havstam *et al.*, 2005; Sommerlad *et al.*, 1994, 2002; Sommerlad, 2005), others several of the multivideofluoroscopic views (Shprintzen, 1989, 1995). Shprintzen wrote 'for the complete clinical diagnosis of velopharyngeal functioning it appears to be absolutely essential to utilize both nasendoscopy and multivideofluoroscopy' (Shprintzen, 1997, p. 387). However, best practice in the diagnosis of VPD is still unknown (Reilly, 2006). Ultimately, this should be determined by the evidence of improved diagnosis and better speech outcomes and the role instrumentation has in this. Sommerlad (2005) also wrote 'the usefulness of investigation methods can only be measured by the outcome of whatever treatment is chosen ... this is a question yet to be answered'.

Most of the research outcome data is surgical and based on retrospective series from single institutions. Guidelines for investigations reflect the experience and opinions of individual practitioners and their surgical protocols (Rudnick and Sie, 2008). Havstam *et al.* (2005) are the only group to have looked at this issue scientifically. They investigated how different visual information influenced the treatment options for VPD in their own centre. They concluded that lateral videofluoroscopy should be recommended as the first step followed by nasendoscopy. Although the sample and treatment options were both small, and they were used to working together as a team, they questioned whether an expensive comprehensive battery of assessments was *always* required to make treatment decisions, suggesting that the historic concept of velopharyngeal function should be reconsidered. This is entirely appropriate, as treatment options have evolved since these diagnostic procedures were developed. Nowadays secondary palate procedures such as the Furlow (1986) or palate re-repair (Sommerlad, 2003) have become popular surgical approaches to VPD, in contrast to the previous frequent option of velopharyngeal surgery in the form of pharyngeal flaps or pharynogoplasties.

Sometimes all that is required to make a surgical decision is a lateral videofluoroscopy, and, furthermore, this is data which can be used as outcome quantifiable evidence. For example, Sommerlad *et al.* (2002) showed that in a study of 85 patients who underwent palate re-repair by a single surgeon, using blind assessment of randomized speech recordings and computerized measurements of velar function from lateral videofluoroscopy images, statistically significant improvements were found for hypernasality, nasal emission, intelligibility, nasal turbulence, closure ratio, velar excursion and gap size at maximum closure. Furthermore, the authors identified several predictive factors of a successful re-repair: a less severe rating of pre-operative hypernasality, a pre-operative gap size of less than 9 mm and a closure ratio of more than 0.45. This would seem to be the evidence Sommerlad suggests is needed to confirm which investigations are required for his protocol in his hands. Of course, the advantage of this approach is that lateral videofluoroscopy alone with no barium insertion can be undertaken on children as young as 2.6 years. What's more, the well-established belief of eliminating glottal/ pharyngeal articulation and encouraging maximum LPW movement is not such an issue when a palate re-repair or Furlow procedure, based on anatomical features, particularly the position of the levators muscles, is a treatment option. This contrasts with the team undertaking midline pharyngeal flaps for example, where, as a minimum, an endoscopic or basal view and frontal view to determine LPW movement are required. Generally this is not possible to undertake on children under 3.6 years of age, and often somewhat older, inevitably delaying surgery.

With increasing evidence of the relationship of speech disorders to literacy development, the achievement of velopharyngeal closure or near-closure at an earlier age is generally considered optimum. Despite this move towards simplification of the surgical approach with secondary palate procedures, maybe the simplification of diagnostics has not kept apace in all centres. Table 8.2 displays protocols involving a palate secondary procedure in three major centres (one in Gothenburg, Sweden, one in Seattle in the USA and the third in London in the UK) and the differences in use and need for investigations can be seen.

In conclusion, probably the investigations, their timing and indeed intervention should be guided by many interacting factors: age and compliance of the patient, diagnosis, stage of language development and cognitive abilities, the hypothesized aetiology,

Table 8.2 Examples of Three Centres' Surgical and Investigations Protocols (Note: Perceptual assessment prefaces investigations in all centres).

Team protocol	Surgical protocol	Assessment protocol
Gothenburg protocol (Havstam et al., 2005)	If a severe VPI: a pharyngeal flap. If a moderate insufficiency: palate re-repair. Authors noted inconsistent choice of surgical method.	Usually, lateral videofluoroscopy followed by a frontal view and nasendoscopy 'if required'. New referrals, suspected diagnosis of SMCP/OSMCP (occult), primary investigation is nasendoscopy
Seattle protocol (Rudnick and Sie, 2008; Sie and Chen, 2007)	If sagittal orientation of the levator veli palatine: Furlow palatoplasty. If transverse orientation of the levator veli palatine: sphincter pharyngoplasty	All patients have nasendoscopy. If levator orientation is transverse or uncertain, non-compliant or suboptimal nasendoscopy, lateral and frontal views with barium are undertaken. Suspected diagnosis of SMCP/OSMCP, primary investigation is nasendoscopy. Videofluoroscopy data not used in planning for Furlow palatoplasty.
London, North Thames Regional Cleft Service (Sommerlad, 2005)	Palate re-repair first option, followed by Hynes pharyngeal wall augmentation if VPI persists; or two-stage repair is planned initally. Where there are concerns that the airway may be compromised by a Hynes procedure, or anatomy is judged to be unfavourable for Hynes, and/or the palate is short looking and maximized with regard to function, buccinator flap lengthening. One-sided defect: Moore pharyngoplasty.	Firstly lateral videofluoroscopy. Nasendoscopy is undertaken when pharyngeal type surgery planned, e.g. Hynes unilateral Moore procedure, buccinator flap lengthening. Suspected diagnosis of SMCP/OSMCP, primary investigation is lateral videofluoroscopy.

relative benefits of each investigation method, the availability of trained staff, the presenting speech disorder, whether this follows failed surgery and, probably above all, the surgical protocol of the surgeons, and its known outcomes. Choice of surgical procedure is often determined by surgeon comfort and experience as well as institutional protocol (Witt and D'Antonio, 1993).

8.7 Future

It may well be possible that as the expertise in investigations spreads to SLTs the responsibility of the diagnostics will increasingly be centralised to this member of the team. With the possibility of comprehensive systematic pre and post intervention, high quality data sets of nasendoscopy, videofluoroscopy and speech recordings, studies of outcome should be used to inform practitioners of the nature of the diagnostics which are necessary for their own protocols. Ideally, the simpler and least invasive the better, as this is often associated with the management of speech disorders at an earlier age. The current gold standard investigations of multiview videofluoroscopy and nasendoscopy have particularly focused on velar elevation and LPW movements. It is possible that real-time MRI will revolutionize this, leading to a re-conceptualization of this whole area of diagnostics and a completely different focus within investigations. Importantly, it is also incumbent on the speech pathology community to address the issue of broader outcome measurements than speech impairment alone, including the impact of the speech problem on the individual's activity and participation in society.

References

Armour, A., Fischbach, S., Klaiman, P. and Fisher, D. (2005) Does velopharyngeal closure pattern affect the success of pharyngeal flap pharyngoplasty? *Plastic and Reconstructuve Surgery*, **115**, 45–52.

Barr, L., Thibeault, S.L., Muntz, H. and de Selles, L. (2007) Quality of life in children with velopharyngeal insufficiency. *Archives of Otolaryngology – Head & Neck Surgery*, **133**, 224–229.

Birch, M., Sommerlad, B.C. and Bhatt, A. (1994) Image analysis of lateral velopharyngeal closure in repaired cleft palates and normal palates. *British Journal of Plastic Surgery*, **47**, 400–405.

Birch, M.J., Sommerlad, B.C., Fenn, C. and Butterworth, M. (1999) A study of the measurement errors associated with the analysis of velar movements assessed from lateral videofluoroscopic investigations. *Cleft Palate-Craniofacial Journal*, **36**, 499–507.

Brunner, M., Stellzig-Eisenhauer, A., Proschel, U. *et al.* (2005) The effect of nasopharyngoscopic biofeedback in patients with cleft palate and velopharyngeal dysfunction. *Cleft Palate-Craniofacial Journal*, **42**, 649–657.

Casper, J., Brewer, D. and Colton, R. (1988) Pitfalls and problems in flexible fiberoptic videolaryngoscopy. *Journal of Voice*, **1**, 347–352.

Croft, C.B., Shprintzen, R.J. and Rakoff, S.J. (1981) Patterns of velopharyngeal valving in normal and cleft palate subjects: a multi-view videofluoroscopic and nasendoscopic study. *Laryngoscope*, **91**, 265–271.

D'Antonio, L.L., Achauer, B.M. and Vander, K.V. (1993) Results of a survey of cleft palate teams concerning the use of nasendoscopy. *Cleft Palate-Craniofacial Journal*, **30**, 35–39.

D'Antonio, L.L., Marsh, J.L., Province, M.A. *et al.* (1989) Reliability of flexible fiberoptic nasopharyngoscopy for evaluation of velopharyngeal function in a clinical population. *Cleft Palate Journal*, 26, 217–225.

D'Antonio, L.L., Muntz, H.R., Marsh, J.L. *et al.* (1988) Practical application of flexible fiberoptic nasopharyngoscopy for evaluating velopharyngeal function. *Plastic and Reconstructive Surgery*, 82, 611–618.

Dudas, J.R., Deleyiannis, F.W., Ford, M.D. *et al.* (2006) Diagnosis and treatment of velopharyngeal insufficiency: clinical utility of speech evaluation and videofluoroscopy. *Annals of Plastic Surgery*, 56, 511–517.

Ettema, S.L., Kuehn, D.P., Perlman, A.L. and Alperin, N. (2002) Magnetic resonance imaging of the levator veli palatini muscle during speech. *Cleft Palate-Craniofacial Journal*, 39, 130–144.

Evans, E. (2007) No Topical Anaesthetic Required. Bulletin of the Royal College of Speech and Language Therapists (March 2007).

Finkelstein, Y., Berger, G., Nachmani, A. and Ophir, D. (1996) The functional role of the adenoids in speech. *International Journal of Pediatric Otorhinolaryngology*, 34, 61–74.

Furlow, L.T. Jr (1986) Cleft palate repair by double opposing Z-plasty. *Plastic and Reconstructive Surgery*, 78, 724–738.

Gilleard, O. (2008) Endoscopic image analysis in submucous cleft palate: an exploratory study. MSc Thesis, Barts and the London Queen Mary's School of Medicine and Dentistry.

Golding-Kushner, K.J., Argamaso, R.V., Cotton, R.T. *et al.* (1990) Standardization for the reporting of nasopharyngoscopy and multiview videofluoroscopy: a report from an International Working Group. *Cleft Palate Journal*, 27, 337–347.

Havstam, C., Lohmander, A., Persson, C. *et al.* (2005) Evaluation of VPI-assessment with videofluoroscopy and nasoendoscopy. *British Journal of Plastic Surgery*, 58, 922–931.

Henningsson, G.E. and Isberg, A.M. (1986) Velopharyngeal movement patterns in patients alternating between oral and glottal articulation: a clinical and cineradiographical study. *The Cleft Palate Journal*, 23 (1), 1–9.

Henningsson, G.E. and Isberg, A.M. (1991) Comparison between multiview videofluoroscopy and nasendoscopy of velopharyngeal movements. *Cleft Palate-Craniofacial Journal*, 28, 413–417.

Henningsson, G.E., Sell, D., Ma, L. *et al.* (1996) *Measuring nasopharyngoscopies: an evaluation of the standardization method proposed by the international working group*, Craniofacial Society of Great Britain, Egham, pp. 13.

Hibi, S., Bless, D., Hirano, M. and Yoshida, T. (1988) Distortions of videofiberoscopy imaging. Reconstruction and correction. *Journal of Voice*, 2, 168–175.

Ibuki, K., Karnell, M.P. and Morris, H.L. (1983) Reliability of the nasopharyngeal fiberscope (NPF) for assessing velopharyngeal function. *Cleft Palate Journal*, 20, 97–107.

Isberg, A. and Henningsson, G. (1987) Influence of palatal fistulas on velopharyngeal movements: a cineradiographic study. *Plastic and Reconstructive Surgery*, 79, 525–530.

Isberg, A., Julin, P., Kraepelien, T. and Henrikson, C.O. (1989) Absorbed doses and energy imparted from radiographic examination of velopharyngeal function during speech. *Cleft Palate Journal*, 26, 105–109.

Kane, A.A., Butman, J.A., Mullick, R. *et al.* (2002) A new method for the study of velopharyngeal function using gated magnetic resonance imaging. *Plastic and Reconstructive Surgery*, 109, 472–481.

Karnell, M. (1994) *Videoendoscopy: From Velopharynx to Larynx*, Singular, San Diego.

Karnell, M.P., Ibuki, K., Morris, H.L. and Van Demark, D.R. (1983) Reliability of the nasopharyngeal fiberscope (NPF) for assessing velopharyngeal function: analysis by judgment. *Cleft Palate Journal*, 20, 199–208.

Karnell, M.P., Rosenstein, H. and Fine, L. (1987) Nasal videoendoscopy in prosthetic management of palatopharyngeal dysfunction. *Journal of Prosthetic Dentistry*, 58, 479–484.

Kuehn, D.P. and Moller, K.T. (2000) Speech and language issues in the cleft palate population: the state of the art. *Cleft Palate-Craniofacial Journal*, 37, 348–383.

Kuehn, D.P., Ettema, S.L., Goldwasser, M.S. *et al.* (2001) Magnetic resonance imaging in the evaluation of occult submucous cleft palate. *Cleft Palate Craniofacial Journal*, 38, 421–431.

Kummer, A. (2008a) *Cleft Palate and Craniofacial Anomalies: Effects on Speech and Resonance*, 2nd edn. Delmar Cencage Learning, Clifton Park, NY.

Kummer, A. (2008b) Videofluoroscopy and other forms of radiography, *Cleft Palate and Craniofacial Anomalies. Effects on Speech and Resonance*, 2nd edn (ed. A. Kummer), Delmar Cencage Learning, Clifton Park, NY, pp. 446–466.

Lam, D.J., Starr, J.R., Perkins, J.A. *et al.* (2006) A comparison of nasendoscopy and multiview videofluoroscopy in assessing velopharyngeal insufficiency. *Otolaryngology – Head and Neck Surgery*, 134, 394–402.

Leder, S.B., Ross, D.A., Briskin, K.B. and Sasaki, C.T. (1997) A prospective, double-blind, randomized study on the use of a topical anesthetic, vasoconstrictor, and placebo during transnasal flexible fiberoptic endoscopy. *Journal of Speech Language and Hearing Research*, 40, 1352–1357.

Liedman-Boshko, J., Lohmander, A., Persson, C. *et al.* (2005) Perceptual analysis of speech and the activity in the lateral pharyngeal walls before and after velopharyngeal flap surgery. *Scandinavian Journal of Plastic and Reconstructive and Hand Surgery*, 39, 22–32.

Loney, R.W. and Bloem, T.J. (1987) Velopharyngeal dysfunction: recommendations for use of nomenclature. *Cleft Palate Journal*, 24, 334–335.

Lotz, W.K., D'Antonio, L.L., Chait, D.H. and Netsell, R.W. (1993) Successful nasoendoscopic and aerodynamic examinations of children with speech/voice disorders. *International Journal of Pediatric Otorhinolaryngoogy*, 26, 165–172.

Malick, D., Moon, J. and Canady, J. (2007) Stress velopharyngeal incompetence: prevalence, treatment, and management practices. *Cleft Palate-Craniofacial Journal*, 44, 424–433.

Mason, R.M. and Warren, D.W. (1980) Adenoid involution and developing hypernasality in cleft palate. *Journal of Speech and Hearing Disorders*, 45, 469–480.

Pannbacker, M., Lass, N.J., Middleton, G.F. *et al.* (1984) Current clinical practices in the assessment of velopharyngeal closure. *Cleft Palate Journal*, 21, 33–37.

Pereira, V., Sell, D., Ponniah, A. *et al.* (2008) Midface osteotomy versus distraction: the effect on speech, nasality and velopharyngeal function in craniofacial dysostosis. *Cleft Palate-Craniofacial Journal*, 45, 353–363.

Pigott, R.W. (1974) The results of nasopharyngoscopic assessment of pharyngoplasty. *Scandinavian Journal of Plastic and Reconstructive Surgery*, 8, 148–152.

Pigott, R.W. (1977) The development of endoscopy of the palatopharyngeal isthmus. *Proceedings of the Royal Society B: Biological Sciences*, 195, 269–275.

Pigott, R.W. and Makepeace, A.P. (1982) Some characteristics of endoscopic and radiological systems used in elaboration of the diagnosis of velopharyngeal incompetence. *British Journal of Plastic Surgery*, 35, 19–32.

Pigott, R.W., Benson, J.F. and White, F.D. (1969) Nasendoscopy in the diagnosis of velopharyngeal incompetence. *Plastic and Reconstructive Surgery*, 43, 141–147.

Reilly, S. (2006) Evidence-based practice and its challenges in speech pathology: the example of cleft management in Children. *Perspectives on Speech Science and Orofacial Disorders*, 16, 9–15.

Rowe, M.R. and D'Antonio, L.L. (2005) Velopharyngeal dysfunction: evolving developments in evaluation. *Current Opinion in Otolaryngology & Head and Neck Surgery*, 13, 366–370.

Rudnick, E.F. and Sie, K.C. (2008) Velopharyngeal insufficiency: current concepts in diagnosis and management. *Current Opinion in Otolaryngology & Head and Neck Surgery*, 16, 530–535.

Sell, D. (2007) Ouch my nose ... or maybe not? Bulletin of the Royal College of Speech and Language Therapists (June, 2007).

Sell, D. and Ma, L. (1996) A model of practice for the management of velopharyngeal dysfunction. *British Journal of Oral and Maxillofacial Surgery*, 34, 357–363.

Sell, D., Mars, M. and Worrell, E. (2006) Process and outcome study of multidisciplinary prosthetic treatment for velopharyngeal dysfunction. *International Journal of Language & Communication Disorders*, 41, 495–511.

Sell, D., Britton, L., Hayden, C. *et al.* (2008) Speech and language therapy and nasendoscopy for patients with velopharyngeal dysfunction. RCSLT Position Paper. Royal College of Speech and Language Therapists, London, UK.

Shprintzen, R.J. (1989) Nasopharyngoscopy, *Communicative Disorders Related to Cleft Lip and Palate*, 3rd edn (ed. K. Bzoch), PRO-ED Inc., Austin, TX, pp. 211–229.

Shprintzen, R.J. (1995) Instrumental assessment of velopharyngeal valving, in *Cleft Palate Speech Management. A Multidisciplinary Approach* (eds R.J. Shprintzen and J. Bardach), Mosby-Year Book, St Louis, Mo, pp. 221–256.

Shprintzen, R.J. (1997) Nasopharyngoscopy, in *Communicative Disorders Related to Cleft Lip and Palate* (ed. K. Bzoch), PRO-ED Inc., Austin, TX, pp. 387–409.

Shprintzen, R.J. and Golding-Kushner, K.J. (1989) Evaluation of velopharyngeal insufficiency. *Otolaryngologic Clinics of North America*, 22, 519–536.

Shprintzen, R.J., Lewin, M.L., Croft, C.B. *et al.* (1979) A comprehensive study of pharyngeal flap surgery: tailor made flaps. *Cleft Palate Journal*, 16, 46–55.

Shprintzen, R. and Marrinan, E. (2009) Velopharyngeal insufficiency: diagnosis and management. *Current Opinion in Otolaryngology & Head and Neck Surgery*, 17, 302–307.

Sie, K.C. and Chen, E.Y. (2007) Management of velopharyngeal insufficiency: development of a protocol and modifications of sphincter pharyngoplasty. *Facial Plastic Surgery*, 23, 128–139.

Sie, K.C., Tampakopoulou, D.A., de Serres, L.M. *et al.* (1998) Sphincter pharyngoplasty: speech outcome and complications. *Laryngoscope*, 108, 1211–1217.

Sie, K.C., Tampakopoulou, D.A., Sorom, J. *et al.* (2001) Results with Furlow palatoplasty in management of velopharyngeal insufficiency. *Plastic and Reconstructive Surgery*, 108, 17–25.

Sie, K.C., Starr, J.R., Bloom, D.C. *et al.* (2008) Multicenter interrater and intrarater reliability in the endoscopic evaluation of velopharyngeal insufficiency. *Archives of Otolaryngology – Head & Neck Surgery*, 134, 757–763.

Siegel-Sadewitz, V.L. and Shprintzen, R.J. (1986) Changes in velopharyngeal valving with age. *International Journal of Pediatric Otorhinolaryngology*, 11, 171–182.

Simpson, R.K. and Austin, A.A. (1972) A cephalometric investigation of velar stretch. *Cleft Palate Journal*, 9, 341–351.

Skolnick, M.L. (1970) Videofluoroscopic examination of the velopharyngeal portal during phonation in lateral and base projections–a new technique for studying the mechanics of closure. *Cleft Palate Journal*, 7, 803–816.

Skolnick, M.L. and Cohn, E.R. (1989) *Videofluoroscopic Studies of Speech in Patients with Cleft Palate*, Springer-Verlag, New York.

Skolnick, M.L. and McCall, G.N. (1972) Velopharyngeal competence and incompetence following pharyngeal flap surgery: video-fluoroscopic study in multiple projections. *Cleft Palate Journal*, 9, 1–12.

Sommerlad, B.C. (1981) Nasendoscopy, in *Recent Advances in Plastic Surgery* (ed. I.T. Jackson), Churchill Livingstone, Edinburgh, pp. 11–27.

Sommerlad, B.C. (2003) A technique for cleft palate repair. *Plastic and Reconstructive Surgery*, 112, 1542–1548.

Sommerlad, B.C. (2005) Evaluation of VPI-assessment with videofluoroscopy and nasoendoscopy. *British Journal of Plastic Surgery*, 58, 932–933.

Sommerlad, B.C., Rowland, N. and Harland, K. (1994) Lateral videofluoroscopy: a modification to aid in velopharyngeal assessment and measurement. *Cleft Palate-Craniofacial Journal*, 31, 134–135.

Sommerlad, B.C., Mehendale, F.V., Birch, M.J. *et al.* (2002) Palate re-repair revisited. *Cleft Palate-Craniofacial Journal*, **39**, 295–307.

Stringer, D.A. and Witzel, M.A. (1989) Comparison of multi-view videofluoroscopy and nasopharyngoscopy in the assessment of velopharyngeal insufficiency. *Cleft Palate Journal*, **26**, 88–92.

Tian, W. and Redett, R.J. (2009) New velopharyngeal measurements at rest and during speech: implications and applications. *Journal of Craniofacial Surgery*, **20**, 532–539.

Trost-Cardamone, J.E. (1989) Coming to terms with VPI: a response to Loney and Bloem. *Cleft Palate Journal*, **26**, 68–70.

Van der Ham, I. and Sell, D. (2000) Positive thinking about nasendoscopy. Presentation to the Craniofacial Society of Great Britain and Ireland.

Vandevoort, M.J., Mercer, N.S. and Albery, E.H. (2001) Superiorly based flap pharyngoplasty: the degree of postoperative 'tubing' and its effect on speech. *British Journal of Plastic Surgery*, **54**, 192–196.

Willging, J.P. (2003) Velopharyngeal insufficiency. *Current Opinion in Otolaryngology & Head and Neck Surgery*, **11**, 452–455.

Witt, P., Cohen, D., Grames, L.M. and Marsh, J. (1999) Sphincter pharyngoplasty for the surgical management of speech dysfunction associated with velocardiofacial syndrome. *British Journal of Plastic Surgery*, **52**, 613–618.

Witt, P.D. and D'Antonio, L.L. (1993) Velopharyngeal insufficiency and secondary palatal management. A new look at an old problem. *Clinics in Plastic Surgery*, **20**, 707–721.

Witzel, M.A. and Posnick, J.C. (1989) Patterns and location of velopharyngeal valving problems: atypical findings on video nasopharyngoscopy. *Cleft Palate Journal*, **26**, 63–67.

Witzel, M.A. and Stringer, D.A. (1990) Method of assessing velopharyngeal function, in *Multidisciplinary Management of Cleft Lip and Palate* (eds J. Bardach and H.L. Morris), WB Saunders, Philadelphia, pp. 763.

Yoon, P.J., Starr, J.R., Perkins, J.A. *et al.* (2006) Interrater and intrarater reliability in the evaluation of velopharyngeal insufficiency within a single institution. *Archives of Otolaryngology – Head & Neck Surgery*, **132**, 947–951.

Ysunza, A., Pamplona, C. and Toledo, E. (1992) Change in velopharyngeal valving after speech therapy in cleft palate patients. A videonasopharyngoscopic and multi-view videofluoroscopic study. *International Journal of Pediatric Otorhinolaryngology*, **24**, 45–54.

Ysunza, A., Pamplona, M., Femat, T. *et al.* (1997) Videonasopharyngoscopy as an instrument for visual biofeedback during speech in cleft palate patients. *International Journal of Pediatric Otorhinolaryngology*, **41**, 291–298.

9

Cross Linguistic Perspectives on Speech Assessment in Cleft Palate

Gunilla Henningsson[1] and Elisabeth Willadsen[2]

[1]Karolinska Institute, Department of Clinical Science, Intervention and Technology, Division of Speech and Language Pathology, SE 141 86 Stockholm, Sweden
[2]University of Copenhagen, Department of Scandinavian Studies and Linguistic, DK 2300 Copenhagen, Denmark

9.1 Introduction

This chapter deals with cross linguistic perspectives that need to be taken into account when comparing speech assessment and speech outcome obtained from cleft palate speakers of different languages. Firstly, an overview of consonants and vowels vulnerable to the cleft condition is presented. Then, consequences for assessment of cleft palate speech by native versus non-native speakers of a language are discussed, as well as the use of phonemic versus phonetic transcription in cross linguistic studies. Specific recommendations for the construction of speech samples in cross linguistic studies are given. Finally, the influence of different languages on some aspects of language acquisition in young children with cleft palate is presented and discussed.

Until recently, not much has been written about cross linguistic perspectives when dealing with cleft palate speech. Most literature about assessment of cleft palate speech has been published in English and has also been based upon studies where both patients and researchers/clinicians talk the same language, usually American or British English.

Cleft Palate Speech: Assessment and Intervention, First Edition. Edited by Sara Howard, Anette Lohmander.
© 2011 John Wiley & Sons, Ltd. Published 2011 by John Wiley & Sons, Ltd.

However, as many people now live in a multicultural and multilingual society, the need to consider cross linguistic issues has been highlighted from a research perspective as well as from a clinical point of view.

9.2   Vulnerable Speech Sounds

In the case of an oral–nasal coupling due to velopharyngeal insufficiency (VPI), a fistula or an unoperated hard and/or soft palate, vowels will inevitably be nasalized to some degree. The other main category of sounds vulnerable to an oral–nasal coupling is pressure consonants (including both voiced and unvoiced sounds) in which the production implies a tight closure of the velopharyngeal port (Watson, Sell and Grunwell, 2001; Peterson-Falzone et al., 2006). Peterson-Falzone, Hardin-Jones and Karnell (2001, p. 171) stated that 'numerous investigations have demonstrated that children with cleft palate have more difficulty with producing pressure consonants than other classes of consonants'. Accordingly, pressure consonants will be labelled vulnerable consonants, and generally, vulnerable consonants along with vowels are thus the sounds to be chosen for assessment of cleft palate speech, regardless of language.

9.2.1   Consonants

Plosives occur in all known languages and at least one bilabial, coronal and dorsal plosive is frequently found. Also, s-like sounds occur in a vast majority of languages (Ladefoged and Maddieson, 1996). In an unpublished study, reported at the 8th International Congress on Cleft Palate and Related Craniofacial Anomalies in Singapore in 1997 (Henningsson and Hutters, 1997), 34 speech and language pathologists (SLPs) with experience in cleft palate speech, representing a great variety of languages in the world, filled in a questionnaire to mark all their individual speech sounds in a form. They were also asked to mark those sounds they considered vulnerable and those used in the speech assessment of cleft palate patients. All SLPs reported the use of labial, coronal (including /s/) and dorsal pressure consonants in their language and marked them as vulnerable. Thus, bilabial, coronal and dorsal plosives and /s/ could probably be included as vulnerable sounds in the speech samples of most cross linguistic studies.

If one language includes more consonants that are vulnerable to the cleft condition than another language, speakers of the former language with cleft palate are at risk of producing more speech errors than speakers of the latter language, other things being equal. Therefore, cleft palate speakers of different languages may be evaluated differently as to their speech quality for that reason alone. For speakers born with a cleft palate, some languages are more difficult to speak 'correctly' according to the norm than others. For example, Hawaiian has two pressure consonants as compared to 16 in English (Hutters and Henningsson, 2004), and Polish has 12 fricatives (Hortis-Dzierzbicka and Steko, 2001) as compared to one in Finnish. It can be speculated that if the speech of a group of Polish and Finnish patients with cleft palate was compared, and both groups demonstrated compensatory production of fricatives, it is most likely that the speech outcome of the Polish patients would be judged worse, as a consequence of language differences. However, it is not only the number of different vulnerable sounds across languages which determines the possible impact on cleft palate speech, but also the frequency of occurrence of vulnerable consonants in a given language.

9.2.2 Vowels

All languages use vowels. Factors such as the overall frequency of occurrence of vowels differ between languages and may have consequences for assessment of cleft palate speech, because hypernasality is mainly perceived on vowels. As an example, Spanish has approximately 48% vowels in conversational speech (Guirao and Jurado, 1990) while English has only 38–40% (Mines, Hanson and Shoup, 1978). Moreover, the distribution of vowel type (high/low/front/back) varies between languages. The height of vowels is of interest in cross linguistic studies of cleft palate speech, because several studies have shown that velar position is higher and the velopharyngeal closure force is greater in high vowels, such as [ɪ] and [u], than in low vowels, such as [a] or [ɑ] (Moon, Kuehn and Huisman, 1994; Kuehn and Moon, 1998). Furthermore, high vowels have a low F1 and as nasality is observed in the low end of a spectrogram, high vowels are more prone to be affected by hypernasality (Philips and Kent, 1984, p. 135). These findings indicate that high vowels are more vulnerable to hypernasality than low vowels.

For the purposes of cross linguistic studies, Hutters and Henningsson (2004) proposed the creation of speech samples with comparable phonetic contexts and the use of similar vowel qualities, in order to obtain as similar an assessment of hypernasality across languages as possible. In the continuing Scandcleft project (which includes Finnish, Norwegian, Danish, Swedish and British English) speech samples were created containing one high vowel in the context of a pressure consonant in singleton words (Lohmander et al., 2009). A similar suggestion with control of vowel height was presented by the 'Speech Parameters Group' (Henningsson et al., 2008). However, a pilot study based on the samples from the Scandcleft study has shown disappointing levels of agreement for inter- and intra-rater judgments based on high vowels in singleton words. As a consequence, the procedure for evaluation of hypernasality in the Scandcleft project is still under development.

9.2.3 Nasal Vowels

Some languages, such as French and Portuguese, also use nasalized vowels phonemically. Cordero (2008) was interested in investigating articulation and resonance in cleft palate speakers of, among other languages, an unfamiliar language Hmong. Hmong is described as a language traditionally spoken by Hmong individuals in some Asian countries (Bliatout, Downing et al., 1988). Heimbach (1980) reports that Hmong has 27 consonants, including some nasals and two phonemically nasalized vowels, which makes it a good example of a language with a sound inventory that may have a very different influence on cleft palate speakers, as compared to languages with no or few nasal consonants and no phonemically nasalized vowels. Unfortunately Cordero was unable to recruit any speakers of Hmong with VPI in her study. So, no studies have yet been published concerning the possible effect of phonetic neutralization of a phonemic contrast due to nasalization, in cleft palate patients. Neither has any study, to our knowledge, been published concerning a possible influence of phonemically nasalized vowels on hypernasality in cleft palate patients.

9.3   Language Background of the Listener Assessing the Speech of Children with Cleft Palate

So far, only a few publications have directly addressed the important question of whether it is possible to make accurate judgments about the cleft palate speech of persons speaking a language of which the assessing SLP is not a proficient speaker (Cordero, 2008; Lee, Brown and Gibbon, 2008). Cordero (2008) investigated this question by having 24 native English speakers judge hypernasality, misarticulations, speech acceptability and velopharyngeal dysfunction (VPD) on a binary (present/absent) scale. The listeners were eight naïve listeners, eight generalist SLPs and eight specialist SLPs, and the balanced speech samples were produced by nine speakers with VPD and 13 controls. Nine of the speakers were English, eight were Spanish and five were Hmong; however, none of the Hmong speakers had VPD. The overall results of the study showed that the listeners were better at judging every speech variable in English speakers than in Hmong speakers. Furthermore, the listeners were better at judging hypernasality and VPD in English than in Spanish, and finally misarticulations were judged more accurately in Spanish than in Hmong. Overall the listeners were better at judging English than Spanish, followed by Hmong, where speech acceptability and misarticulations were especially difficult to judge. Moreover, Cordero found an advantage of specialist SLPs at all levels of judgments.

Lee, Brown and Gibbon (2008) investigated hypernasality in Cantonese speakers as judged by English and Cantonese listeners. Their overall findings, using a DME (direct magnitude estimate) procedure, showed that English listeners assigned higher values than Cantonese listeners to the female Cantonese speakers. But they also found that the English and Cantonese listeners ranked the Cantonese speech samples in a similar order. This finding is somewhat contradictory to the finding of Cordero (2008) but could be partly explained by the different procedures used, such as the use of professional versus untrained listeners. Certainly, more research is needed in this area.

Prior to the above mentioned studies, three studies were carried out in the 1970s and 1980s with American SLPs evaluating the speech of Slovak (Morris, 1978), German (Bardach, Morris and Olin, 1984) and Swiss German speakers with cleft palate (Van Demark et al., 1989). These studies reported an acceptable level of agreement regarding an overall judgement of VPD function of the speakers evaluated using a three-point scale (competent, marginal, incompetent) and accepting a one point difference. However, the study by Van Demark et al. (1989) only reported agreement between American judges, whereas no information was provided about agreement with the Swiss German SLPs for this variable. Regarding agreement of articulation scores between the American and native SLPs, the results were even more difficult to interpret. Van Demark *et al.* (1989) compared judgments of correct/incorrect realizations of target consonants and found an agreement of 88% between the American and Swiss German SLPs, whereas Bardach, Morris and Olin (1984) only found an agreement of 65% for judgement of correct/incorrect realizations of a target word. Morris (1978) refrained from evaluating articulation, because he was not a speaker of Slovak. In a similar vein Sell (2008) pointed out, on the basis of extensive experience in evaluating Sinhala – a language spoken in Sri Lanka, the importance of using a structured speech sample of repeated words and sentences at the assessment of an unfamiliar language. She also stated that intelligibility cannot be evaluated in cleft palate patients speaking a native language that is unfamiliar to the SLP involved (Chapter 5 gives a more elaborate description).

The finding that misarticulations are difficult to evaluate for speakers of a different language (Morris, 1978; Bardach, Morris and Olin, 1984; Cordero, 2008), is also supported by the experience reported from the Eurocleft speech project (Brøndsted *et al.*, 1994) including five Germanic languages (Swedish, Norwegian, English, Dutch and Danish). In that study it was decided that the speech analyses should be carried out cross linguistically. However, in the pilot study it became obvious that phonetic transcription of target sounds of cleft palate patients with a different language than the SLP was not possible. Instead, a set of common cross-linguistic descriptive phonetic categories that identified the characteristics of cleft palate speech was used. Similarly, systematic differences due to different language backgrounds of listeners have been observed in a continuing training project within the Scandcleft trial. This training project aims to develop acceptable levels of agreement for transcription of target sounds in order to be able to evaluate speech outcome as a function of surgery (Lohmander *et al.*, 2009). One example of a systematic difference observed between listeners is the fact that Danish listeners often transcribe a target [b] realized with some degree of nasalization as [m], whereas the majority of speakers of Norwegian, English and Swedish transcribe it as [b̃]. This difference is most likely due to the fact that Danish has no voicing contrast for plosives but an aspiration contrast, as opposed to Norwegian, English and Swedish. This means that Danish listeners perceiving a bilabial consonant that is voiced and nasalized will only have one possible match in their phonemic inventory, that is [m]. Another example is a difference observed between listeners concerning the evaluation of target Swedish aspirated plosives realized without accompanying nasal emission. In this case, Norwegian, Danish and English listeners often judge the realization as correct, as opposed to the native Swedish speakers who judge the same realization as weak. This systematic difference is probably due to the fortis realization of aspirated plosives in Swedish, as opposed to a lenis realization of similar plosives in Norwegian, English and Danish.

When phonetic transcription of target sounds is used as recommended (Sell, Harding and Grunwell, 1994; Hutters and Henningsson, 2004; Henningsson *et al.*, 2008) in cross linguistic studies, it is not possible to evaluate speech outcome in cleft palate patients with a different native language than the SLP. This means that for research projects speech outcome has to be assessed by native speakers of the same language as the cleft palate patient being evaluated.

For clinical purposes, however, it seems plausible that SLPs can evaluate the presence or absence of VPD and misarticulations if the language under evaluation is not too typologically different from the native language of the SLP. Such assessments should be based on standardized speech samples developed according to principles similar to the ones mentioned earlier in this chapter.

9.3.1 Phonemic versus Phonetic Transcription

In traditional assessment of cleft palate speech, consonant errors of a speaker may be described in general terms without taking specific target sounds into consideration. This procedure certainly elicits information about a speaker's articulation and may sometimes be sufficient for clinical purposes. However, in research, and particularly when comparing the speech outcome cross linguistically, the phonological level of a speech sound is not specific enough for describing small but important differences between two seemingly alike target sounds (Chapter 7). The difference between the phonetic and the phonological level can be illustrated by comparing plosives in two of the languages involved in the Scandcleft project, Norwegian and Finnish. As described in the example below, Finnish only has one series of plosives whereas Norwegian has two. At the phonological level the two Norwegian series of plosives are normally symbolised by /p t k/ and /b d g/. In contrast, Finnish only has one series of plosives /p t k/. Thus, judging from the phoneme symbols three of the plosives /p t k/ are similar in the two languages. However, at the phonetic level the three plosives differ. In Finnish /p t k/ are realised as unaspirated, unvoiced and fortis plosives, whereas in Norwegian the series /p t k/ are realised as aspirated, unvoiced and lenis plosives. The /b d g/ are realised as unaspirated, voiced and lenis plosives. As a consequence of the different realization of plosives in Finnish and Norwegian, plosives can be influenced to a different degree by a coupling between the oral and nasal cavity, such as velopharyngeal insufficiency, a fistula, or an unoperated hard palate, as in delayed hard palate closure procedures. This is because the production of aspirated plosives requires a higher level of intraoral air pressure than unaspirated plosives do. Accordingly, aspirated plosives may be regarded as even more vulnerable to a coupling between the oral and nasal cavity as unaspirated plosives, and they may more easily be realised with either accompanying nasal emission/turbulence or reduced air pressure than their unaspirated counterparts. These examples would neither have been possible to illustrate, nor of interest to explain, had the plosives only been treated as phonemes.

The other difference between the realization of plosives in Finnish and Norwegian is that the Norwegian plosives /b d g/ are realised voiced as opposed to unvoiced in Finnish /p t k/. In the presence of a coupling between the oral and nasal cavity, a voiced plosive is realised with some degree of nasalization and this may, in more severe cases, lead to the perception by the listener of the nasal cognate of the target sound. This means that for example an intended [b] may be perceived as [m], and in that case the realization of the target sound has crossed a phonemic boundary. Such a situation might also influence speech intelligibility.

As shown in the example above, the sound inventory of a language may have an influence on speech assessment. However, it should be pointed out that the phonetic differences between Finnish and Norwegian do not automatically imply that Finnish and Norwegian plosives may not be similar with regard to the effect of a coupling between the oral and nasal cavity. But this can only be decided by comparing the consonant errors for the plosives of the two languages and including many speakers to take into account individual variations of the speakers.

In cross linguistic studies there is no choice; the speech error must be related to the target sound because it is part of the procedure to provide comparable speech data. Or, to put it differently, with traditional articulatory descriptions it is impossible to eliminate the language specific factor, a process that is crucial for cross linguistic speech outcome comparisons. It is also now strongly suggested that the speaker's consonant production should be described in relation to the target sounds (Sell, Harding and Grunwell, 1994; Hutters and Henningsson, 2004; Henningsson *et al.*, 2008).

9.4   What Is Known about More Unfamiliar Languages?

Shahin (2002) has reported speech data from Arabic speakers with cleft palate. This report is interesting because Arabic has phonemic use of pharyngeal and glottal obstruents (/ħ ʕ ʔ h/), that is speech sounds classified as compensatory articulations in cleft palate speakers of languages without these phonemes in their sound inventory (Trost, 1981; Harding and Grunwell, 1996). As stated by Shahin (2002), compensatory use of pharyngeal and glottal articulations in Arabic would lead to phonetic neutralization of phonemic contrasts. The speech sample included in this study was single word naming of about 80 pictures, but the speech sample was not balanced and not the same for the participants. The participants were three children with cleft palate between 3¼ and 5½ years. Target sounds were analysed using narrow phonetic transcription and the analysis revealed that two children produced glottal compensatory articulations, and one child produced compensatory pharyngeal articulations. The author described some speech characteristics found in these children that had not been reported prior to her study (implosive airstream, oral plosive devoicing, and labiodental stopping for /f/). However, the main findings led her to conclude that: 'the abundant neutralization resulting from the backed (uvular and pharyngeal) and glottal replacements seem to indicate that the children's productions were insensitive to the phonemics of the language. This is consistent with the conclusion of previous studies that the characteristics of cleft speech stem from the nature of the organic condition and are largely universal' (Shahin, 2002, p. 8).

The discussion of universality of cleft speech characteristics/errors is limited to the languages reported so far, which are, apart from Arabic, not very different from each other typologically. Languages in which cleft palate speech mode is not known in detail may add more types of consonants to this category, as for example phonemic use of glottal stop, pharyngeal fricatives or even clicks.

9.5   Cross Linguistic Speech Samples

To compare speech results as a function of treatment obtained from different cleft palate centres, it is mandatory that the same assessment procedure is used. Furthermore, in case of inclusion of different languages in speech outcome studies, some important methodological implications have to be considered. In cross linguistic studies a standardized battery of speech samples is indispensible to ensure validity of intra- and inter-subject comparisons. So, in order to compare speech outcome as a function of treatment, other factors which influence speech outcome have to be eliminated. Since the nature of the effect of the cleft condition on a speech sound is influenced by the phonetic characteristics of the individual sound, sounds to be compared must be similar. Single words comprise the type of speech sample fulfilling these recommendations that so far has been tested.

The number of sounds which are comparable in cross linguistic studies dealing with speech outcome depends on: (i) the total number of sounds in each language, which determines the upper limit of comparable sounds; (ii) the number of sounds that are phonetically similar across the languages; (iii) the type of similar sounds, that is whether they are considered vulnerable or not, which determines the lower limit of comparable sounds. It is thus recommended to establish a specification of vulnerable speech sounds for a given language.

9.5.1 Specific Recommendations for Single Words and Sentences Regardless of Language

The specific recommendations for the structure of the speech samples in terms of the single words and sentences presented are basically the same (Hutters and Henningsson, 2004; Henningsson *et al.*, 2008; the Eurocran Speech Project (http://www.eurocran.org, recently moved to http://www.clispi.org). Such speech samples are also recommended to be used within individual languages. Some of the most important recommendations for single word and sentence stimuli are as follows: (i) the test word should include only one target pressure consonant per word; (ii) no nasals, (iii) the target consonant of the word should occur in the so-called 'strong position'; (iv) if other pressure consonants have to be used because of lack of suitable test words, the same consonant should be used, as for instance 'cake' in case of /k/ as a target consonant.

Similar recommendations exist for sentences: each word in a sentence should focus on one pressure consonant target only, but the speech samples should include samples of all positions of the target consonant appropriate to the language. It should be pointed out that these recommendations emerge from a theoretical framework and it has so far not been tested whether every recommendation is necessary in every study.

9.5.2 Specific Recommendations for Single Words and Sentences in Cross Linguistic Comparisons

For cross linguistic comparisons, there are even more specific recommendations for constructions of speech samples. Firstly, the target consonants should be of similar phonetic content; secondly, the target consonants must occur in a similar phonetic context, that is in 'strong position'. Further, as expressed in the Eurocran speech project (www.eurocran.org): 'the language specific word lists from each country/language should be compared in order to identify words which include target sounds that meet these two criteria. This should result in a word list presumably smaller and including only words with comparable target sounds'. Based upon a comparison between the language specific matrices, a corpus of similar consonants can be established for particular languages in a comparative speech outcome study. They will be consonants from the same basic category and similar in terms of their error specifications. From a minimum standard point of view only minimum corpora of similar relevant consonants need to be determined. However, if more than a minimum corpus of similar consonants can be established, it should be done in order to make the results more reliable. Also, as stated in the Eurocran speech project (http://www.eurocran.org., recently moved to http://www.clispi.org): 'In practice, the requirements for the speech samples stated above may not totally be met, which should be taken into account in interpretation of data'.

The principle of using single words as part of the speech samples can hardly be in question, but where use of sentences loaded with pressure consonants is concerned, it is more complicated when small children are assessed. Traditionally such sentences are often articulatorily tricky, because they tend to focus on one specific target sound at a time, such as: 'buy baby a bib' (target sounds are in bold); and this also causes the sentences to be semantically forced or even far-fetched. It might be preferable to produce sentences that are easier to articulate for children but at the same time meet the criteria mentioned above, as for example 'buy Sue a car'. This would allow assessment of the target sounds in question and at the same time avoid a possible influence on the results of articulatory difficulties that are unrelated to the cleft condition.

9.5.3   Speech Samples Developed According to Recommendations for Cross Linguistic Comparisons

In 1997 it was decided to start a multicentre study (the Scandcleft project) with the purpose of comparing treatment outcomes as a function of surgical treatment methods in patients with unilateral cleft lip and palate. This project involves five different languages and at the time it became obvious that a methodology for comparisons of cleft palate speech without influence of the languages did not exist, and that it was thus necessary to develop one.

Within the framework of the Scandcleft project, speech samples for cross linguistic speech assessment of the five involved languages were implemented (Lohmander *et al.*, 2009). The construction of the speech samples was initially influenced by GOS. SP.ASS'98 (Sell, Harding and Grunwell, 1999) and later by Hutters and Henningsson (2004).

At the CLISPI (2010) web site (http://www.clispi.org), word lists created according to the recommendations described are found for Polish, Swedish, Norwegian, Danish and Finnish. Recently, Portuguese has also been added as part of a new RCT study on Timing Of Primary Surgery for cleft palate, the so-called TOPS project. Furthermore, speech samples following the principles outlined above have also been published in German (Neumann, 2010), suggestions for Spanish have been presented (Cleves *et al.*, 2009) and an American English speech sample is in the process of being constructed (Trost-Cardamone J., personal communication).

Henningsson *et al.* (2008) recommended that SLPs in cleft palate teams adapt the methodology suggested and construct speech samples in accordance with their specific language.

9.6 Influence on Assessment of Language Acquisition in the Young Child with Cleft Palate

From a cross linguistic point of view, comparisons between measures of language development in youngsters with cleft palate growing up in different language surroundings are a special challenge. This is because different languages have, for example, different sound inventories, and different phonotactic and syntactic rules. Imagine the different task for a baby with cleft palate having to acquire a language with a wealth of obstruents, as compared to a language with only a few obstruents, and/or with phonemically nasalized vowels. Different sounds are acquired at different ages in normally developing children. As reported by Edwards and Beckman (2008, p. 126) some developmental traits seem to be universal, such as the fact that 'children produce unaspirated unvoiced plosives before they produce either aspirated plosives or voiced plosives in English (Macken and Barton, 1980a), French (Allen, 1985), Spanish (Macken and Barton, 1980b), Thai (Gandour et al., 1986), Taiwanese (Pan, 1994) and Hindi (Davis, 1995)'. However, acquisition of plosives is also language specific to some degree, as shown in a longitudinal study of children acquiring Korean, which has a three way contrast for plosives (Minjung and Stoel-Gammon, 2009).

These findings must be expected to hold true for children with cleft palate as well. Another interesting parameter to look at regarding phonological development is the errors typically produced by children, with, for example, 'backing' of anterior obstruents being described as a universal characteristic of cleft palate patients (Brøndsted et al., 1994). Interestingly, however, normally developing Japanese children show the same pattern with twice as many children producing /k/ for target /t/ as opposite, and this pattern is the reverse of what is observed in English speaking children (Edwards and Beckman, 2008). Similarly, in Putonghua and Japanese alveo-palatal and post alveolar fricatives and affricates are mastered earlier than dental and alveolar fricatives, and, furthermore, backing errors with these sounds are more frequent than fronting errors. These findings contrast with English where the opposite pattern is found (Edwards and Beckman, 2008) and strongly emphasize the caution needed when evaluating and comparing, for example, percentage of phonemes produced correctly by youngsters with cleft palate growing up in different language surroundings.

From the age of 10 months it has been shown that the frequency of different sound classes in babbling is different in children growing up in different language surroundings (Boysson-Bardies and Vihman, 1991). This means that even pre-linguistically, differences exist between the sound productions of babies due to their different language backgrounds. Consequently, differences observed in sound inventories of babbling between children with cleft palate growing up in different language environments may also be highly related to language and not for example just to different surgical protocols. Furthermore, differences in babbling productions as a consequence of language background have some implications for the development of the early lexicon. This relationship is described in more detail in Chapter 2 on the development of speech in children with cleft palate.

Recently, Bleses et al. (2008) published an article comparing lexical development in babies from 14 different language backgrounds based on parent questionnaires, using the so-called MCDI (MacArthur-Bates Developmental Inventory). That comparative study showed quite extensive differences in lexical development, in terms of word comprehension and word production, between the languages, with a median score of comprehended words of 4–42 words at eight months and of 82–190 at 13 months of age. The productive vocabulary varied between a median score of 0–4 at eight months and of 17–100 at 16 months. These pronounced differences in lexical development due to different language backgrounds underline the importance of caution in cross linguistic comparisons of different measures of vocabulary size as a consequence of, for example, surgical treatment. Accordingly, inclusion of a control group of children without cleft palate is necessary in cross linguistic studies including measures of vocabulary size. Inclusion of a control group will make it possible to evaluate *differences* between children with and without cleft palate within each language, and these differences can then be compared between languages.

9.7 Conclusion

During the last decades it has become obvious that the differences between languages, in terms of both structure and acquisition, must be highlighted when assessing speech in persons with cleft palate. In the ideal world, well selected speech samples in cross linguistic studies allow for evaluation of speech as a function of treatment outcome as well as a function of language. In publications of speech outcome of cleft palate patients (Chapter 4), it is recommended that an overview of the speech sound inventory of the language investigated should be included, even if the study only addresses a single language. This will enable the reader to compare the results reported to the speech outcome results of his/her own language, and to better understand the results reported.

Today the knowledge of cleft palate speech errors is mainly based upon Germanic languages. New knowledge will hopefully become available about the vulnerability of speech sounds in cleft palate in less familiar or less well evaluated languages, which will teach us more about universal speech errors.

References

Allen, G.D. (1985) How the young French child avoids the pre-voicing problem for word-initial voiced stops. *Journal of Child Language*, **12**, 37–46.

Bardach, J., Morris, H.L. and Olin, W.H. (1984) Late results of primary veloplasty: the Marburg project. *Plastic Reconstructive Surgery*, **73**, 207–215.

Bleses, D., Vach, W., Slott, M. *et al.* (2008) Early vocabulary development in Danish and other languages: a CDI-based comparison. *Journal of Child Language*, **35**, 619–650.

Bliatout, B., Downing, B., Lewis, J. and Yang, D. (1988) Handbook for Teaching Hmong-Speaking Students, Southeast Asia Community Resource Center, Rancho Cordova, CA.

Boysson-Bardies, B. and Vihman, M.M. (1991) Adaptation to language: evidence from babbling and first words in four languages. *Language*, **67**, 297–319.

Brøndsted, K., Grunwell, P., Henningsson, G. *et al.* (1994) A phonetic framework for cross linguistic analysis of cleft palate speech. *Clinical Linguistics & Phonetics*, **8**, 109–125.

Cleves, M., Hanayama, M., Tavena, M.C. *et al.* (2009) Reliability of the perceptual evaluation of MP3 speech samples. Presentation at the 11th International congress on cleft lip and palate and related craniofacial anomalies. Fortaleza, Brazil (September, 2009).

CLISPI (2010) Cleft palate international speech issues. http://www.clispi.org (accessed 2010).

Cordero, K.N. (2008) Assessment of cleft palate articulation and resonance in familiar and unfamiliar languages: English, Spanish, and Hmong. PhD thesis: University of Minnesota, USA.

Davis, K. (1995) Phonetic and phonological contrasts in the acquisition of voicing: voice onset time production in Hindi and English. *Journal of Child Language*, 22, 275–305.

Edwards, J. and Beckman, M.E. (2008) Some cross linguistic evidence for modulation of implicational universals by language-specific frequency effects in phonological development. *Language Learning and Development*, 4, 122–156.

Gandour, J., Holasuit Petty, S., Dardarananda, R. et al. (1986) The acquisition of the voicing contrast in Thai: a study of voice onset time in word-initial stop consonants. *Journal of Child Language*, 13, 561–572.

Guirao, M. and Jurado, M.A.G. (1990) Frequency of occurrence of phonemes in American Spanish. *Revue Quebecoise de Linguistique*, 19, 135–150.

Harding, A. and Grunwell, P. (1996) Characteristics of cleft palate speech. *European Journal of Disorders of Communication*, 31, 331–357.

Heimbach, E. (1980) *White Hmong-English Dictionary*, Southeast Asia Program Publications, Ithaca, NY.

Henningsson, G. and Hutters, B. (1997) Perceptual assessment of cleft palate speech – with special reference to minimum standards for inter-centre comparisons of speech outcome, in *Transactions of the 8th International Congress on Cleft Palate and Related Craniofacial Anomalies* (ed. S.T. Lee), Stamford Press Pte Ltd, Singapore, pp. xxxiii–xxxvii.

Henningsson, G., Kuehn, D.P., Sell, D. et al. (2008) Universal parameters for reporting speech outcomes in individuals with cleft palate. *Cleft Palate-Craniofacial Journal*, 45, 1–17.

Hortis-Dzierzbicka, M. and Steko, E. (2001) Cleft and Polish language – neurophysiological and anatomical considerations. Transactions from the 9th International Congress on Cleft Palate and Related Craniofacial Anomalies, Gothenburg, Sweden, 427–428.

Hutters, B. and Henningsson, G. (2004) Speech outcome following treatment in cross linguistic cleft palate studies: methodological implications. *Cleft Palate-Craniofacial Journal*, 41, 544–549.

Kuehn, D.P. and Moon, J.P. (1998) Velopharyngeal closure force and levator veli activation levels in varying phonetic context. *Journal of Speech, Language and Hearing Research*, 41, 51–62.

Ladefoged, P. and Maddieson, I. (1996) *The Sounds of the World's Languages*, Blackwell, Oxford.

Lee, A., Brown, S. and Gibbon, F.E. (2008) Effect of listeners' linguistic background on perceptual judgments of hypernasality. *International Journal of Communication Disorders*, 43, 487–498.

Lohmander, A., Willadsen, E., Persson, C. et al. (2009) Methodology for speech assessment in the Scandcleft project – an international randomized clinical trial on palatal surgery: experiences from a pilot study. *Cleft Palate-Craniofacial Journal*, 46, 347–362.

Macken, M.A. and Barton, D. (1980a) The acquisition of the voicing contrast in English: a study of voice onset time in word-initial stop consonants. *Journal of Child Language*, 7, 41–74.

Macken, M.A. and Barton, D. (1980b) The acquisition of the voicing contrast in Spanish: a phonetic and phonological study of word-initial stop consonants. *Journal of Child Language*, 7, 433–458.

Mines, M., Hanson, B. and Shoup, J. (1978) Frequency of occurrence of phonemes in conversational English. *Language and Speech*, 21, 221–241.

Minjung, K. and Stoel-Gammon, C. (2009) The acquisition of Korean word-initial stops. *Journal of the Acoustic Society of America*, 125, 3950–3961.

Moon, J.B., Kuehn, D.P. and Huisman, J.J. (1994) Measurement of velopharyngeal closure force during vowel production. *Cleft Palate-Craniofacial Journal*, 31, 356–363.

Morris, H.L. (1978) *The Bratislava Project: Some Results of Cleft Palate Surgery*, University of Iowa Press, Iowa City.

Neumann, S. (2010) *Sprachtherapeutische Diagnostik Bei Menschen Mit Lippen-Kiefer-Gaumen-Fehlbildung*, Verlag Dr. Kovac, Hamburg.

Pan, H.-H. (1994) The voicing contrasts of Taiwanese (Amoy) initial stops: data from adults and children. PhD thesis, Ohio State University, USA.

Peterson-Falzone, S.J., Hardin-Jones, M.A. and Karnell, M.P. (2001) *Cleft Palate Speech*, 3rd edn. Mosby, St. Louis.

Peterson-Falzone, S.J., Trost-Cardamone, J.E., Karnell, M.P. and Hardin-Jones, M.A. (2006) *The Clinician's Guide to Treating Cleft Palate Speech*, Mosby-Elsevier, St Louis.

Philips, B.J. and Kent, R.D. (1984) Acoustic-phonetic descriptions of speech production in speakers with cleft palate and other velopharyngeal disorders, in *Speech and Language: Advances in Basic Research and Practice* (ed. N. Lass), Academic Press, New York, pp. 132–160.

Sell, D. (2008) Speech in the unoperated or late operated cleft lip and palate patient, in *Management of Cleft Lip and Palate in the Developing World* (eds M. Mars, D. Sell and A. Habel), John Wiley & Sons Ltd, Chichester, pp. 177–192.

Sell, D., Harding, A. and Grunwell, P. (1994) A screening assessment of cleft palate speech (Great Ormond Speech assessment). *European Journal of Disorders of Communication*, **29**, 1–15.

Sell, D., Harding, A. and Grunwell, P. (1999) Revised GOS.SP.ASS'98: an assessment for speech disorders associated with cleft palate and/or velopharyngeal dysfunction. *International Journal of Language & Communication Disorders*, **34**, 17–33.

Shahin, K. (2002) Remarks on the speech of Arabic-speaking children with cleft palate. *California Linguistic Notes*, **27**, 1–10.

Trost, J.E. (1981) Articulatory additions to the classical description of the speech of persons with cleft palate. *Cleft Palate Journal*, **18**, 193–203.

Van Demark, D.R., Gnoinski, W., Hotz, M. *et al.* (1989) Speech results of the Zurich approach in the treatment of unilateral cleft lip and palate. *Plastic Reconstructive Surgery*, **83**, 605–613.

Watson, A.C.H., Sell, D.A. and Grunwell, P. (eds) (2001) *Management of Cleft Lip and Palate*, Whurr, London.

10

Voice Assessment and Intervention

Lesley Cavalli

Great Ormond Street Hospital NHS Trust, Speech & Language Therapy Department, London, WC1N 3JH, UK

10.1 Introduction

This chapter aims to provide an overview of those voice difficulties most frequently found in the child with a cleft palate and to discuss the assessment and management principles most relevant to this group of children. It assumes a solid knowledge base that includes the normal anatomy, physiology and growth of the vocal tract, with specific reference to the larynx. More detailed reference to specific disorders, assessments and treatment techniques can be found in dedicated voice texts (Aronson and Bless, 2009; Shewell, 2009; Hartnick and Boseley, 2008; Hunt and Slater, 2003; Colton, Casper and Leonard, 2006; Andrews and Summers, 2002; Mathieson, 2001).

10.2 Defining a Voice Disorder

Abnormal voice is present when there is an alteration to voice quality, pitch, vocal loudness and/or vocal flexibility that calls attention to the child's voice and that is

Cleft Palate Speech: Assessment and Intervention, First Edition. Edited by Sara Howard, Anette Lohmander.
© 2011 John Wiley & Sons, Ltd. Published 2011 by John Wiley & Sons, Ltd.

inappropriate to the child's age, gender, stature and/or the communicative situation (adapted from Aronson and Bless, 2009). All voices are variable and affected by many normally occurring factors, including fluctuations in general health, physical fatigue, voice use and emotional state. There can, therefore, be an overlap between normal and abnormal voice and it can be helpful to consider any voice as moving along a continuum between normal and disordered (Mathieson, 2001). Disordered voice (dysphonia) may therefore be consistent or intermittent and may also be accompanied by symptoms of vocal fatigue and discomfort. The threshold for judging a voice as clinically disordered (i.e. as warranting clinical investigation and potential management), is not always easy to agree.

A severely abnormal voice or an absence of voice (aphonia) is typically obvious to listener, child and carers. In this context the need for investigation is usually clear cut, in order both to exclude pathology and also to identify targets for intervention. A less severe voice problem may be apparent to some listeners but not necessarily obvious to the child or the main carers, whose expectations of normal voice may differ from the wider norm. Clinically, however, concern regarding potential pathology is also very relevant here, although unlike in adults, laryngeal carcinoma in children is very rare. It is also important in these milder cases to consider the impact of the voice disorder (dysphonia) on the child's educational and social functioning, emotional well-being and overall speech intelligibility in everyday situations. A voice disorder may have a direct impact on a child's ability and, sometimes, desire to participate fully in educational and social activities and may contribute to low self-esteem. Adverse judgements can be made of the dysphonic child by both their peers and adults (Lass *et al.*, 1991).

10.2.1   Prevalence of Dysphonia

There is controversy in the literature as to whether children and adults with a history of cleft palate (CP) with, or without cleft lip, are more vulnerable to dysphonia than the normal population. Studies in the cleft palate and cleft lip and palate (CLP) population have suggested figures between 17% and 41% (D'Antonio, Muntz and Province, 1988; Sell *et al.*, 2001; Hamming, Finkelstein and Sidman, 2009) with a decline in prevalence towards puberty. Recently, researchers have suggested that this relatively high prevalence of dysphonia in CP and CLP populations is similar to that found in the normal population (Hamming, Finkelstein and Sidman, 2009). However, a close look at the literature makes it clear that direct comparison with other non-cleft groups is not as straightforward as might sometimes be suggested. The prevalence of voice disorders in the United Kingdom primary-school-aged population is reported as being approximately 6% in the large epidemiological study by Carding, Roulstone and Northstone (2006). Smaller, yet still important, European studies have noted differences in urban and rural school-aged children, with prevalence increasing to as much as 44% for children growing up in towns and cities (Multinovic, 1994).

There is disagreement in the literature as to whether children with CP are less vulnerable to dysphonia that those with CLP. Hocevar-Boltezar, Jarc and Kozelj (2006) reported prevalence figures of 12.5% for both isolated CP and unilateral cleft lip and palate groups; however, Timmons, Wyatt and Murphy (2001) found a higher prevalence of dysphonia for CLP (41%) than for CP (30%). There is no reported difference in prevalence between unilateral and bilateral CLP groups (Van Lierde *et al.*, 2004). As with the normal population, boys with a history of CP are likely to be more vulnerable to dysphonia than their female counterparts (Van Lierde *et al.*, 2004).

10.2.2   Nature of the Voice Disorder

The reported vocal characteristics of the dysphonic child with CP vary considerably and are not condition specific. The literature reports alterations to voice quality that include hoarseness, breathiness and strain. There is also no consensus as to likely changes to vocal fundamental frequency. The author has experience of some additional unreported vocal features in the clinical perceptual evaluation of dysphonic patients with cleft palate that include pharyngeal constriction, close jaw posturing, raised larynx, clavicular breathing, reduced breath control, vocal fatigue and vocal discomfort, but these features are also not restricted to cases with CP.

Although neither a uniform nor a comprehensive description exists currently of the presenting dysphonia in children with cleft palate, there is overall consensus that the majority of dysphonic children with CP or CLP will present with a muscle tension voice disorder, with or without reactive mucosal changes such as vocal fold nodules and diffuse inflammation/oedema (Hocevar-Boltezar, Jarc and Kozelj, 2006; Van Lierde *et al.*, 2004; Lewis *et al.*, 1993). As this is also true of the normal paediatric population, it is difficult to confirm whether children with isolated CP or CLP are more prone to laryngeal pathology associated with vocal hyperfunction than those children without such a history. Syndromic CP, however, may be associated with a wide range of organic laryngeal disorders, including calcification of the larynx in Apert Syndrome, cleft larynx in Opitz-G Syndrome, vocal fold paralysis and glottic web in 22q11.2 deletion syndrome.

10.2.3   Causes of Voice Disorder in CLP and Classification

The literature suggests a wide range of causes for the muscle tension dysphonia found in adults and children with CP and CLP. One of the most compelling arguments is that the child learns to use increased laryngeal adductory and respiratory forces to compensate for air leak through an incompetent velopharyngeal port (Leder and Lerman, 1985; Warren, 1986). Other authors have theorized that voice difficulties arise from hyperfunction associated with speech articulations, such as pharyngeal and glottal stops, laryngeal fricatives and affricates and posterior tongue posturing (Tanimoto *et al.*, 1994; Kido *et al.*, 1992). Kawano, Isshiki, *et al.* (1997) showed that such articulations involved the epiglottis, arytenoids, aryepiglottic folds and vocal folds. Such laryngeal involvement may not always be evident from perceptual evaluation despite the efforts to undertake narrow phonetic transcription by specialist speech and language therapists (SLTs).

There is disagreement as to whether the severity of the child's velopharyngeal insufficiency (VPI) impacts on the vulnerability to dysphonia. Hamming, Finkelstein and Sidman (2009) found no relationship between VPI and hoarseness. Leder and Lerman (1985), however, reported acoustic evidence of laryngeal hyperfunction only in those patients with significant hypernasality. Lohmander-Agerskov *et al.* (1995) report significant improvements in the severity of dysphonia in patients at eight years of age, following closure of the hard palate, suggesting a link between structural palatal anomaly and dysphonia. Clinical observation by the author suggests that learned physiological hyperfunctional laryngeal gestures, including false fold and vocal fold hyperconstriction and supraglottic narrowing, can persist even when the VPI is resolved, a view supported by D'Antonio, Muntz and Province (1988).

Important attention has been given more recently to the relationship between conductive hearing loss and dysphonia in the cleft palate population. Hocevar-Boltezar, Jarc and Kozelj (2006) found that two thirds of cleft children with muscle tension dysphonia had a history of protracted middle ear difficulties with over half presenting with hearing loss of >30 dB together with associated ear pathology. The incidence of nocturnal nasal breathing was also noted in the same study to be high (17.5% of CP and 49% of CLP children) and considered to arise from rhinitis and deviated septum. It could therefore be possible, as it is for the general dysphonic population, that nasal breathing adds to vocal vulnerability through the drying of laryngeal secretions.

In addition to all of the above, it is important to remember that a child or adult with a CP/CLP may also present with a voice difficulty arising from a cause unrelated to the history of palatal cleft, for example psychogenic voice loss or change, acquired vocal fold paralysis, papillomatosis, vocal fold cysts and intubation injuries, allergy, asthma or laryngo-pharyngeal reflux. In addition, muscle tension voice disorders in children may also occur as a consequence of other speech disorders, including dyspraxia and dysfluency or vocal misuse.

The causes of voice disorder in the cleft palate population, as with many other patient groups, are thus likely to be wide ranging and potentially multifactorial in any single patient. Identifying the relevance of the VPI to the presenting dysphonia can be particularly difficult when there are multiple aetiological factors all having the potential to impact on laryngeal functioning. As in the management of all voice disorders, it is therefore essential that the speech and language therapist (SLT) and otolaryngologist work jointly during both assessment and treatment stages and that there is involvement with other professionals, for example respiratory and audiology, as required.

10.3   Assessment

Examination and management of any child with a voice disorder has inherent challenges. The components to comprehensive voice assessment are shown schematically in Figure 10.1 and outlined in more detail below. Comprehensive assessment should include ENT (ear, nose and throat) laryngeal examination carried out in conjunction with a detailed case history, an oro-motor examination; a perceptual assessment that allows evaluation not only of voice quality but also of pitch, loudness, resonance, breathing for speech and articulation, and which is supported by instrumental analyses; evaluation of posture and muscle tension; and a measure of the perceived vocal handicap. A screening assessment of cognitive and language levels is necessary when voice therapy or surgical management is being considered, as knowledge of a child's learning levels allows tasks and techniques to be delivered appropriately and with realistic expectation.

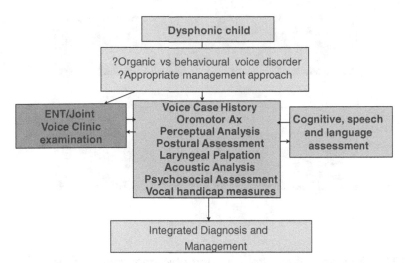

Figure 10.1 Schematic representation of the assessment pathway for the child referred with dysphonia. Contributed by Professor Adrian Fourcin.

10.3.1 ENT Examination

Early on in management, it is important that the child with a cleft palate is seen by the otolaryngologist to evaluate both the larynx, airway and hearing levels. Oral, nasal and aural examination should be undertaken, as well as visualization of the larynx. Videolaryngostroboscopy, as in adults, is the gold-standard examination tool for the accurate diagnosis of vocal fold pathology/anomaly, combined with an appreciation of the vocal fold dynamics. The Joint Voice Clinic (Papsin, Pengilly and Leighton, 1996; Harris *et al.*, 1998) combines the skills of an otolaryngologist and specialist SLT and provides the necessary equipment and tools for an effective laryngeal examination. Currently, the majority of United Kingdom voice clinics do not specialize in the management of children, but many accept referral and are very able to develop an appropriate management plan.

Whether or not the child has access to a specialist Voice Clinic, it remains important that an attempt is made in ENT outpatients to visualize the larynx, in order to exclude or clarify the presence of laryngeal pathology/anomaly and any muscle tension behaviours. The 70° rigid laryngoscope can be used successfully in the examination of children from approximately six years of age (Papsin, Pengilly and Leighton, 1996; Wolf, Primov-Fever and Jedwab, 2005). Flexible laryngoscopy via the nose is important for examining laryngeal movement within speech tasks (Hartnick, Umeno and Nakashima, 2005), can be used with young children and can be used to trial therapy techniques with biofeedback (Rattenbury, Carding and Finn, 2004). One accepted drawback of using the flexible scope has been that there may be insufficient light for accurate diagnosis of small laryngeal pathology. However, the latest generation of flexible distal chip nasendoscopes may provide an effective compromise between ease of examination and accuracy of diagnostic information. For some children with CP/CLP, it may be appropriate to

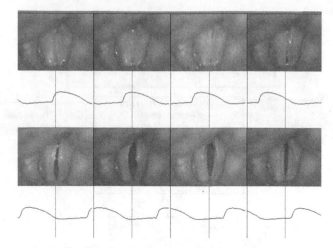

Figure 10.2   Simultaneous electrolaryngographic and laryngostroboscopic images acquired in a Voice Clinic Setting. Contributed by Professor Adrian Fourcin.

combine velopharyngeal and laryngeal endoscopy examinations within the same procedure. This combined evaluation reduces the number of endoscopies for the child and allows appreciation of the physiological partnership and interaction between laryngeal and velopharyngeal valving mechanisms. However, in reality this can be difficult to organize and is not common practice. Whichever endoscope is used, it is desirable to record and store the endoscopy images, as captured views are likely to be relatively short and therefore use of a playback facility aids interpretation, as well as augmenting the subsequent education of the child and carer with regard to the nature of their voice difficulty and the rationale behind management.

Stroboscopy should ideally be available to allow detailed visualization of the vocal folds and their movement and so minimize misdiagnosis (Woo *et al.*, 1991). Interpretation of the stroboscopic laryngeal images is difficult in young children due to the short phonation time and frequency of vibration but can be facilitated by simultaneous use of electrolaryngography/glottography during live recording. Figure 10.2 demonstrates how a sequence of images of the vocal folds captured during sustained phonation can be interpreted using the corresponding electrolaryngographic trace, showing the point of capture with reference to the closed versus open phase of vocal fold vibration.

The decision as to whether to proceed to microlaryngoscopy (ML) assessment under general anaesthesia is taken by the ENT professional. Microlaryngoscopy may be necessary for a number of reasons. For example, for those children who are unable to tolerate outpatient examination, particularly when the perceptual voice signs and the case history indicate the need to clarify the status of the vocal folds, and/or where outpatient laryngeal examination indicates questionable pathology, for example cyst versus nodular lesion. It must be noted that any child with a consistent voice difficulty accompanied by a history of worsening breathing difficulties and/or stridor should be referred to ENT as a priority, to exclude potentially life-threatening pathology such as papillomatosis.

10.3.2   The Case History

The purpose of the SLT voice case history is to help identify factors that may have predisposed the child to a voice disorder and that may be contributing to its maintenance. The history also helps to identify whether a child needs to be prioritized for otolaryngology assessment, if this has not already occurred. History taking should involve the child as well as the parent. Even the young child is often able to communicate whether he/she feels physical effort or laryngeal discomfort when talking and to give a realistic picture of the amount and nature of vocal activity (e.g. the child who referred to his voice as 'my weapon'). Children may also have some awareness of whether the voice tires and which activities they find vocally challenging. Areas in a standard voice history include details regarding the onset of the dysphonia, progression of and consistency of vocal characteristics (including whether the voice is ever normal) and whether there are any associated airway/breathing problems. It is important to remember that the concept of normal voice varies culturally and in the case of a chronic voice disorder, the child and carers may have lost sight of what normal voice is. However, if present at least some of the time, normal voice is a positive prognostic factor.

Information about daily voice should be sought and include: educational demands and after school activities, play preferences, family and social make-up, styles of communication, environmental noise levels, sleep, eating and drinking routines and exposure to environmental irritants such as smoke and dust. This is all important in order to determine opportunities for vocal and physical rest and whether there is a need to improve vocal care and hygiene as part of the management programme. In addition, the medical history must refer back to the birth history and the neonatal period in order to identify possibilities for laryngeal injury via intubation and emergency delivery procedure. Early feeding difficulties must also be explored to identify vulnerability to reflux and any suggestion of early and potentially continuing developmental neuromuscular/coordination difficulties. Current swallowing difficulties need investigation, and findings may inform knowledge of laryngeal functioning. Medications such as asthma drugs, antihistamines and treatments for gastro-oesophageal reflux (GORD) must be noted. The SLT must liaise with the child's GP (General Practitioner)/paediatrician about the potential need for any changes to pharmacological routines or treatment plans. Previous planned and emergency surgical procedures including cardiac, respiratory and gastroenterology procedures should be recorded and any change in voice around such procedures noted for their potential to indicate possible trauma (e.g. dislocation of the arytenoids, laryngeal paresis/palsy etc.). Tonsillectomy and adenoidectomy, frequency of upper respiratory tract infections, sleep disturbance and signs of nasal congestion should be noted alongside the audiology history. If there is any doubt about hearing status then this needs to be followed up via ENT/Audiology at the earliest opportunity and before direct voice therapy commences.

Alongside the voice history it is important to collate accurate screening information about the child's developmental history, including gross and fine motor milestones, speech and language history and overall cognitive development. This is in order to obtain information about attention, behaviour and linguistic development, as well as signs of dysfluency, dysarthria or dyspraxia, and will help ensure that therapy is planned at an appropriate level and with appropriate targets.

It is also important to understand the significance of any stressors in the child's life and to explore, if necessary, whether these might be impacting on the presentation of hyperfunctional voice production. Areas to explore include family dynamics and relationships, friendships, bereavements, changes to routine and performance pressures. Questioning about the child's personality, position and role in the family and how he/she deals with challenging situations and exhibits anxiety may all be relevant (Andrews, 1999). A profile that includes anxiety and stress does not in itself indicate a psychological aetiology but rather the need to exclude a psychogenic diagnosis through more detailed psychosocial assessment (Butcher, Elias and Cavalli, 2007) and to consider the need for psychosocial/lifestyle management support and stress management techniques within the treatment plan.

10.3.3   Perceptual Evaluation

The literature has suggested a varied vocal presentation within the CP and CLP population and thus, as with all dysphonic patients, it remains necessary to evaluate each patient individually and comprehensively. To be comprehensive, perceptual evaluation must include all of the following vocal parameters: voice quality, pitch, loudness, resonance, airflow/breathing and muscle tension/effort, which combined can give rise to an overall severity rating. Rating voice *quality* is universally accepted as challenging (Mathieson, 2001). The SLT is the most qualified professional to provide a comprehensive perceptual evaluation of the child's speech and voice. In the child with co-existing VPI this task is particularly complex due to the impact on perception that the coupling effects within the vocal tract have on the speech signal. Nasality affects the voice signal in a number of ways, for example by shifting the first formant, providing extra resonances and antiresonances, as well as noise between the formants, less distinct formant transitions and reduced overall intensity. D'Antonio, Muntz and Province (1988) found that in 11% of patients with CP, the dysphonia was masked perceptually by a co-occurring marked hypernasality. The implication of this is that a voice problem may not be identified until rehabilitation of the VPI is underway.

The most commonly used voice *quality* rating scale in the United Kingdom is the GRBAS (grade, roughness, breathiness, asthenia and strain) (Hirano, 1981). The GRBAS is recognized as 'the absolute minimum standard of vocal perceptual analysis for all practising SLTs in the UK' (Carding *et al.*, 2000, p. 1), is relatively quick to learn and indeed training is relatively easy to access. It is limited, however, in that it provides a measure of only one vocal parameter, that of voice quality, and thus takes no account of parameters such as pitch and vocal loudness. Such a rating scheme is therefore inadequate for judging the full extent of any voice disorder. More comprehensive scales do exist, for example the Buffalo III Voice Profile (Wilson, 1987) and the instrument recommended by ASHA, the CAPE-V (Consensus Auditory Perceptual Evaluation of Voice) (Kempster *et al.*, 2009). Carding *et al.* (2000) make a recommendation that the Vocal Profile Analysis Scheme (Wirz and MacKenzie Beck, 1995) be used by voice specialists in the United Kingdom. Although training in this scheme is currently difficult to source, it is the author's view that this system remains unsurpassed both as an assessment and management tool. It also translates neatly to the VoQS (Voice Quality Symbols) system used in clinical phonetic transcription (Chapter 7). Importantly for the cleft palate population, it evaluates dimensions that may influence the final percept, such as tongue posturing for speech (backed versus fronted, high versus low), jaw posturing (close versus open), pharyngeal constriction and laryngeal height.

Perceptual evaluation should also evaluate breathing and muscle tension behaviours. It needs to differentiate between clavicular and abdomino-diaphragmatic breathing, talking on residual air, inappropriate breath grouping, audible inspiration during speech and excessive involvement of the neck strap muscles during voice production. This assessment may also include palpation of the extrinsic laryngeal musculature. Clinical evaluation suggests that children and adults with CLP and CP may use a variety of tensioning postures to augment speech intelligibility and compensate for valving insufficiency at the velopharyngeal port. In some cases, elimination of some of these behaviours as a target for voice therapy may increase the perception of nasality and a compromise may need to be reached between management of the dysphonia versus the child's nasality. Ratings of vocal discomfort and vocal fatigue are also helpful, although formal systems designed for children do not currently exist to evaluate these.

The voice sample required for both perceptual and instrumental evaluation is similar to that recommended for adults (Abberton, 2005; McGlashan and Fourcin, 2008) and is ideally collected simultaneously for both purposes. The sample includes sustained high and low vowels, a neutral schwa vowel, pitch glides and counting from one to twenty at varying rates and increased loudness levels. Continuous speech is typically assessed using a standardized reading passage of approximately 45 seconds. Where the child's literacy skills do not allow this, it is recommended that the clinician encourages narration of a familiar fairy tale, for example Goldilocks and the three bears. A sample of conversational speech is also desirable. In addition, voice therapists may record the patient's maximum phonation time (MPT), that is how long they can sustain a vowel on a single breath, and measure the length of breath groups in spontaneous speech. A good quality simultaneous audio recording should be acquired either digitally or via a DAT recorder using a pressure sensitive non-directional microphone (Royal College of Speech and Language Therapists, 2005).The recording environment needs to be controlled as much as possible, with noisy siblings occupied elsewhere and intrusive 'noise' from additional equipment reduced.

10.4   Instrumental Assessment

The complexity of perceptual speech evaluation in the case of the child with features of both nasality and dysphonia has already been discussed. Instrumental analysis can assist the assessment process by extracting out specific components of speech production for interpretation but in itself is not diagnostic of vocal pathology. The reader is referred elsewhere, for more in-depth discussion of the different types of instrumental measures, technical and procedural considerations and paediatric normative data (Baken and Orlikoff, 2000; McGlashan and Fourcin, 2008; Hartnick and Boseley, 2008).

Routine specialist voice assessment may include reference to the following measures:

- Vocal fundamental frequency (Fo) measured in Hz – corresponds with the rate of vocal fold vibration and is a primary factor, but not the only one, in the perception of pitch.

- Perturbation – is a measure of the average cycle to cycle variation. This is most often applied to frequency (jitter) and amplitude (shimmer) but vocal fold contact duration (Qx) is now also beginning to be of clinical use.

- Speech intensity (e.g. dB, SPL) – is the physical correlate of loudness and may vary as a result of changes to subglottic pressure and amplitude of vocal fold vibration.

- Phonetogram – is a visual display of intensity versus fundamental frequency ranges.

- Spectral measures – provide a plot of intensity against frequency.

- Contact quotient – can be acquired using electrolaryngography/glottography, which measures electrical conductance across the neck at the level of the vocal folds using two electrodes placed on the thyroid lamina. High conductance is associated with complete vocal fold contact and low conductance with an absence of contact. The contact quotient (Qx) is a measure of the duration of contact against the total duration of the vibratory cycle.

- Subglottal pressure (P_s) – is the amount of force per unit area exerted at the level of the lower surfaces of the vocal folds and with normal velopharyngeal closure can be measured indirectly as intraoral pressure, using sequenced bilabial plosives at a constant intensity, fundamental frequency and rate. In the population with VPI, however, such measures will be difficult to extract due to difficulties generating intraoral pressure.

As with all assessment, selection of any instrumental measure should be made on a case by case basis, using the case history information and perceptual assessment to decide on the essential data set for acquisition. Measures may be extracted from the acoustic waveform and/or the electrolaryngographic/glottographic signal. Traditionally, sustained vowels are used; more recently, however, the trend is to use samples of connected speech as being more representative of patient need and more relevant to accurate analysis.

It may be possible for the clinician specialising in VPI disorders to acquire at least some of the above measures using instrumentation already in the clinic (e.g. Perci Sars: Chapter 11). However, dedicated voice instrumentation such as the electrolaryngograph will allow more comprehensive acquisition. In all cases age appropriate normative data should be referred to when interpreting results.

10.5   Vocal Handicap Measures

It is important to gain insight from the patient as to how he or she is affected by their dysphonia. It is the author's experience that vocal handicap can increase as the child gets older and develops increased awareness of themselves and others, even when the voice perceptually remains static or improves in part. Thus it is possible that, although perceptual and acoustic measures indicate an improved voice profile after voice intervention, the child or young person's perceptions of the negative impact of any residual voice difficulty may increase. Critical periods are likely to exacerbate this awareness, for example, often around eight years of age with developing self and peer awareness of differences, and also when transitioning to secondary school.

There are currently two validated tools available for use with children with voice disorders, both of which have been devised in the form of a parent proxy questionnaire. The Paediatric Voice Related Quality of Life Survey (PV-RQOL) (Boseley et al., 2006; Merati et al., 2008) is a 10 item instrument that uses a six-point rating scale. It has been shown to have good consistency and validity and can be completed relatively quickly by parents. The Paediatric Vocal Handicap Index (pVHI) (Zur et al., 2007) is a 23 item parent proxy version of the widely used VHI for adults. It looks at the functional, physical and emotional impact of the voice disorder and is again completed by the parent. The child's perception of the vocal handicap should also be obtained wherever possible; for example 'Are there things you can't do because of your voice?', 'Do other children talk about your voice? How does that make you feel inside?', 'Does it feel hard work to talk? Are there places you don't like to go because of your voice?' Children with a reading age of 10–12 years and over are usually ready to complete the adult version of the VHI and some younger children do so very capably (with the exclusion of at least one question which asks about income!).

10.6   Treatment

Comprehensive multidisciplinary assessment determines whether a paediatric clinical voice disorder is best managed by voice therapy, surgery, medicine/pharmacology or a combined approach. Organic voice disorders (Mathieson, 2001) most often require surgical or medical treatments as the primary intervention, although voice therapy may also be appropriate where the child has learned additional maladaptive patterns of voice production that complicate the vocal efficiency or effectiveness. Voice therapy will be the treatment of choice for almost all voice disorders identified as having a hyperfunctional or psychogenic aetiology, including vocal fold nodules. As the child with a cleft palate and dysphonia most frequently presents with a hyperfunctional voice disorder, with or without mucosal changes such as nodules, voice therapy is typically very relevant to include within the child's overall speech and language therapy management programme.

The goals of voice therapy intervention are, firstly, to prevent further deterioration of the voice and, secondly, to restore or at least improve voice function. Alongside these goals will be anticipated improvements in the level of laryngeal discomfort, vocal efficiency and effectiveness in vocal activities of everyday living. Normal voice production may also be an appropriate goal for some organic based paediatric voice disorders, for example laryngopharyngeal reflux and fungal infection, but with many other organic based voice disorders, for example vocal fold palsy, laryngeal scarring, sulcus and laryngeal web, the goal is to maximize the communicative potential rather than restore normal voice.

Voice therapists distinguish between direct and indirect treatment approaches. Examples of these two approaches are shown in Table 10.1

Table 10.1   Examples of indirect and direct treatment approaches.

Indirect approaches
Education around the voice disorder and normal voice production.
Vocal hygiene/voice care advice.
Voice rest and voice conservation, for example creating opportunities for
    non-vocal play.
Management of the environment, for example appropriate positioning of the
    child in the classroom and reducing levels of background noise.
Counselling and support.
The use of augmentative/alternative communication devises, for example voice
    amplifiers.
Direct approaches *(altering the vocal physiology)*
Speech breathing exercises.
Adjustment to vocal fold onset/vibratory patterns.
Postural realignment.
Muscle relaxation/deconstriction techniques.

10.6.1   Which Approach?

Firstly, when considering voice therapy intervention with any child it is critical to select
an approach that is developmentally appropriate. Voice is a relatively abstract concept
(Andrews and Summers, 2002) and arguably less tangible than oral and articulatory/
phonological work. It is usual to consider a child of eight years and over as developmentally ready to work directly on changing physiological vocal concepts and to be
capable of mastering the necessary skills to generalize task based vocal activities into
everyday speech. However, each child's readiness must be evaluated separately and other
confounding factors considered, for example, parental involvement, frequency of attendance and home rehearsal (Trani *et al.*, 2007). Younger children may respond better to
an indirect approach that involves all significant carers, siblings and peers and one that
helps them to grasp the cause–effect relationship between vocal behaviour and their
symptoms.

Age also impacts on physiological and anatomical maturity. This is most obvious
at puberty when one tends to anticipate lowering of the vocal fundamental frequency
in both sexes, temporary vocal shifts/breaks in boys and increased vocal loudness,
pitch range and resonance in both sexes (Harries *et al.*, 1996). The literature suggests
that there is generally a resolution of vocal fold nodules in a significant percentage
of boys at puberty, although voice problems may persist due to the habitualization
of hyperfunctional patterns. Girls with nodules are less likely to see nodule improvement
as a result of puberty, and should therefore be judged as a more at risk group for
chronic hyperfunctional voice disorder beyond adolescence (De Bodt, Ketelslagers
and Peeters, 2007). The trend to improvement in laryngeal status at puberty has
also been noted in children with cleft palate (McWilliams, Lavorato and Bluestone,
1973).

10.6.2   When to Intervene?

Voice therapy intervention for adults with hyperfunctional voice disorder has been well substantiated. There is less evidence in paediatrics but those few papers that have looked at outcomes suggest a number of key prognostic factors, which include parental involvement, intensity of sessions and home rehearsal (Mori, 1999; Lee and Son, 2005; Trani *et al.*, 2007). For the child with a history of cleft palate, it is most important that timing of voice therapy intervention be considered alongside the child's overall medical, surgical and speech and language therapy management. If the origin of the voice disorder is judged to relate to laryngeal hypervalving as a consequence of VPI, it may be very appropriate to defer direct therapy for the voice until control of airflow through the upper respiratory tract is optimized via surgical or prosthetic management. If nasal congestion and hearing are influential, then early management of these areas is a priority and in most cases should precede direct voice work. Management of attention and behaviour difficulties/delay that give rise to excessively loud/strained vocalizations may also indirectly improve vocal behaviour and optimize conditions for achieving an effective voice therapy outcome later on. It may also be the case that intervention on articulatory compensations and co-occurring speech diagnoses such as dyspraxia may reduce laryngeal hyperfunction and that specific voice therapy is not required. Voice therapy targets should ideally be integrated within the programme aimed at speech sound development. The clinician should not feel pressured to step in too early with active voice intervention before such compounding factors have been accounted for and an integrated management plan developed.

Other factors to consider when deciding on the treatment approach and timing of intervention include:

a) Laryngeal status: that is the nature of any pathology and size of any lesion.

b) Severity and chronicity of the dysphonia.

c) Medical history.

d) Results of stimulability/trial therapy.

e) Resources available, timing of appointments, skill base and so on.

10.6.3   Designing the Treatment Programme

Traditional voice therapy treatment programmes include an initial focus on voice care and vocal hygiene and move on to addressing postural adjustment, targeted relaxation of muscle tension, breathing behaviour for speech and then patterns of vocal fold vibration (e.g. hard versus soft onsets, pitch, loudness etc.). Treatment should also include a focus on any psychosocial/emotional aspects identified through the voice assessment as impacting on vocal physiology (Butcher, Elias and Cavalli, 2007). How much time is allocated to each of these areas will be determined by the assessment. It may well be possible to combine some areas within a single focus so as to simplify the child's cognitive task; for example, posture and breathing can be worked on concurrently in some children, as can breathing and vocal fold approximation work.

It is not within the remit of this chapter to describe in detail specific techniques and treatment approaches. However, there are three key stages to achieving an effective voice outcome in children.

Stage 1: Developing general awareness of voice and voice production. This stage must critically include a whole family approach and is essential to governing the necessary motivation required for commitment to change.

Stage 2: Developing auditory discrimination and vocal control of the targeted vocal behaviour(s).

Stage 3: Developing self-monitoring and vocal control in generalized speech activities.

Children will progress at different rates through the three stages of treatment and it is likely in younger children that more than one contract of therapy may be required to reach the important target of generalization. In some cases, there may also be a need to include management of those psychosocial/emotional factors judged to be significant in contributing to muscle tension behaviours.

There are many reasons why voice therapy targets may not be achieved. Many of these have already been referred to elsewhere in the text, that is:

• Insufficient/inaccurate diagnostic information.

• Developmental limitations.

• Differing priorities/Reduced motivation – child and or carer.

• Unrealistic/inappropriate goals/approach.

• Clinician skill base and/or resources available.

• Cultural/language barriers.

• Additional factors, for example other communication problems, health, psychosocial factors.

Where the reasons for limited progress are clear, it is important to be overt in communications with the child, family and other professionals as to the likely reasons why.

A review by ENT is important when the SLT has been in the position of working with a child who has not had a complete laryngeal examination, due perhaps to poor compliance or the method of examination used, and who then does not go on to recover normal voice as anticipated. It is also very relevant when examination has taken place but recovery does not proceed as expected and the explanation for this is unclear.

10.6.4 Surgical and Medical Management Options

Phonosurgery for vocal nodules in pre-pubertal children is rarely considered appropriate. This largely relates to a lack of knowledge about the impact surgery may have on the developing lamina propria and the risk of permanent scarring. (McMurray, 2008). Other factors that impact on surgical outcome include failure to comply with post-surgical voice rest and persisting hyperfunctional vocal behaviours. It should also be remembered that a significant percentage of boys will 'grow out' of their nodules at puberty, although their dysphonia may still persist due to continuing hyperfunctional voice production (De Bodt, Ketelslagers and Peeters, 2007). Studies often quoted in support of surgical correction of vocal nodules in children suggest early improvements in voice, that is at one month follow-up (Mori, 1999) but do not follow-up children beyond this early recovery period. An early study looking at surgical removal of nodules in children with cleft palate (McWilliams, Lavorato and Bluestone, 1973) found it to be an ineffective treatment, although it is likely that phonosurgical procedures have advanced since the date of the study.

Surgery for organic laryngeal disorders (e.g. glottic web, vocal fold palsy, papillomatosis) aims to restore/preserve both an adequate airway and vocal fold vibration. Surgical procedure and technique will depend on the lesion type, severity of symptoms and disease progression. When the young child's dysphonia is judged to be having limited functional, emotional and or participatory consequences, surgery for some benign lesions (e.g. an intra-cordal cyst), may be deferred until such time as post-surgical compliance for voice rest and conservation can be better assured. This is to minimize the possibility of a lesion being replaced with scar tissue as a result of poor post-operative healing. Surgery for symptomatic tonsillar/adenoid hypertrophy may ease congested symptoms but may impact on VPI and must, therefore, be approached via careful evaluation and consultation between professionals and family (Chapters 1 and 3).

Medical management for voice may include a trial of anti-reflux medication over a four to six month period, pharmacological management of nasal congestion and post-nasal drip and allergy treatments (Hocevar-Boltezar, Jarc and Kozelj, 2006; Hocevar-Boltezar, Radsel and Zargi, 1997) as indicated by the case history and ENT examination. Further information on surgical and medical ENT management is available in more comprehensive texts (Gleeson, 2008; Hartnick and Boseley, 2008; Lennox, 2001).

10.7 Conclusion

Voice management for the child/adolescent with a history of cleft palate requires close collaboration between child, parent and a team of professionals that may include SLT, ENT and plastic surgeons, audiologist, psychologist and school teacher. Comprehensive assessment is essential and results of the voice evaluation should be interpreted alongside knowledge of the velopharyngeal dysfunction and other medical symptomology. Voice therapy should not be considered as a stand-alone treatment. Therapy management of the dysphonia is best integrated into the overall speech and language therapy programme with goals evaluated and prioritized against other target areas for treatment. Voice therapy can be effective when carefully planned and when realistic goals are set out. The impact of a dysphonia on a child's self-image and social functioning should not be overlooked.

Where a clinician does not specialize in voice management, it is advised that a close relationship is established with a voice specialist centre where advice and access to specialist skills and equipment are available.

References

Abberton, E. (2005) Phonetic considerations in the design of voice assessment material. *Logopedic Phoniatrics Vocology*, 30, 175–180.

Andrews, M. (1999) *Manual of Voice Treatment. Paediatrics through Geriatrics*, 2nd edn. Singular Publishing Group, San Diego.

Andrews, M. and Summers, A. (2002) *Voice Treatment for Children & Adolescents*, Singular-Thomson Learning, San Diego.

Aronson, A. and Bless, D. (2009) *Clinical Voice Disorders*, 4th edn. Thieme, New York.

Baken, R.J. and Orlikoff, R.F. (2000) *Clinical Measurement of Speech and Voice*, 2nd edn. Singular-Thomson Learning, San Diego.

Boseley, M., Cunningham, M., Volk, M. and Hartnick, C. (2006) Validation of the paediatric voice-related quality of life survey. *Archives of Otolaryngology – Head & Neck Surgery*, 132, 717–720.

Butcher, P., Elias, A. and Cavalli, L. (2007) *Understanding and Treating Psychogenic Voice Disorder: A CBT Framework*, John Wiley & Sons Ltd, Chichester.

Carding, P., Carlson, E., Epstein, R. *et al.* (2000) Formal perceptual evaluation of voice quality in the UK. *Logopedics Phoniatrics Vocology*, 25, 133–138.

Carding, P., Roulstone, S., Northstone, K. and The ALSPAC Study Team (2006) The prevalence of childhood dysphonia: a cross-sectional study. *Journal of Voice*, 20, 623–630.

Colton, R.H., Casper, J.K. and Leonard, R. (2006) *Understanding Voice Problems – A Physiological Perspective for Diagnosis and Treatment*, 3rd edn. Lippincott, Williams and Wilkins, Baltimore.

D'Antonio, L., Muntz, H. and Province, M. (1988) Laryngeal/voice findings in patients with velopharyngeal dysfunction. *Laryngoscope*, 98, 432–438.

De Bodt, M., Ketelslagers, K. and Peeters, T. (2007) Evolution of vocal fold nodules from childhood to adolescence. *Journal of Voice*, 21, 151–156.

Gleeson, M. (ed.) (2008) *Scott-Brown's Otorhinolaryngology, Head and Neck Surgery*, 7th edn. Edward Arnold, London.

Hamming, K., Finkelstein, M. and Sidman, J. (2009) Hoarseness in children with cleft palate. *Archives of Otolaryngology – Head and Neck Surgery*, 140, 902–906.

Harries, M., Griffith, M., Walker, J. and Hawkins, S. (1996) Changes in the male voice during puberty: speaking and singing voice parameters. *Logopedics Phoniatrics Vocology*, 21, 95–100.

Harris, T., Harris, S., Rubin, J. and Howard, D. (1998) *The Voice Clinic Handbook*, Whurr, London.

Hartnick, C. and Boseley, M. (2008) *Paediatric Voice Disorders*, Plural Publishing, San Diego, CA.

Hartnick, C., Umeno, H. and Nakashima, T. (2005) Pediatric video laryngostroboscopy. *International Journal of Pediatric Otorhinolaryngology*, 69, 215–219.

Hirano, M. (1981) *Clinical Examination of Voice*, Springer-Verlag, Vienna.

Hocevar-Boltezar, I., Jarc, A. and Kozelj, V. (2006) Ear, nose and throat problems in children with orofacial clefts. *The Journal of Laryngology and Otology*, **120**, 276–281.

Hocevar-Boltezar, I., Radsel, Z. and Zargi, M. (1997) The role of allergy in the aetiopathogenesis of laryngeal mucosal lesions. *Acta Otolaryngologica (Suppl.)*, **527**, 134–137.

Hunt, J. and Slater, A. (2003) *Working with Children's Voice Disorders*, Speechmark, London.

Kawano, M., Isshiki, N., Honjo, I. *et al.* (1997) Recent progress in treating patients with cleft palate. *Folia Phoniatrica et Logopaedica*, **49**, 117–138.

Kempster, G., Gerratt, B., Verdolini-Abbott, K. *et al.* (2009) Consensus auditory-perceptual evaluation of voice: development of a clinical protocol. *American Journal of Speech-Language Pathology*, **18**, 124–132.

Kido, N., Kawano, M., Tanokuchi, F. *et al.* (1992) Glottal stop in cleft palate. *Studia Phonologica*, **26**, 34–41.

Lass, N., Ruscello, D., Stout, L. and Hoffman, F. (1991) Peer perceptions of normal and voice disordered children. *Folia Phoniatrica et Logopaedica*, **43**, 29–35.

Leder, S. and Lerman, J. (1985) Some acoustic evidence for vocal abuse in adult speakers with repaired cleft palate. *Laryngoscope*, **95**, 837–840.

Lee, E. and Son, Y.-I. (2005) Muscle tension dysphonia in children: voice characteristics and outcome of voice therapy. *International Journal of Pediatric Otorhinolaryngology*, **69**, 911–917.

Lennox, P. (2001) Hearing and ENT management, in *Management of Cleft Lip and Palate* (eds A.C.H. Watson, D. Sell and P. Grunwell), Whurr, London, pp. 210–225.

Lewis, J., Andreassen, M., Leeper, H. and Macrae, D. (1993) Vocal characteristics of children with cleft lip/palate and associated velopharyngeal incompetence. *The Journal of Otolaryngology*, **22**, 113–117.

Lohmander-Agerskov, A., Soderpalm, E., Friede, H. and Lilja, J. (1995) A longitudinal study of speech in 15 children with cleft lip and palate treated with late repair of the hard palate. *Scandinavian Journal of Plastic and Reconstructive Surgery and Hand Surgery*, **29**, 21–31.

Mathieson, L. (2001) *Greene and Mathieson's The Voice and Its Disorders*, 6th edn. Whurr, London.

McGlashan, J. and Fourcin, A. (2008) Objective evaluation of voice, *Scott-Brown's Otorhinolaryngology, Head and Neck Surgery*, 7th edn. (ed. M. Gleason), Hodder Arnold, London.

McWilliams, B., Lavorato, A. and Bluestone, C. (1973) Vocal cord abnormalities in children with velopharyngeal valving problems. *Laryngoscope*, **83**, 1745–1753.

McMurray, J.S. (2008) Benign lesions of the pediatric vocal folds, in *Pediatric Voice Disorders* (eds C. Hartnick and M. Boseley). Plural Publishing, San Diego, CA, pp. 171–190.

Merati, A., Keppel, K., Braun, N. *et al.* (2008) Pediatric voice-related quality of life: findings in healthy children and in common laryngeal disorders. *Annals of Otology, Rhinology & Laryngology*, **117**, 259–262.

Mori, K. (1999) Vocal fold nodules in children: preferable therapy. *International Journal of Pediatric Otorhinolaryngology*, **49** (Suppl.):S303–S306.

Multinovic, Z. (1994) Social environment and incidence of voice disturbances in children. *Folio Phoniatrica et Logopaedica*, **46**, 135–138.

Papsin, B., Pengilly, A. and Leighton, S. (1996) The developing role of a paediatric voice clinic: a review of our experience. *The Journal of Laryngology and Otology*, **110**, 1022–1026.

Rattenbury, H., Carding, P. and Finn, P. (2004) Evaluating the effectiveness and efficiency of voice therapy using transnasal flexible laryngoscopy: a randomised trial. *Journal of Voice*, **18**, 522–533.

Royal College of Speech and Language Therapists (2005) *RCSLT Clinical Guidelines: Clinical Voice Disorders*, Speechmark, London.

Sell, D., Grunwell, P., Mildenhall, S. *et al.* (2001) Cleft lip and palate care in the United Kingdom (UK) – The Clinical Standards Advisory Group (CSAG) Study. Part 3 – Speech outcomes. *Cleft Palate-Craniofacial Journal*, **38**, 30–37.

Shewell, C. (2009) *Voice Work: Art and Science in Changing Voices*, John Wiley & Sons Ltd, Chichester.

Tanimoto, K., Henningsson, G., Isberg, A. and Ren, Y.-F. (1994) Comparison of tongue position during speech before and after pharyngeal flap surgery in hypernasal speakers. *Cleft Palate-Craniofacial Journal*, **31** (4), 280–286.

Timmons, M., Wyatt, R. and Murphy, T. (2001) Speech after repair of isolated cleft palate and cleft lip and palate. *British Journal of Plastic Surgery*, **54**, 377–384.

Trani, M., Ghidini, A., Bergamini, G. and Presutti, L. (2007) Voice therapy in pediatric functional dysphonia: a prospective study. *International Journal of Pediatric Otorhinolaryngology*, **71**, 379–384.

Van Lierde, K., Claeys, S., De Bodt, M. and Van Cauwenberge, P. (2004) Vocal quality characteristics in children with cleft palate: a mutiparameter approach. *Journal of Voice*, **18**, 354–362.

Warren, D. (1986) Compensatory speech behaviours in individuals with cleft palate: a regulation/control phenomenon? *Cleft Palate Journal*, **23**, 251–259.

Wilson, K. (1987) *Voice Problems of Children*, 3rd edn. Williams and Wilkins, Baltimore.

Wirz, S. and MacKenzie Beck, J. (1995) Assessment of vocal quality- The vocal profile analysis scheme, in *Perceptual Approaches to Communication Disorders* (ed. S. Wirz), Whurr, London, pp. 39–55.

Wolf, M., Primov-Fever, A.O. and Jedwab, D. (2005) The feasibility of rigid stroboscopy in children. *International Journal of Pediatric Otorhinolaryngology*, **69**, 1077–1079.

Woo, P., Colton, R., Casper, J. and Brewer, D. (1991) Diagnostic value of stroboscopic examination in hoarse patients. *Journal of Voice*, **5**, 231–238.

Zur, K., Cotton, S., Kelchner, L. *et al.* (2007) Paediatric Voice Handicap Index (pVHI): a new tool for evaluating paediatric dysphonia. *International Journal of Pediatric Otorhinolaryngology*, **71**, 77–82.

11

Nasality – Assessment and Intervention

Triona Sweeney

The Children's University Hospital, Speech and Language Therapy Department, Dublin 1, Republic of Ireland

11.1 Introduction

Nasality and nasal airflow errors are distinctive speech problems that are often synonymous with cleft palate and/or velopharyngeal dysfunction. These parameters have remained challenging for Speech and Language Therapists working on the cleft team due to a lack of standardized terminology to describe nasality and nasal airflow, variations in approaches to their assessment and management and poor reliability in ratings of nasality and nasal airflow errors. This chapter reviews some of the issues regarding poor reliability, presents definitions of terms used to describe nasality, including nasal airflow errors, and highlights some of the controversies regarding terminology. A detailed assessment protocol is proposed using perceptual and instrumental techniques and the interpretation of results are discussed. The issues regarding speech therapy intervention for nasality and nasal airflow errors are considered, while a brief overview of prosthetic management is presented.

Nasality is a type of resonance present in normal voice production and is defined as the balance between oral and nasal resonance. It refers to perceived nasal resonance

Cleft Palate Speech: Assessment and Intervention, First Edition. Edited by Sara Howard, Anette Lohmander.
© 2011 John Wiley & Sons, Ltd. Published 2011 by John Wiley & Sons, Ltd.

during production of multisegmental units resulting from the coupling of the oral and nasal resonating cavities. In English, nasality typically occurs on nasal consonants /n, m, ŋ/ and on adjacent vowels. A vital factor in inducing nasal resonance is the ratio of nasopharyngeal port size to the oropharyngeal port size (Laver, 1980), thus producing a balance between oral and nasal resonance. Normal nasal resonance has a range of acceptability and is perceived along a continuum (Peterson-Falzone, Hardin-Jones and Karnell, 2010), while nasal resonance disorders can be associated with cleft palate, velopharyngeal disorders and nasal obstruction, resulting in nasality problems and nasal airflow errors. *Nasal airflow error* is a generic term to describe any inappropriate escape of air through the nasal cavity during the production of high pressure sounds. The most common cause of nasality problems and nasal airflow errors is velopharyngeal dysfunction and/or the presence of a fistula in the hard palate. Velopharyngeal dysfunction (VPD), which includes velopharyngeal insufficiency (VPI) (structural aetiology), velopharyngeal incompetency (neurological aetiology) and velopharyngeal mislearning (functional aetiology), is described in detail by Sell and Pereira (Chapter 8.)

Nasality and nasal airflow errors are perceptual phenomena and research to date indicates substantial variations in the reliability of listener judgements of these parameters (Sweeney, 2000). This variation may be due to the use of different types of assessment scales measuring the parameters, and the use of different statistics to evaluate the reliability of these assesment scales. Also, a number of factors have been found to influence the reliability of perceptual assessment of nasality and nasal airflow. These include terminology used to describe speech (Kent, 1996), the speech sample used to analyse speech (Henningsson *et al.*, 2008; Sell *et al.*, 2009), linguistic background of the rater (Lee, Brown and Gibbon, 2008), listening conditions (Sell *et al.*, 2009,) listener training (Lee, Whitehill and Ciocca, 2009) and the presence of associated articulation/phonation problems (McWilliams, Morris and Shelton, 1990).

It has been reported that listeners have different internal standards when rating voice quality (Kreiman *et al.*, 1993; Lohmander *et al.*, 2009). Experienced clinicians who frequently assess a specific type of disorder may develop their own standard references, which are stored in long-term memory (Kuehn, 1982). This internal standard may explain why experienced listeners have better reliability than inexperienced listeners (Hayden and Klimacka, 2000; Sweeney and Fennell, 2009). Equally, there is limited evidence regarding the validity of perceptual assessments. Although the general consensus is that perceptual assessment is the gold standard, there may be questions regarding the validity of the Speech and Language Therapists' assessment. Some studies have reported high validity by comparing perceptual assessments with clinical outcomes (John *et al.*, 2006) or with instrumental assessments (Watterson, McFarlane and Wright, 1993; Watterson, Lewis and Deutsch, 1998; Sweeney and Sell, 2008). However, Brunnegard, Lohmander and Van Doorn (2009) compared perceptual ratings of nasality and nasal airflow errors by lay listeners with ratings by Speech and Language Therapists and found that lay listeners were less sensitive to mild nasal airflow errors, therefore casting some doubt on the validity of this aspect of the Speech and Language Therapist's assessment. Thus they suggest that the significance of the error in everyday life needs to be considered as part of the clinical assessment.

Some steps can be taken to reduce factors influencing reliability and validity, specifically defining terminology, standardising the speech sample, obtaining high quality audio and/

or video recordings, and using a standardized rating scale with definitions of the scalar points.

The need for definition of the terms used to describe these types of speech problems and the standardization of these terms is essential, as the imprecise use of terminology can lead to erroneous assumptions regarding a patient and inappropriate clinical actions (Peterson-Falzone, Hardin-Jones and Karnell, 2010), and render the interpretation of speech outcome data difficult. Resonance disorders include hypernasality, hyponasality, cul de sac resonance and mixed nasality. The degree and consistency of resonance disorders can vary in speech.

Hypernasality is the occurrence of excessive nasal resonance perceived during speech production. It results from an abnormal coupling of oral and nasal resonating cavities when the velopharyngeal sphincter is in an open position. According to Laver's (1980) classification, hypernasality occurs when there is an increase in the ratio of nasopharyngeal port to oropharyngeal port size, thus shifting the balance to produce increased nasal resonance. A diagrammatic representation of the vocal tract during hypernasal speech production, with phonetic transcription, is presented in Figure 11.1 (Sell *et al.*, 2009).

Hyponasality is the reduction or absence of expected nasal resonance associated with nasal consonants and their adjacent vowels in English. This is usually due to the reduction of the size of the velopharyngeal port and/or nasal airway, as might be expected if adenoids are enlarged (Peterson-Falzone, Hardin-Jones and Karnell, 2010). According to Laver's (1980) classification, there is a decrease in the ratio of the nasopharyngeal

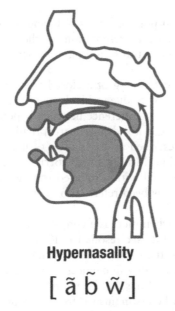

Hypernasality

[ã b̃ w̃]

Figure 11.1 Diagrammatic representation of vocal tract during hypernasal speech production, with phonetic transcription. (Reproduced with permission from Sell *et al.*, 2005; Appendix B in Sell *et al.*, 2009.)

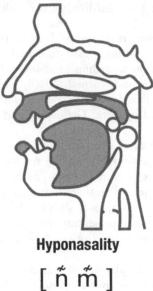

Hyponasality

[n̊ m̊]

Figure 11.2 Diagrammatic representation of vocal tract during hyponasal speech production, with phonetic transcription. (Reproduced with permission from Sell *et al.*, 2005; Appendix B in Sell *et al.*, 2009.)

port size to the oropharyngeal port size, thus reducing nasal resonance and increasing oral resonance. A diagrammatic representation of the vocal tract during hyponasal speech production, with phonetic transcription, is presented in Figure 11.2 (Sell *et al.*, 2009).

Cul de sac resonance is the coupling of a closed nasal resonating cavity to the oral resonating cavity. It is thought to be due to blockage of the anterior section of the nasal cavity. Auditorily, there is a subtle difference between hyponasality and cul de sac resonance. Although this difference is not defined perceptually or acoustically in detail, cul de sac resonance has been described as a variation of hyponasality, which differs only in the place of nasal obstruction (McWilliams, Morris and Shelton, 1990). Perceptually, cul de sac resonance is associated with a muffled tone which is often heard when the speaker has a head cold and has been referred to as 'potato in the mouth' quality (Sell and Grunwell, 2001).

Mixed Nasality can occur when there is a combination of hypernasality and hyponasality or hypernasality and cul de sac resonance. Kummer (2008) states that if there is coexisting velopharyngeal insufficiency and nasal blockage, such as enlarged tonsils and adenoids, there may be hypernasality in connected speech with some evidence of hyponasality during the production of nasal consonants.

Disorders of nasality must be distinguished from disorders of nasal airflow. Sweeney *et al.* (1996) proposed the term *nasal airflow error* in order to discriminate between perceptual and instrumental measures of nasal airflow. In the literature on aerodynamics, nasal airflow is a well recognized physical measurement of the rate of airflow through the nasal cavity (Warren, 1989). In perceptual assessment the term *nasal airflow error* is defined as any inappropriate escape of air through the nasal cavity during the production of voiced and voiceless pressure consonants and includes nasal emission and nasal turbulence (Sweeney *et al.*, 1996). The purpose of this generic definition is to perceptually differentiate between sound distortion associated with nasal escape of air and the distortion of the voice quality on vowels and voiced sounds due to hypernasality which, according to Bzoch (1989), is critical for differential diagnosis of VPD. Some authors classify nasal airflow errors as patterns of misarticulation (Whitehill and Lee, 2008; Peterson-Falzone, Hardin-Jones and Karnell, 2010) or sound error distortions (Kuehn and Moller, 2000), while others classify nasal airflow errors independently, as they can coexist with either nasality problems and/or articulatory errors (John *et al.*, 2006; Sweeney and Sell, 2008). It is important to define and distinguish the nasal airflow errors in order to plan future management.

Nasal emission is the inappropriate audible escape of air through the nasal cavity accompanying production of oral pressure consonants. It is usually due to incomplete closure of the velopharyngeal sphincter and/or the presence of a fistula in the palate. A frictional sound is produced when the airflow is sufficiently strong and the constriction is sufficiently narrow to create noisy random vibrations in the airstream. Nasal emission has a frictional but no turbulent or snorting quality. During consonant production there is oral and nasal release of air, as the nasal emission accompanies the consonant (Sell, Harding and Grunwell, 1999). Figure 11.3 presents a diagrammatic representation of

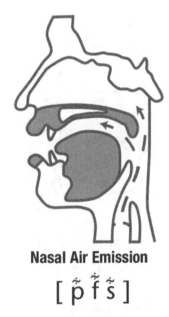

Nasal Air Emission

$$[\, \tilde{p}\, \tilde{f}\, \tilde{s}\,]$$

Figure 11.3 Diagrammatic representation of vocal tract during nasal emission on sounds, with phonetic transcription. (Reproduced with permission from Sell *et al.*, 2005; Appendix B in Sell *et al.*, 2009.)

the vocal tract during nasal emission on consonants, with phonetic transcription. Inaudible nasal emission may also exist. This occurs when there is escape of air through the nasal cavity during the production of high pressure sounds but it is not perceived by the listener. It can be associated with nasal flare or nasal grimace and can be detected by placing a mirror under the nose while looking for misting on the mirror during sound production.

Nasal turbulence is defined as a 'snorting' or turbulent noise, which may be a result of the approximation but inadequate closure of the superior border of the velum and the posterior pharyngeal wall (Duckworth *et al.*, 1990). It accompanies oral consonants resulting in oral and nasal release of air. This has been described by Kummer *et al.* (1992) as a 'nasal rustle', which is associated with a small velopharyngeal gap. Nasal turbulence has also been associated with incomplete velar–adenoidal closure where the adenoidal pad is irregular, resulting in a velar–adenoidal seal that is not tight. Trost (1981) described an audible resistance to nasal airflow that is produced within the nasal cavity and this has been referred to as intra-nasal turbulence (Sweeney, 2000). Hence the exact cause of nasal turbulence is still not fully understood and may vary from patient to patient. Perceptually it is possible to distinguish between nasal turbulence and nasal emission. Figure 11.4 presents a diagrammatic representation of the vocal tract during nasal turbulence on consonants, with phonetic transcription.

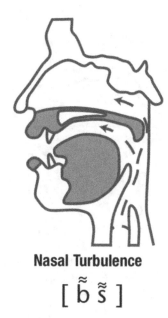

Nasal Turbulence

[b̃̃ s̃̃]

Figure 11.4 Diagrammatic representation of vocal tract during nasal turbulence on sounds. (Reproduced with permission from Sell *et al.*, 2005; Appendix B in Sell *et al.*, 2009.)

It is crucial to distinguish between nasal emission/nasal turbulence accompanying an oral consonant and nasal emission/nasal turbulence replacing an oral consonant. The latter is referred to as a *Nasal Fricative* (Sweeney *et al.*, 1996; John *et al.*, 2006). During the production of a nasal fricative, there is no audible oral release of the target sound. It has been described as the realization of an oral target consonant as a nasal, with airflow through the nasal cavity creating friction (Harding and Grunwell, 1998). Harding and Grunwell (1998) differentiated between *active nasal fricatives,* which are produced by actively directing the airflow nasally and stopping the oral release of the sound, and *passive nasal fricatives*, where the air passively escapes through the nasal cavity and oral airflow is not stopped but is inaudible. Active nasal fricatives are usually associated with velopharyngeal mislearning, while passive nasal fricatives are usually a result of velopharyngeal insufficiency.

Terms used to describe nasal airflow errors in the literature vary considerably, in fact Sell (2005) reported eleven different terms. Peterson-Falzone, Hardin-Jones and Karnell (2010) describe nasal turbulence as a severe form of audible nasal emission, while Kummer (2008) describes three types of nasal emission ranging from inaudible nasal emission to audible nasal emission to nasal rustle (turbulence). Sell, Harding and Grunwell (1999), Sweeney *et al.* (1996) and John *et al.* (2006) classify nasal emission and nasal turbulence separately and consider that nasal emission and nasal turbulence can coexist in patients with velopharyngeal insufficiency and/or a palatal fistula. This use of different terminology to describe the perceptual features of nasality and nasal airflow highlights the need for future collaboration of experts in the field to agree on the definition of terms.

Assessment of nasality and nasal airflow errors can be divided into perceptual and instrumental investigations. Perceptual investigations depend on the listeners' ability to perceive nasality and nasal airflow during speech production, while the instrumental investigations of acoustic and aerodynamic assessments are indirect measures of these speech parameters.

11.2   Perceptual Assessment of Nasality and Nasal Airflow Errors

Perceptual measurement is a vital part of the assessment protocol, as client management decisions are based on subjective judgements and, as Kuehn and Moller (2000) note, there is currently no instrumental assessment of nasality that is sufficiently related to perceived nasality. It is considered the gold standard for speech evaluation and is integral to assessment of cleft speech (Sell, 2005; John *et al.*, 2006). The importance of assessing different levels or complexity of speech has been highlighted in the literature (Kuehn and Moller, 2000; http//clispi.org; Sell *et al.*, 2009). Hence, the speech sample for the perceptual assessment of nasality and nasal airflow should include single word utterances, standardized sentences, automatic speech and conversational speech. A detailed phonetic/phonological analysis of single words using narrow phonetic transcription will help identify speech patterns, which may facilitate perception of nasality, nasal airflow and/or articulation errors.

Standardized speech samples have been developed for clinical assessment of nasality and nasal airflow errors and articulation in the United Kingdom (The GOS.SP.ASS'98; Sell, Harding and Grunwell, 1999), Ireland (Temple Street Scale; Sweeney, 2000) and Sweden (SVANTE; Lohmander *et al.*, 2005)). Automatic speech, which includes counting and rote speech such as nursery rhymes, is a useful method of obtaining a speech sample from younger children (Peterson-Falzone, Hardin-Jones and Karnell, 2010; http//clispi.org). It also provides an opportunity to listen to and rate vulnerable high pressure targets and high and low vowels in connected speech. Finally, it is important to rate conversational speech, as this yields the most representative sample of a patient's speech performance (Kuehn and Moller, 2000). Variability in speech performance between single word utterances and conversational speech may be indicative of inconsistency of velopharyngeal function and has implications for future management. For evaluation of hyponasality, the use of an additional nasally loaded sentence sample may be beneficial.

Descriptive category judgments and equal-appearing interval (EAI) scaling have been the favoured approach to the perceptual assessment of nasality (Sell, 2005). However, Whitehill (2002) reported that EAI ratings of nasality are not valid and have poor reliability. Other assessment scales include direct magnitude estimation (DME), which has been found to have good reliability in the assessment of hypernasality (Whitehill, 2002). But, as Folkins and Moon (1990) point out, the differences between the two procedures may not always justify the amount of work required for DME procedures in the clinic. More recently, Whitehill (2010) reported good reliability for a visual analogue scale and, although this approach shows promise for research, visual analogue scales like EAI and DME scales make clinical reporting of nasality and nasal airflow errors difficult, as all members of the multidisciplinary team may not understand the ratings.

A descriptive scale for assessing nasality and nasal airflow, the Temple Street Scale (TSS), has been tested for validity, reliability and acceptability (Sweeney, 2000; Sweeney and Sell, 2008; Sweeney and Fennell, 2009). This approach assesses nasality and nasal airflow errors, using detailed definitions of terms and descriptive definitions of scalar points. The descriptive hypernasality and hyponasality scales have subsequently been adopted in the Cleft Audit Protocol for Speech–Augmented (John *et al.*, 2006). The TSS is divided into two sections: Nasality and Nasal Airflow errors, which include the parameters of hypernasality, hyponasality, cul de sac resonance, nasal emission, nasal turbulence and nasal fricatives. Each parameter is rated after listening to and transcribing a standard speech sample (Appendix 11.A).

It is necessary for inexperienced raters to make either an audio or video record of the speech sample, as this allows repeated listening in a quiet environment. High quality digital audio recording has been suggested for assessment of cleft speech and found to have adequate quality for voice analysis (Winholtz and Titze, 1998), although Vogel and Morgan (2009) state that this equipment may be unavailable in the future due to advances in technology. They reported on different types of audio recording equipment for speech and voice analysis and provide good recommendations for equipment in terms of quality, portability, ease of use and budget. A professional condenser microphone with a 'uni'-directional pick up pattern should be mounted on a stable stand. When recording speech, if the microphone is placed too close to the mouth there is the possibility of distortion referred to as 'popping' associated with airflow blasting the microphone, particularly on plosive sounds. To reduce the risk of this, it is common practice in the broadcast industry to place the microphone approximately 30 centimetres from the mouth and to the side (Sell *et al.*, 2009). For video recording, good lighting in a quiet room and a plain background has been recommended (http//clispi.org), with the microphone positioned as indicated above.

Listening conditions may also affect ratings of audio and video recorded speech samples. The choice of amplifier and speaker can significantly alter the frequency content of a well-recorded speech sample. Therefore, professional amplifier/speaker combinations, or high quality headphones (such as 90 Sennheiser or similar specification) should be used when analysing speech from recordings. Where possible, listening and rating should be completed in a quiet environment. There are conflicting findings in the literature regarding the use of audio versus audio/video recordings for speech analysis in speakers with cleft palate. Moller and Starr (1984) found no difference in perceptual assessment of audio and audiovisual samples. Sell *et al.* (2009) found there were no statistically significantly differences in speech ratings between the audio and audio/video recordings, but video analysis tended to produce more critical ratings of hypernasality and nasal turbulence.

11.3   Instrumental Assessment of Nasality and Nasal Airflow Errors

Instrumental measurements supplement the perceptual assessment of nasality and nasal airflow and can provide additional information, aid in diagnosis of the speech problems and increase confidence regarding assessment outcomes. The Nasometer (Kay PENTAX, Lincoln Park, NJ) has been used both clinically and in research studies to measure the acoustic correlate of nasality. It consists of a headset, containing a sound separator with microphones on either side, which detects oral and nasal components of the patient's speech. The sound signal is filtered and digitized and a computer processes the data. The resultant signal is the ratio of nasal to nasal-plus-oral acoustic energy and is expressed as a Nasalance score. This system is non-invasive and provides a graphic as well as quantitative result. The patient wears the headset and repeats a standardized set of sentences, which are recorded on the system and analysed. Figure 11.5 illustrates the position of the head set during data collection and Figure 11.6 illustrates the Nasometer set up when assessing children.

Previous studies have indicated that factors such as language, dialect and the speech stimuli influence the scores obtained on the Nasometer (Seaver *et al.*, 1991; Karnell, 1995;). To date, normative data have been published for several languages and dialects (see Brunnegard and Van Doorn, 2009, for a comprehensive list). It is essential, therefore, to compare the patient's clinical nasalance scores to normative data representing the patient's dialect. Standard speech samples should also be used in data collection and some are provided in the Nasometer manual (Kay Elemetrics Corporation, 2003). However, some of the proposed speech samples for nasalance data are too complex for children, are culturally biased (Sweeney, Sell and O'Regan, 2004) or are devoid of nasal consonants (Watterson, Hinton and McFarlane, 1996), which are not representative of normal conversational speech and may lack validity in the assessment of hypernasality (Sweeney and Sell, 2008). Karnell (1995) hypothesized that a speech sample devoid of

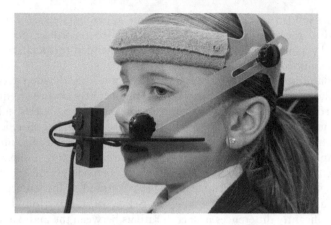

Figure 11.5 Placement of the Nasometer headset, indicating the nasal microphone above the sound separator and the mouth microphone beneath it. The sound separator should not interfere with lip movement.

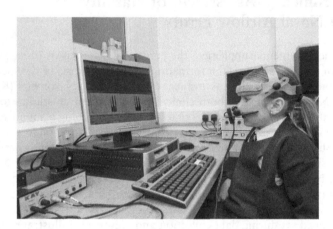

Figure 11.6 Nasometer set-up for data collection. The child is repeating two of the test sentences.

nasal consonants and high pressure oral consonants (i.e. low pressure consonant sample) would enable measurement of nasal acoustic energy that is due to nasal resonance and not influenced by turbulent nasal airflow. He proposed the use of additional low pressure consonant sentences for nasometric assessment.

Standardized speech samples have been developed for both perceptual and instrumental assessment of nasality and nasal airflow error in different languages, including Dutch (Keuning *et al.*, 2002), English (Sweeney, 2000) and Swedish (Brunnegard & Van Doorn, 2009). The samples can then be divided according to consonant type, and separate

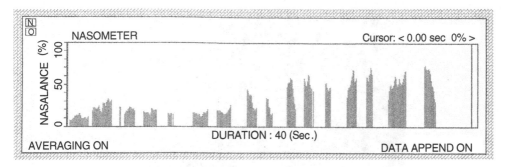

Figure 11.7 Nasometer graph of 16 test sentences for normal speaker. Nasalance (%) is indicated on X axis and time is indicated on the Y axis.

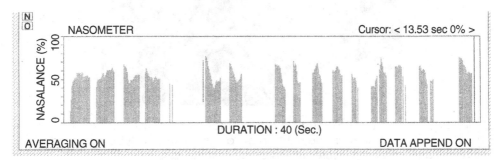

Figure 11.8 Nasometer graph of 16 test sentences for a hypernasal speaker. Nasalance (%) is indicated on X axis and time is indicated on the Y axis.

nasalance scores can be obtained for mixed consonant sentences, high pressure consonant sentences and, in English, low pressure consonant sentences. Figures 11.7 and 11.8 indicate a nasometry graph for a normal speaker and a hypernasal speaker, respectively, during the production of the English sample containing all consonants. For assessment of hyponasal speech, a separate speech sample containing nasally loaded sentences/passage is recommended (Brunnegard and Van Doorn, 2009).

Much of the research on acoustic analysis of nasality in the last decade has evaluated the clinical use of the Nasometer. However, there are other similar instruments which provide nasalance scores (Whitehill and Lee, 2008). These include the Nasality Visualization System (Glottal Enterprises Inc., Syracuse, NY) and the NasalView (Tiger Electronics Inc., Seattle, WA), both of which are not widely used clinically. Bressmann, Klaiman and Fischbach (2006) found that there are differences between nasalance scores obtained by the different instruments and concluded that the nasalance scores from these systems are not interchangeable. Spectrographic analysis of hypernasal speech has developed considerably in the last decade and recently attempts have been made to quantify the degree of hypernasality. Whitehill and Lee (2008) reviewed the most recent approaches to evaluating hypernasality using Linear Predictive Coding (LPC) analysis, formant

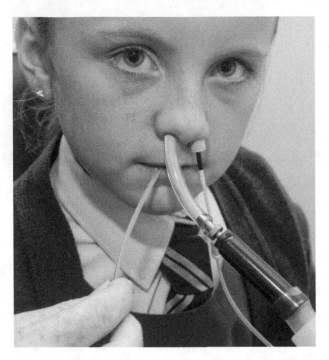

Figure 11.9   Position of oral and nasal tubes for pressure/flow data collection. A nasal flow tube is placed in the right nostril, a nasal pressure tube is placed in the left nostril and an oral pressure tube is placed at the lips.

analysis and one-third-octave spectral analysis and reported that the measures are vowel dependant. Although these approaches might be suitable for clinical assessment in the future, further research into this area is required.

Warren (1979) developed a pressure/flow technique for measuring the velopharyngeal orifice area during sound production. It is based on a modification of the theoretical hydraulic principle, which assumes that the area of an orifice can be determined if the differential pressure across the orifice is measured simultaneously with the rate of flow through it. The PERCI SARS (Speech Aero-Dynamic Research System, MicroTronics, Inc., Chapel Hill, NC) is a computer software/hardware interface for in-depth assessment of speech aeromechanics and nasal airway patency (Figures 11.9 and 11.10).

This computer based system allows for measurements of oral pressure, nasal pressure, oral flow, and nasal flow. Using these measurements, differential pressure and velopharyngeal port area can be calculated. For clinical assessment using PERCI SARS, an appropriately sized nasal flow tube is placed in the most patent nostril and connected to a heated pneumotachograph transducer. The nasal pressure catheter is placed in the least patent nostril and is connected to a pressure transducer. The oral pressure catheter is placed in the patient's mouth ensuring that the tongue does not obstruct the tube and is connected to a pressure transducer. The rate of nasal airflow is measured in litres per

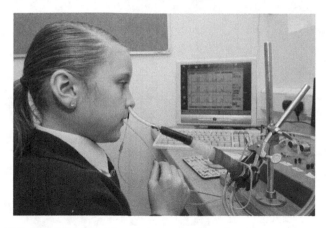

Figure 11.10 PERCI SARS set-up for data collection for measurements of nasal flow and velopharyngeal port area.

second, and nasal and oral pressures are measured in cm H_2O (Zajac, 2008). Figure 11.9 indicates the position of the tubes during assessment, while Figure 11.10 shows the assessment set up for pressure/flow measurements. The patient produces the syllable and word repetitions with the tubes *in situ*, while simultaneous audio recordings of the speech sample are taken.

Pressure/flow measurements are displayed on three separate channels, indicating oral pressure, nasal pressure and nasal flow (Microtronics Corporation, 1994). Audio speech playback permits accurate identification of the peak oral pressure for the /p/ sound. The six highest oral pressure peaks (excluding initial and final peaks) are selected using a cursor, while simultaneous nasal pressure and nasal flow are automatically marked, allowing calculation of mean nasal flow (ml/s) and mean velopharyngeal port area (cm^2) (Microtronics Corporation, 1994). Figure 11.11 indicates oral pressure, nasal pressure and nasal flow during the repetitions of /p/ in 'pa', when produced by a speaker with nasal emission. The pressure flow system can be adapted for assessment of /s/ and an in-depth description of the system has been described by Zajac (2008). Good reliability of the PERCI SARS has been found on test re-test analysis for nasal flow (0.88) and velopharyngeal port area (0.77) using Generalizability Theory (Sweeney, 2000), while Zajac and Mayo (1996) reported good intra-rater agreement for analysis of two normal speakers.

11.4 Interpreting Results

All perceptual and instrumental assessment results must be interpreted in the context of the individual's functioning within their environment. Clinically, assessment results focus on the individual's level of impairment but it is also important to assess the impact of the impairment on the individual's functional performance that is activity and the social consequences. Sell (2005, p. 117) reports on patients who 'had low impairment scores

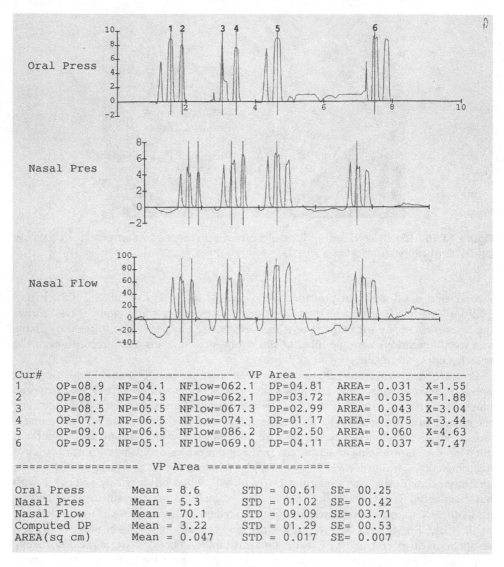

Figure 11.11   Pressure/flow graph indicating oral pressure, nasal pressure and nasal flow during the repetitions of /p/ in 'pa', when produced by a speaker with nasal emission. **Oral press** indicates highest oral peak pressure (cm H_2O) on X axis and time on Y axis. **Nasal pres** indicates nasal pressure (cm H_2O) at peak oral pressure. **Nasal flow** indicates nasal flow in ml/sec during highest peak oral pressure. The section **VP Area** indicates oral pressure, nasal pressure, nasal flow, differential pressure and velopharygeal area measurements at each of the six cursors. The last column **VP Area** presents the mean measurements during the six productions of /p/.

on the perceptual scales but high scores on disability/activity, with observations such as worse when not very well, worse when tired, limiting talking in front of a large group of people, and avoidance of speaking on the telephone. In other words, their speech disorders had significant limiting consequences, disadvantaging them socially'. The same level of impairment can have different consequences for different individuals. Such factors may well influence future management of patients.

Perceptual data must form the basis of all assessment results despite the recognized problems associated with perceptual assessments. The central role of perception in the assessment of disordered speech is not surprising considering that the ultimate goal of speech is communication, and the ultimate test of acceptability of speech involves the perceptual acceptability to the listener (Gerratt *et al.*, 1993). Nasality ratings should be evaluated in the context of the phonological and phonetic repertoire, given that the patient's sound system may influence the perception of nasality.

The relationship between perceptual and instrumental scores needs to be examined while considering that each assessment measures a different characteristic of nasality and/or nasal airflow errors. The instrumentation described in this chapter measures acoustic and aerodynamic correlates of nasality and nasal airflow, while providing additional indirect information regarding velopharyngeal function. There is considerable variation in the literature regarding the relationships between instrumental and perceptual scores (Whitehill and Lee, 2008). This is largely due to the methodological differences in the various studies (Dalston and Warren, 1986; Watterson, Hinton and McFarlane, 1996; Keuning *et al.*, 2002; Dotevall *et al.*, 2002).

However, using the assessment protocol presented in this chapter, good relationships have been found between nasalance scores for the sentence sample containing all consonant types and perceptual ratings of nasality and between nasalance scores for high pressure consonant sentences and perceptual ratings of nasality (Sweeney and Sell, 2008). While good relationships between perceptual ratings of nasal emission and pressure/flow measurements were found, specificity of the pressure/flow measurements was weak. This may be due to the system's capability of detecting inaudible nasal emission (Sweeney, 2000). Interestingly, this study also found a weak non-significant relationship between ratings of nasal turbulence and pressure/flow measurements. Certain factors can influence the relationship between perceptual and instrumental measurements, including the coexistence of nasality and nasal airflow errors (Karnell, 1995), consistency of nasality (Sweeney and Sell, 2008), the acoustic restrictions of the Nasometer (Watterson, McFarlane and Wright, 1993), the presence of articulation or voice problems, the use of a limited speech sample for pressure/flow measurements and the presence of inaudible nasal emission (Sweeney, 2000).

Cut-off scores for nasometry and pressure/flow measurements have been recommended to differentiate between normal and abnormal speakers, by comparing patient scores with mean normal instrumental scores (statistically determined cut-off score), and by comparing the patient's scores with instrumental scores from a clinical population (clinically determined cut-off scores) (Watterson, Lewis and Deutsch, 1998). A combination of statistically and clinically determined cut-off values has been found to produce the best overall efficiency ratings for nasometry and pressure/flow measurements (Sweeney, 2000). A combined perceptual and instrumental assessment protocol provides a valid and reliable assessment of nasality and nasal emission. When both perceptual and instrumental measurements agree, the examiner can have confidence that the findings provide a valid, reliable measurement of speech. When the perceptual and instrumental measurements disagree, the examiner needs to investigate the causes of discrepancies in their results.

The active nasal fricative associated with velopharyngeal mislearning is usually easily perceived during the production of isolated words and at sentence level. Here it usually replaces an oral target, such as /s/ and /z/, but can also be present for /ʃ/ /tʃ/ and /dʒ/. The nasometer may show an unusually high spike on the graph during the production of an active nasal fricative, but it will not distinguish between a nasal fricative and nasal turbulence accompanying a sound. When velopharyngeal mislearning is present the patient has phoneme specific errors and there is usually no evidence of hypernasality or nasal emission/nasal turbulence accompanying oral targets, although in a cleft population it may co-exist with mild hypernasality with perhaps borderline velopharyngeal closure. Nose holding is a good way of distinguishing between an active and a passive nasal fricative (Harding and Grunwell, 1998).

Perceptual data can determine if hypernasality and/or nasal airflow errors are present but it cannot identify the cause of the problem. To differentiate between velopharyngeal insufficiency and velopharyngeal incompetency direct assessment of the velopharyngeal sphincter is required. This usually involves nasendoscopy and palatal videofluoroscopy (Chapter 8). Pressure/flow measurements can help identify timing errors in palatal function, which may be associated with velopharyngeal incompetency. In normal speech production of 'mp' in the word 'hamper', the peak nasal flow is evident before the peak oral pressure indicating the /m/ sound prior to the release of the /p/. Problems in the timing of velopharyngeal closure may result in overlap between nasal flow and oral pressure graphs. Warren, Dalston and Mayo (1993) found that speakers with timing errors had shorter time gaps between the beginning, peak and end of the nasal flow graphs and the beginning, peak and end of the oral pressure graphs than normal speakers. The identification of timing errors using in pressure/flow measurements requires further research.

11.5 Intervention

Speech therapy for nasality and/or nasal airflow errors is not usually appropriate if the cause of the speech disorder is structural, such as velopharyngeal insufficiency, a palatal fistula, or blockage in the nasal cavity where medical or surgical intervention is recommended. It is now generally agreed that patients with moderate to severe hypernasality and/or nasal airflow errors will require further investigations of velopharyngeal function, as these perceptual phenomena are usually indicative of a structural problem, which will not resolve with speech therapy alone and will usually require surgical or prosthetics management (Sell, Mars and Worrell, 2006; Ruscello, 2008).

Speech therapy is recommended for active nasal fricatives due to velopharygeal mislearning, even if there are additional symptoms of VPI. There is a great deal of anecdotal evidence from clinical practice that active nasal fricatives can be eliminated using traditional articulation therapy; however, there is only a small body of research evidence in the literature. Ruscello, Shuster and Sandwisch (1991) presented a single case study of an adult with active nasal fricatives for /s/ and /z/ and reported a successful outcome using conventional articulation therapy and biofeedback with a pressure/flow device. Harland and Albery (1994) reported that 98% of their cohort presenting with velopharyngeal mislearning were successful in eliminating active nasal fricatives with speech therapy alone. In the treatment of active nasal fricatives occlusion of the nostrils can facilitate oral airflow while establishing oral airflow and encouraging correct placement for sounds. Initially, the nostrils are occluded fully; then, pressure on the nostril is reduced gradually so the child can begin to control airflow him/herself. An oral target may also be elicited by encouraging the child to produce an approximation to the target phoneme. For example, /s/ can be elicited from /θ/ or /tsss/ and /tʃ/ can be elicited from /tj/.

Patients with mild hypernasality and/or nasal airflow errors may develop an increase in symptoms following adenoidal atrophy or maxillary advancement surgery as there is an increase in velopharyngeal port size. Thus, patients require speech monitoring for a number of years. Occasionally, therapy for articulation errors is recommended for children who are awaiting velopharyngeal investigations or surgery (Kummer, 2008; Peterson-Falzone, Hardin-Jones and Karnell, 2010). When a child presents with cleft speech characteristics, such as glottal and pharyngeal realizations, limited use of oral pressure consonants and/or the child is stimulable on oral targets, articulation therapy may improve velopharyngeal function, as Henningsson and Isberg (1991) found that velopharyngeal movements were worse when these speech errors were produced. However, additional surgical management is usually required. This trial period of therapy has the advantage of potentially improving placement for oral sounds and increasing velopharyngeal function; however, there is no evidence in the literature regarding efficacy of this approach.

There has been much controversy regarding training programmes for modifying velopharyngeal closure in an effort to improve resonance and eliminate nasal airflow errors. Three main approaches to therapy are oral motor training, such as Talk Tools (Rosenfield-Johnson, 1999), Continuous Positive Airway Pressure (CPAP) therapy (Kuehn *et al.*, 2002) and biofeedback of velopharyngeal function. Oral motor training programmes, with and without speech activities, have been used clinically for the treatment of hypernasality and nasal airflow errors associated with velopharyngeal insufficiency and incompetency despite the lack of evidence to support efficacy (Ruscello, 2008; Peterson-Falzone, Hardin-Jones and Karnell, 2010). In fact, there is a body of evidence that non-speech activities induce velopharyngeal closure patterns that are different from those required for speech (Kummer, 2008), and that these exercise treatments were not successful in changing velopharyngeal function for speech (Ruscello, 2008).

Kuehn *et al.* (2002) describe a muscle resistance therapy known as Continuous Positive Airway Pressure (CPAP) therapy. This approach aims to strengthen the velopharyngeal muscles by applying progressive resistance to the velopharyngeal muscles, using continuous positive airway pressure applied to the nasal cavity, while the patient is speaking. They evaluated changes in hypernasality following eight weeks of therapy using CPAP in 43 patients at eight centres. Results were inconclusive due to various methodological issues and lack of data regarding inter-rater reliability. Biofeedback techniques using nasometry, aerodynamics and nasendoscopy for the treatment of hypernasality and nasal airflow errors are described in the literature (Sell and Grunwell, 2001; Kummer, 2008; Peterson-Falzone, Hardin-Jones and Karnell, 2010) but there is limited evidence of the effectiveness of these treatments. Ysunza *et al.* (1997) reported that videonasendoscopy feedback was useful in changing patterns of velopharyngeal closure and cleft articulatory errors. However, this approach did not eliminate hypernasality and/or nasal airflow errors and all the patients in this cohort required surgical management of VPI.

In summary, there may be some benefits in the use of Continuous Positive Airway Pressure (CPAP) and biofeedback techniques for a small number of patients who have the structural capability to achieve velopharyngeal closure during speech (Ruscello, 2008). It is possible that these patients had evidence of velopharyngeal incompetency rather than insufficiency and it is imperative to differentiate between the different types of VPD when evaluating treatment outcomes.

Prosthetic speech appliances, mainly palatal lifts and speech bulbs, can be used for the treatment of hypernasality and/or nasal airflow errors associated with velopharyngeal insufficiency and incompetency in a small number of patients (Golding-Kushner, Cisneros and LeBlanc, 1995). A palatal lift is a prosthetic appliance that elevates the soft palate into the velopharyngeal sphincter, thereby placing it in a raised position. The device has been used occasionally in the treatment of patients with cleft palate in whom the palate is intact but deficient in movement (Sell, Mars and Worrell, 2006). A speech bulb consists of a dental appliance with an extension which projects behind the palate and terminates in an acrylic bulb, which is positioned in the velopharynx (Sell, Mars and Worrell, 2006). A review of these two speech appliances has been presented elsewhere (Peterson-Falzone, Hardin-Jones and Karnell, 2010). Sell, Mars and Worrell (2006) found significant improvement in hypernasality and nasal emission in a cohort of 16 patients with VPD using a speech bulb. They found that 63% of the group presented with normal nasality, and 55% eliminated nasal emission following intervention. Hyponasality was evident in 19% of the group. They concluded that prosthetics could be effective in treating hypernasality and nasal emission as a permanent solution in carefully selected complex VPD cases or when surgery is not an option.

11.6   Conclusion

Detailed perceptual and instrumental assessment is required in order to identify nasality and nasal airflow problems in patients with repaired cleft palate. Perceptual, acoustic and aerodynamic investigations can provide reliable and valid information regarding the patient's speech status, when specific steps are taken to consider factors that influence nasality and nasal airflow errors. These assessments identify patients who require velopharyngeal investigation and/or speech therapy intervention. To decide on the appropriate intervention the cause of the speech problem must be ascertained, while the impact of the problem on the patient's life must be considered. Although the general consensus is that surgery is the best option for patients with moderate to severe hypernasality and nasal airflow errors of structural aetiology, there is an urgent need for more rigorous research on speech outcomes following surgery. There is much anecdotal evidence that speech therapy is successful for treatment of velopharyngeal mislearning but further research is required to provide evidence to identify those patients that do and those that do not benefit from intervention. These details of speech outcomes will be vital for future evidence based practice.

Appendix 11.A Temple Street Scale of Nasality and Nasal Airflow Errors

Temple street scale – Nasality

Hypernasality:	Present	Absent

a) Mild – evident but acceptable.
b) Mild/Moderate – unacceptable distortion, evident on close vowels.
c) Moderate – evident on close and open vowels.
d) Moderate/Severe – evident on all vowels and some consonants.
e) Severe – evident on all vowels and most voiced consonants.

	Consistent	Inconsistent
Hyponasality:	Present	Absent

a) Mild – evident, but acceptable.
b) Moderate – all vowels reduced nasality.
c) Severe – total denasal production of nasal consonants.

	Consistent	Inconsistent
Cul de Sac:	Present	Absent

Temple street scale – Nasal airflow

Nasal emission:	Frequent	Infrequent
	Consistent	Inconsistent
Nasal turbulence:	Frequent	Infrequent
	Consistent	Inconsistent
Nasal fricative	Present	Absent
	Phoneme specific	

References

Bressmann, T., Klaiman, P. and Fischbach, S. (2006) Same noses, different nasalance scores: data from normal subjects and cleft palate speakers for three systems for nasalance analysis. *Clinical Linguistics & Phonetics*, **20**, 163–170.

Brunnegard, K. and Van Doorn, J. (2009) Normative data on nasalance scores for Swedish as measured on the Nasometer: influence of dialect, gender and age. *Clinical Linguistics & Phonetics*, **23**, 58–69.

Brunnegard, K., Lohmander, A. and Van Doorn, J. (2009) Untrained listeners' ratings of speech disorders in a group with cleft palate: a comparison with speech and language pathologists, ratings. *International Journal of Language and Communication Disorders*, **44**, 656–674.

Bzoch, K.R. (1989) *Communication Disorders Related to Cleft Lip and Palate*, 3rd edn. Little Brown and Co, Boston.

Dalston, R. and Warren, D. (1986) Comparison of Tonar ll, Pressure-Flow, and listener judgements of hypernasality in assessment of velopharyngeal function. *Cleft Palate Journal*, **23**, 108–115.

Dotevall, H., Lohmander-Agerskof, A., Ejnell, H. and Bake, B. (2002) Perceptual evaluation of speech and velopharyngeal function in children with and without cleft palate and the relationship to nasal airflow patterns. *Cleft Palate-Craniofacial Journal*, **39**, 409–423.

Duckworth, M., Allen, G., Hardcastle, W. and Ball, M. (1990) Extensions to the International Phonetic Alphabet for the transcription of atypical speech. *Clinical Linguistics & Phonetics*, **4**, 273–280.

Folkins, J.W. and Moon, J.B. (1990) Approaches to the study of speech production, in *Multidisciplinary Management of Cleft Lip and Palate* (eds J. Bardach and H.L. Morris), W.B. Saunders & Co, Philadelphia, pp. 707–717.

Gerratt, B., Kreiman, J., Antonanzas-Barroso, N. and Berke, G.S. (1993) Comparing internal and external standards in voice quality. *Journal of Speech and Hearing Research*, **36**, 14–20.

Golding-Kushner, K.J., Cisneros, G.J. and LeBlanc, E. (1995) Speech bulbs, in *Cleft Palate Speech Management: A Multidisciplinary Approach* (eds R.J. Shprintzen and J. Bardach), Mosby, St Louis, pp. 352–363.

Harding, A. and Grunwell, P. (1998) Active versus passive cleft-type speech characteristics. *International Journal of Language and Communication Disorders*, **33**, 329–352.

Harland, K. and Albery, E. (1994) Management of 100 cases of phoneme-specific nasal emission: a two centre audit. Presented at the Annual Meeting of the Craniofacial Society of Great Britain and Ireland, Cambridge, UK (April 1994).

Hayden, C. and Klimacka, L. (2000) Inter-rater reliability in cleft palate speech assessment. *Journal of Clinical Excellence*, **2**, 269–173.

Henningsson, G. and Isberg, A. (1991) A cineradiographic study of velopharyngeal movements for deviant versus nondeviant articulation. *Cleft Palate-Craniofacial Journal*, **28**, 115–117.

Henningsson, G., Kuehn, D., Sell, D. *et al.* (2008) Universal parameters for reporting speech outcomes in individuals with cleft palate. *Cleft Palate-Craniofacial Journal*, **45**, 1–17.

John, A., Sell, D., Sweeney, T. *et al.* (2006) The cleft audit protocol for speech- augmented: a validated and reliable measure for auditing cleft speech. *Cleft Palate-Craniofacial Journal*, **43**, 272–288.

Karnell, M.P. (1995) Discrimination of hypernasality and turbulent nasal airflow. *Cleft Palate-Craniofacial Journal*, **32**, 145–148.

Kay Elemetrics Corporation (2003) Nasometer II Model 6400 Instruction manual. Kay Elemetrics Corporation, New Jersey.

Kent, R.D. (1996) Hearing and believing: some limits to the auditory-perceptual assessment of speech and voice disorders. *American Journal of Speech – Language Pathology*, **5**, 7–23.

Keuning, K., Wieneke, G., van Wijngaarden, H. and Dejonckere, P. (2002) The correlation between nasalance and a differential perceptual rating of speech of Dutch patients with velopharyngeal insufficiency. *Cleft Palate-Craniofacial Journal*, **39**, 277–284.

Kreiman, J., Gerratt, B.R., Kempster, G.B. *et al.* (1993) Perceptual evaluation of voice quality: review, tutorial, and a framework for future research. *Journal of Speech and Hearing Research*, **36**, 21–40.

Kuehn, D.P. (1982) Assessment of resonance disorders, in *Speech, Language and Hearing. Vol. 11, Pathologies of Speech and Language* (eds N.J. Lass, L.V. McReynolds, J.C. Northam and D.E. Yoder), W. B. Saunders Co, Philadelphia, pp. 499–524.

Kuehn, D.P. and Moller, K.T. (2000) Speech and language issues in the cleft population: the state of the art. *Cleft Palate-Craniofacial Journal*, **37**, 348–383.

Kuehn, D.P., Imrey, P.B., Tomes, L. *et al.* (2002) Efficacy of continuous positive airway pressure for treatment of hypernasality. *Cleft Palate-Craniofacial Journal*, **39**, 267–276.

Kummer, A.W. (2008) *Cleft Palate and Craniofacial Anomalies: Effects on Speech and Resonance*, 2nd edn. Thomson Delmar Learning, New York.

Kummer, A.W., Curtis, C., Wiggs, M. *et al.* (1992) Comparison of velopharyngeal gap size in patients with hypernasality, hypernasality and nasal emission, or nasal turbulence (rustle) as the primary speech characteristic. *Cleft Palate-Craniofacial Journal*, **29**, 152–156.

Laver, J. (1980) *The Phonetic Description of Voice Quality*, Cambridge University Press, Cambridge.

Lee, A., Brown, S. and Gibbon, F.E. (2008) Effect of listeners' linguistic background on perceptual judgements of hypernasality. *International Journal of Language and Communication Disorders*, **43**, 487–498.

Lee, A., Whitehill, T.L. and Ciocca, V. (2009) Effects of listener training on perceptual judgements of hypernasality. *Clinical Linguistics & Phonetics*, **23**, 319–334.

Lohmander, A., Borell, E., Henningsson, G. *et al.* (2005) *SVANTE: Svenskt Articulations Och Nasalitets Test (Swedish Test of Articulation and Nasality)*, Pedagogisk Design, Malmö.

Lohmander, A., Willadsen, E., Persson, C. *et al.* (2009) Methodology for speech assessment in the Scandcleft project – an international randomized clinical trial on palatal surgery: experiences from a pilot study. *Cleft Palate-Craniofacial Journal*, **46**, 347–363.

McWilliams, B.J., Morris, H. and Shelton, R. (1990) *Cleft Palate Speech*, 2nd edn. B.C. Decker Inc, Philadelphia.

Microtronics Corporation (1994) PERCI Speech-Aeromechanics Research System: system manual. Microtronics Corporation, Chapel Hill, NC.

Moller, K.T. and Starr, C.D. (1984) The effects of listening conditions on speech ratings obtained in a clinical setting. *Cleft Palate Journal*, **21**, 65–69.

Peterson-Falzone, S.J., Hardin-Jones, M.A. and Karnell, M.P. (2010) *Cleft Palate Speech*, 4th edn. Mosby, St Louis.

Rosenfield-Johnson, S. (1999) Horns as therapy tools. Published in ADVANCE magazine. http//www.talktools.net (accessed 29 October 2009).

Ruscello, D.M. (2008) An examination of nonspeech oral motor exercises for children with velopharyngeal inadequacy. *Seminars in Speech and Language*, **39**, 294–303.

Ruscello, D.M., Shuster, L.J. and Sandwisch, A. (1991) Modification of context-specific nasal emission. *Journal of Speech and Hearing Research*, **34**, 27–32.

Seaver, E.J., Dalston, R.M., Leeper, H.A. and Adams, L.E. (1991) A study of nasometric values for normal nasal resonance. *Journal of Speech Hearing Research*, **34**, 715–721.

Sell, D. (2005) Review of issues in perceptual speech analysis in cleft palate and related disorders. *International Journal of Language and Communication Disorders*, **42**, 103–121.

Sell, D. and Grunwell, P. (2001) Speech assessment and therapy, in *Management of Cleft Lip and Palate* (eds A.C.H. Watson, D. Sell and P. Grunwell), Whurr, London, pp. 258–285.

Sell, D., Harding, A. and Grunwell, P. (1999) GOS.SP.ASS'98. An assessment for speech disorders associated with cleft palate and/or velopharyngeal dysfunction (revised). *International Journal of Language and Communication Disorders*, **34**, 17–33.

Sell, D., Mars, M. and Worrell, E. (2006) Process and outcome study of multidisciplinary prosthetic treatment for velopharyngeal dysfunction. *International Journal of Language and Communication Disorders*, **41**, 495–511.

Sell, D., John, A., Harding-Bell, A. and Sweeney, T. (2005) Cleft Speech Diagrams with Phonetic Transcription. Produced for the Cleft Audit for Speech-Augmented training package, Department of Medical Illustrations, Great Ormond Street Hospital, London.

Sell, D., John, A., Harding-Bell, A. *et al.* (2009) CAPS-A: outcomes of a training package for speech and language therapists. *International Journal of Language and Communication Disorders*, **44**, 529–548.

Sweeney, T. (2000) The perceptual and instrumental assessment of nasality and nasal airflow errors associated with velopharyngeal dysfunction. PhD thesis, Trinity College, Dublin, Ireland.

Sweeney, T. and Fennell, G. (2009) Temple Street Scale for assessment of nasality and nasal airflow errors in speech: inter-rater reliability and acceptability. Presented at the 11th international cleft palate and craniofacial congress. Fortaleza, Brazil (September 2009).

Sweeney, T. and Sell, D. (2008) Relationship between perceptual ratings of nasality and nasometry in children/adolescents with cleft palate and/or velopharyngeal dysfunction. *International Journal of Language and Communication Disorders*, **43**, 265–282.

Sweeney, T., Grunwell, P., Leahy, M. *et al.* (1996) Nasality and nasal airflow – definition of terms. *Journal of Clinical Speech and Language Studies*, 6, 65–76.

Sweeney, T., Sell, D. and O'Regan, M. (2004) Nasalance scores for normal-speaking Irish children. *Cleft Palate-Craniofacial Journal*, 41, 168–174.

Trost, J.E. (1981) Articulatory additions to the classic description of the speech of persons with cleft palate. *Cleft Palate Journal*, 18, 193–198.

Vogel, A. and Morgan, A. (2009) Factors affecting the quality of sound recording for speech and voice analysis. *International Journal of Speech-Language Pathology*, 11, 431–437.

Warren, D.W. (1979) Perci: a method for rating palatal efficiency. *Cleft Palate-Craniofacial Journal*, 16, 279–285.

Warren, D.W. (1989) Aerodynamic assessment of velopharyngeal performance, *Communication Disorders Related to Cleft Lip and Palate*, 3rd edn (ed. K.R. Bzoch), Little Brown & Co, Boston, pp. 195–210.

Warren, D.W., Dalston, R.M. and Mayo, R. (1993) Hypernasality in the presence of 'adequate' velopharyngeal closure. *Cleft Palate-Craniofacial Journal*, 30, 150–154.

Watterson, T., McFarlane, S. and Wright, D.S. (1993) The relationship between nasalance and nasality in children with cleft palate. *Journal of Communication Disorders*, 26, 13–28.

Watterson, T., Hinton, J. and McFarlane, S. (1996) Novel stimuli for obtaining nasalance measures in young children. *Cleft Palate-Craniofacial Journal*, 33, 67–73.

Watterson, T., Lewis, K.E. and Deutsch, C. (1998) Nasalance and nasality in low pressure and high pressure speech. *Cleft Palate-Craniofacial Journal*, 35, 293–298.

Whitehill, T.L. (2002) Assessing intelligibility in speakers with cleft palate: a critical review of the literature. *Cleft-Palate-Craniofacial Journal*, 39, 50–58.

Whitehill, T.L. (2010) Rating hypernasality: current challenges and future directions. Presented at the Annual meeting of the speech & language therapy cleft and craniofacial special interest group. Liverpool, UK (April 2010).

Whitehill, T.L. and Lee, A. (2008) Instrumental analysis of resonance in speech impairment, in *Handbook of Clinical Linguistics* (eds M.J. Ball, M.R. Perkins, N. Müller and S. Howard), Blackwell, Oxford, pp. 332–343.

Winholtz, I.R. and Titze, W. (1998) Suitability of Minidisc (MD) recording for voice perturbation analysis. *Journal of Voice*, 12, 138–142.

Ysunza, A., Pamplona, M., Femat, T. *et al.* (1997) Videonasopharyngoscopy as an instrument for visual feedback during speech in cleft palate patients. *International Journal of Pediatric Otorhinolaryngology*, 41, 291–298.

Zajac, D.J. (2008) Speech aerodynamics, *Cleft Palate and Craniofacial Anomalies: Effects on Speech and Resonance*, 2nd edn (ed. A.W. Kummer), Thomson Delmar Learning, New York, pp. 415–445.

Zajac, D.J. and Mayo, R. (1996) Aerodynamic and temporal aspects of velopharyngeal function in normal speakers. *Journal of Speech and Hearing Research*, 39, 1199–1207.

12

Articulation – Instruments for Research and Clinical Practice

Fiona E. Gibbon and Alice Lee

University College Cork, Department of Speech and Hearing Sciences, Cork, Republic of Ireland

12.1 Introduction

Instruments play a relatively minor role in the assessment and treatment of articulation disorders in individuals with cleft palate at the present time. The limited use of instruments for articulation contrasts starkly with their much more widespread use for investigating velopharyngeal function in this clinical population. The value of techniques such as nasendoscopy and videofluoroscopy is undisputed and their routine use in research and specialist cleft palate clinics is testament to this fact. At first sight the underuse of instruments for articulation is puzzling because they have much to offer. Speech involves fast and complex movements of organs located within the vocal tract that are, therefore, largely hidden from view. Our knowledge and understanding of articulation can be greatly enhanced if, in addition to listening to speech, we are able to 'see' what is happening inside the vocal tract space when we speak. The main advantage that instruments have over other techniques is their capacity to provide images and traces of the articulators during speech.

Cleft Palate Speech: Assessment and Intervention, First Edition. Edited by Sara Howard, Anette Lohmander.
© 2011 John Wiley & Sons, Ltd. Published 2011 by John Wiley & Sons, Ltd.

Further advantages lie in instruments' capacity to measure the articulators directly and objectively. Direct measurement reveals details about articulation that are not available from other routine analyses, such as acoustic or perceptual approaches. In reality, the phenomena that instruments measure are much more than the term 'details' implies; they are, more accurately, 'fundamentals' of speech production. Examples of these fundamentals are: location of major constriction; speed and velocity of movement; lateral bracing of the tongue; shape and position of the articulators; tongue grooving; timing and coordination of articulators; and coarticulation. Disruption to any of these functions may occur in cleft palate speech and will lead to diminished speech intelligibility.

This chapter describes a number of instruments that can be used to record articulation in speakers with cleft palate. It is worth mentioning at this point that most techniques were not developed originally for this purpose. Some were developed to investigate normal speech and were subsequently used for disordered speech. Others were developed to investigate different body parts and were later applied to the articulators. In all cases, however, researchers saw the potential value of applying techniques to clinical populations and individuals with cleft palate were an obvious choice. In terms of intervention, the visual feedback provided by some instruments can help children unlearn abnormal compensatory articulations and relearn more normal patterns. Altogether, these factors create a well-defined need in research and clinical practice for instruments applied to the diagnosis and treatment of articulation in cleft palate speech.

The techniques discussed are: electropalatography; imaging techniques (X-ray, ultrasound, magnetic resonance imaging); and motion tracking (electromagnetic articulography, optoelectronic). Although advantages and disadvantages for research and clinical use are suggested, detailed technical descriptions of the instruments are not given; there are excellent surveys available that give comprehensive coverage for the interested reader (Baken and Orlikoff, 2000; Stone, 1997; Thompson-Ward and Murdoch, 1998; Wood and Hardcastle, 2000). Although all the instruments discussed record articulatory data, only two – electropalatography and ultrasound – have a facility to provide visual feedback and the evidence that this type of intervention is effective is reviewed.

12.2   Electropalatography (EPG)

At the forefront of instruments for articulation is electropalatography (EPG). In terms of research and clinical applications, EPG is the most widely used instrument for studying articulation associated with cleft palate. EPG is a technique that detects the tongue's contact against the hard palate during speech and creates a visual display of the resulting patterns. EPG data provide clinically relevant information, such as place of articulation, lateral bracing and groove formation. EPG is ideally suited to recording abnormal articulation in individuals with cleft palate who often have particular difficulties with alveolar speech sounds. In addition to its diagnostic role, a highly attractive feature of EPG is its facility to provide visual feedback. During EPG therapy, children's abnormal articulation patterns are revealed to them on the computer screen and they can use this dynamic visual feedback display to help them produce normal contact patterns.

12.2.1 The Technique

A component of all EPG systems is a custom-made artificial plate moulded to fit the speaker's hard palate. Embedded in the artificial plate are sensors exposed to the lingual surface that detect tongue contact. A number of different EPG systems have been developed although three have dominated over the past 40 years. A British system – developed originally at the University of Reading – was used in the majority of studies conducted in Europe and Hong Kong (Gibbon and Wood, 2010; Hardcastle and Gibbon, 1997). A new Windows® version of the Reading EPG has been developed more recently (WinEPG™, Articulate Instruments Ltd, 2008). The Kay Palatometer was used most widely in the United States (Fletcher, 1983) although there is now a new EPG system manufactured by CompleteSpeechTM, which was formerly known as by Logometrix® (Schmidt, 2007). The Rion EPG was most widely used in Japan (Fujimura, Tatsumi and Kagaya, 1973) but this system has not been available commercially since 1996 (Fujiwara, 2007). All EPG systems share some common general features, but differ in details such as the construction of the plates, number and configuration of sensors, as well as hardware and software specifications (Hardcastle and Gibbon, 1997).

The traditional Reading plates are still manufactured; they are made from a relatively rigid acrylic and are held in place by metal clasps that fit over the upper teeth. There are 62 sensors placed according to identifiable anatomical landmarks. A newer version – the Articulate EPG plate – has a similar design to the Reading plate and is compatible with the Reading EPG systems. It is made using thermoforming and flexible circuits sealed between layers of acrylic plastic (Wrench, 2007). Although it is relatively time consuming and expensive to construct EPG plates, one advantage of being custom made is that they can be tailored to fit individuals with abnormally shaped hard palates, dental anomalies as well as those who wear dental braces or dentures. These types of structural differences frequently occur in individuals with cleft palate, so tailoring of plates to individuals helps to ensure a snug and comfortable fit. A drawback of plates, however, is that they are invasive to the extent that an intraoral device such as this might interfere with natural speech production. Most speakers adapt to wearing the plate in a short period, allowing them to speak naturally with it in place (McLeod and Searl, 2006), although some people have sensitive mouths and find the plate uncomfortable to wear.

Figure 12.1 shows two Reading plates, one for an adult speaker with a normal palatal arch (Figure 12.1a) and one for an adult with a repaired cleft palate (Figure 12.1b). The figure shows how the sensors are arranged in a standard configuration of eight horizontal rows. The sensors are spaced so that the distance between the front four rows is half that of the back four rows. The high concentration of sensors in the alveolar region allows features of tongue-tip articulation, such as grooving during sibilants, to be recorded in detail. In the posterior region, the sensors extend to the junction of the hard and soft palates and in the lateral margins they extend to the gingival border. With the recent modification of the EPG plate design – advancing the first row of sensors by 1 mm and placing the last row of sensors straight across the soft palate – the Articulate EPG plate can now capture linguo-dental articulation and relatively more posterior velar contact (Wrench, 2007).

Figure 12.1c shows a single EPG palatogram, with row numbers 1–8 indicated. Palatograms are schematic displays, which are standard for every speaker regardless of individual differences in the shape and size of the EPG plate. The contact pattern

(a)
(b)

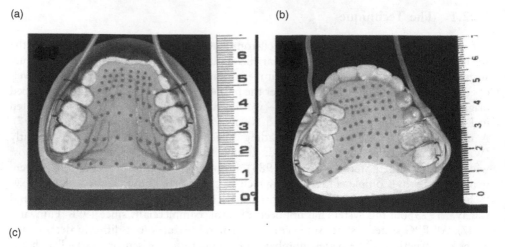

(c)

	Row		
0 0 0 0 0 0	1	Alveolar	Anterior
0 0 0 . . 0 0 0	2		(tongue
0 . . . . . 0 0	3	Post-alveolar	tip/blade)
0 0	4		
0 0	5		
0 0	6	Palatal	Posterior
0 0	7		(tongue
0 0	8	Velar	dorsum)
Lat Cen Lat			

Figure 12.1 Photographs of two artificial plates for the Reading EPG system, placed on top of the plaster model of the hard palate and upper teeth of an adult with normal craniofacial anatomy (a) and an adult with repaired cleft palate who wore a partial denture (b). A schematic palatogram is shown in (c), where tongue palate contact is indicated by zeros; no contact is indicated by dots. (c) shows how palatograms correspond to alveolar, post-alveolar, palatal and velar regions and the tongue tip and tongue body.

displayed in Figure 12.1c is sometimes referred to as a 'horseshoe' shape. This shape reflects contact in the lateral and alveolar regions of the palate and is a typical pattern observed to occur during alveolar stops /t/, /d/ and /n/. Figure 12.1c also indicates how the schematic palatograms broadly correspond to the phonetic regions of the palate (i.e. alveolar, post-alveolar, palatal and velar) and to the relevant active articulators (i.e. tongue tip and tongue body). Dynamic sequences of EPG frames are shown later in Figure 12.2.

(a) /k/ produced as [ǂ] by a 14-year-old girl with velocardiofacial syndrome.

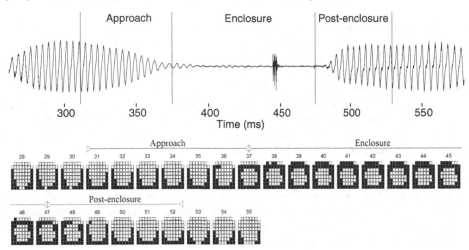

(b) /k/ produced as [k] by a 7-year-old girl with normal velopharyngeal function.

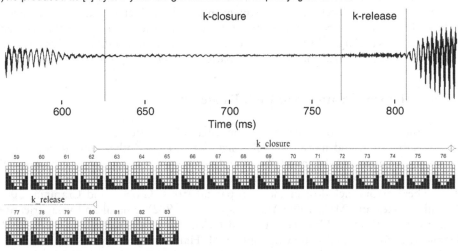

Figure 12.2 EPG printouts for two children's productions of /k/ in the word 'cheeky'. These are full EPG printouts with a sample interval of 10ms. The individual palatograms are numbered and read from left to right. In this printout, the frames occur at 10ms intervals, and tongue contact is indicated by filled black squares along the eight horizontal rows.

12.2.2 Normal Patterns

EPG records characteristic patterns in normal speakers for all English lingual phoneme targets /t/, /d/, /k/, /g/, /s/, /z/, /ʃ/, /ʒ/, /tʃ/, /dʒ/, the palatal approximant /j/, nasals /n/, /ŋ/, and the lateral /l/. Varying amounts of contact are registered during bunched and retroflex varieties of /r/, relatively close vowels, such as /i/, /ɪ/, /e/, /u/, /ʊ/ and rising diphthongs, such as /eɪ/, /aɪ/, /ɔɪ/, /aʊ/, /əʊ/. There is, however, usually minimal contact during open vowels, such as /ɑ/ and /ɒ/. Normative data from adults and children are helpful in identifying abnormal EPG patterns in cleft palate speech and are useful when devising appropriate target patterns when EPG is used for visual feedback therapy (Gibbon and Wood, 2010; Cheng et al., 2007; McLeod and Singh, 2009).

Although previous studies have identified characteristic EPG patterns for consonants and vowels, a consistent finding is that typical speakers vary in the overall amount of contact they produce. Some speakers have twice, or even three times, as much contact as others. Caution is needed when comparing normal and cleft palate data, however. The hard palates of those with cleft palate (at least those who have a cleft of the alveolus) tend to be smaller, narrower and more irregular in shape than those of normal speakers. Further, abnormal dental conditions (e.g. maxillary collapse, dental malalignment, missing teeth, ectopic eruption of teeth, supernumerary teeth and protrusion of the maxilla) as well as malocclusion are frequent in people with cleft palate. These factors will have direct effects on the amount and overall configuration of tongue–palate contact. The above points highlight the importance of taking into account individuals' craniofacial anatomy as well as normal tongue contact patterns when interpreting EPG data.

12.2.3 Abnormal Patterns in Cleft Palate Speech

Overall, the body of knowledge about abnormal EPG patterns associated with cleft palate is substantial and more comprehensive than for any other clinical population. Two studies – Gibbon (2004) and Gibbon and Lee (2010) – summarized approximately 25 articles about abnormal tongue–palate contact in children and adults with cleft palate. These errors included: middorsum palatal stops (Gibbon and Crampin, 2001; Whitehill, Stokes and Man, 1996; Yamashita et al., 1992); palatal and velar fricatives and affricates (Howard, 2004; Howard and Pickstone, 1995; Yamashita et al., 1992); velar plosives (Gibbon, Ellis and Crampin, 2004; Hardcastle, Morgan Barry and Nunn, 1989); lateral fricatives and affricates (Yamashita et al., 1992); lateral release of lingual plosives (Gibbon and Crampin, 2001); labial–velar double articulations (Gibbon and Crampin, 2002); alveolar-velar double articulations (Gibbon, Ellis and Crampin, 2004); pharyngeal and glottal fricatives and stops (Gibbon, 2004); clicks (Gibbon et al., 2008); vowels (Gibbon, Smeaton-Ewins and Crampin, 2005; Yamashita and Michi, 1991); and posterior nasal fricatives (Yamashita et al., 1992).

Collectively, EPG studies have added to our knowledge about the articulation difficulties experienced by individuals with cleft palate. In some studies, the EPG data were able to confirm inferences made about articulation from listener judgments. Here, EPG and listener perceptions were consistent (e.g. the middorsum palatal stops reported by Gibbon and Crampin, 2001). In other studies, the EPG data revealed a higher level of detail about articulator location and timing than could be gained from a perceptual or acoustic analysis. An example comes from an EPG study of clicks (Gibbon *et al.*, 2008). The studies that have really caught the attention of researchers and clinicians, however, are those that have identified new types of compensatory articulations, which are often not detected reliably using perceptually based analysis and, therefore, not described previously in the literature. These studies have stimulated the most debate and created the biggest impact on clinical practice. Three examples where incongruent data led to new insights into cleft palate speech are: labial–velar double articulations; covert contrasts; and complete contact during vowels (Gibbon and Crampin, 2001; Gibbon and Crampin, 2002; Gibbon, Smeaton-Ewins and Crampin, 2005).

Dynamic EPG data illustrating abnormal EPG patterns for the target /k/ in 'cheeky' are shown in Figure 12.2a. For comparison, normal patterns for the same target are in Figure 12.2b. The abnormal production, which was heard as a click, comes from the speech of an adolescent with velocardiofacial syndrome and repaired cleft palate. The sequence of patterns is extracted from a time frame around click production (for a more complete account of clicks; Gibbon *et al.*, 2008). The EPG data in Figure 12.2a reveal that the click involved two articulatory closures, one in the anterior and the other in the posterior region of the palate. The occurrence of two closures is clearly abnormal when compared to the normal data in Figure 12.2b, which shows one closure located in the posterior region of the palate. The data in Figure 12.2a show how the two closures are timed precisely to produce the click sound in a manoeuvre similar to clicks that occur in southern African languages. This example demonstrates the high level of detail available from EPG data, revealing exact tongue position and movement over time.

12.2.4   Visual Feedback Therapy

A principal feature of EPG is its facility to provide real time visual feedback of tongue–palate contact. This moment-to-moment feedback makes EPG unique and distinct from other approaches to therapy for articulation disorders. Under normal circumstances, individuals do not have precise knowledge or awareness about how their tongues move when they speak; the associated internal cues (e.g. tactile, kinaesthetic) are too subtle to perceive clearly or accurately. EPG therapy derives its effectiveness from enabling individuals to develop conscious control of the internal cues associated with tongue activity. Detailed knowledge and awareness about the precise details of their own tongue movements help those who are receiving feedback therapy to change abnormal articulations so that they more closely approximate normal patterns. Using EPG to provide visual feedback is described in numerous previous studies and has been summarized by Gibbon and Wood (2010).

In a typical EPG therapy set up, a person receiving EPG therapy and a speech and language therapist sit side-by-side in front of a computer screen, as shown in Figure 12.3. EPG has the facility for two multiplexers to be connected, one for the child or adult receiving therapy and one for the clinician, with a switch to toggle between the two. When the clinician is connected, it is possible to demonstrate normal contact patterns on the dynamic display. It is also possible to capture or freeze the normal pattern onto the static display. When a person is connected to the EPG equipment, they can see their own tongue patterns. The target EPG pattern used as a model for the child or adult to

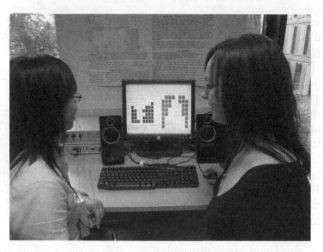

Figure 12.3 Photograph of a typical EPG therapy set up, where the clinician (on the right) uses the EPG feedback function in therapy.

copy in therapy will resemble a normal pattern. However, target patterns are tailored for each individual to ensure that the best perceptual result is achieved.

12.2.5 Empirical Basis

Researchers in Japan pioneered the application of EPG to treating cleft palate speech. In the late 1980s, when researchers in Europe first published some single case studies using EPG with cleft palate speakers, researchers in Japan had already used the technique with nearly 300 individuals (Suzuki, 1989). Over the past 20 years EPG has been used with many clinical populations, although its most frequent application as a treatment tool remains with cleft palate (Gibbon and Wood, 2010). A number of studies have reported positive therapy outcomes in single cases or small groups (Michi *et al.*, 1986; Hardcastle, Morgan Barry and Nunn, 1989; Michi *et al.*, 1993; Whitehill, Stokes and Man, 1996). Although a large number of EPG therapy studies exist, there are limitations in the quality of the evidence about effectiveness. Lee, Law and Gibbon (2009) recently conducted a Cochrane systematic review of studies on EPG therapy for individuals with cleft palate and found that definite conclusions about the efficacy of EPG could not be drawn until high quality, randomized controlled trials were undertaken in the future (Lee, Law and Gibbon, 2009).

12.3 Imaging Techniques

This section covers three techniques: X-ray; ultrasound; and magnetic resonance imaging (MRI). As the name implies, these techniques are capable of recording visual images of the human body primarily for medical diagnosis and have subsequently been used to record the movement and position of the articulators, in particular the tongue. Collectively, these techniques have the advantage of creating the most realistic images of the vocal tract, or parts of it. They also involve minimum disruption to natural speech and some are capable of providing an extensive view of the vocal tract. X-ray has a long history of imaging the vocal tract in people with cleft palate, but so far there are only a few studies of the applications of ultrasound and MRI to this clinical population.

12.3.1 X-Ray

X-ray uses ionizing radiation to obtain images, which makes it possible to view most of the vocal tract, including the moving articulators (e.g. tongue, lips) contrasted against the fixed structures (e.g. hard palate). X-ray presents a composite two-dimensional image of a three-dimensional structure, namely the head. The two-dimensional view can make identifying the soft tissues of the tongue difficult because the bony structures of the jaw and teeth may obscure the view (Stone, 1997). It can also be difficult to identify which part of the tongue (lateral or midline) is being imaged unless a contrast medium is used to mark the midline (Stone, 1997). Images may be still or cine, with static X-ray images of a single posture or vocal tract configuration usually taken from the side of the head in order to create a lateral image. Serial or cineradiography can record dynamic events and was widely used for investigating articulator motion up until the early 1970s (Hiiemae and Palmer, 2003). Fluoroscopic and fluorographic techniques consist of an X-ray image intensifier linked to photographic and video cameras. Videofluorography became widely used in the late 1980s for diagnostic radiological purposes and had the advantage of having lower radiation levels.

X-ray is still used in clinical contexts for imaging the activity of the velum and pharyngeal wall during speech in individuals with cleft palate who may need to undergo surgery to improve velopharyngeal function. Although the primary purpose is to view the velopharyngeal mechanism, it is possible to view at the same time the actions of the tongue, lips and jaw and to observe abnormal behaviour, such as compensatory movements of the tongue. Indeed, a number of previous studies have used X-ray to investigate tongue behaviour in individuals with cleft palate (Brooks, Shelton and Youngstrom, 1965; Powers, 1962; Tanimoto et al., 1994; Trost, 1981). For example, X-ray techniques have been used to investigate pharyngeal or glottal substitutions in cleft palate speech. Trost (1981) used radiography to describe how the pharyngeal stop can be produced at various locations in the pharynx, from high (oropharynx) to low (epiglottis). Kawano et al. (1997) used fluorovideoradiographic data to detect features of the pharyngeal stop in speakers with cleft palate. They found that a higher site (with the tongue base contacting the oropharynx) was observed more frequently in older children and adults and a lower site (at the oro- and laryngopharynx) more frequently in younger children. Secondly, as with previous studies, they noted that the pharyngeal stop is greatly influenced by phonetic context, in other words by preceding and following sounds (Brooks, Shelton and Youngstrom, 1965; Honjo and Isshiki, 1971; Kawano et al., 1997; Trost, 1981). These studies showed that pharyngeal stops occur primarily in the context of low, back vowels, such as /a/, but not high, front vowels such as /i/ (/k/ in these contexts was often produced correctly or as other types of errors). Their explanation of the vowel effect was that the production of pharyngeal stops involves the base of the tongue, and the pharyngeal location is too distal anatomically from that of the high vowels. Nowadays, due to radiation exposure, X-ray techniques are used only for essential medical purposes and not for routine investigation of articulation. The fact that this technique is not biologically safe means that alternative methods are used in research and clinical practice to investigate articulation in individuals with cleft palate.

12.3.2   Ultrasound

Unlike X-ray, ultrasound is biologically safe and although not yet widely applied to cleft palate speech, it is becoming a popular technique to investigate tongue shape and movements in normal speech and swallowing (Chi-Fishman, 2005; Stone, 1991, 1997, 2005). Like EPG, ultrasound has the added attraction of a facility to provide visual feedback, which can be used in speech therapy to modify abnormal articulations. Using ultrasound for imaging the tongue in speech has been pioneered by Maureen Stone and her colleagues over the past 15 years and the reader is directed to Stone (2005) for a description of the technical details and principles of ultrasound and its application to imaging the tongue.

Essentially, ultrasound creates images of body tissue using ultra high frequency sound waves, which create visual images of tongue shape and movement during lingual consonants and vowels of speech (Lundberg and Stone, 1999; Stone, 2005; Stone and Lundberg, 1996). When imaging the tongue, a probe that emits and receives ultrasound waves is placed below the chin and the beam angled upwards. The sound waves travel up through the tongue, and when they reach the boundary between soft tissue and air at the tongue surface, some of the sound waves, or echoes, are reflected back to the probe and are picked up by the probe. A specially designed helmet is usually worn during recordings to stabilize the head and probe. The reflected sound waves are recorded and displayed as real-time visual images of lengthwise (sagittal) or cross-sectional (coronal) views of the tongue.

Figure 12.4 depicts sagittal and coronal ultrasound images of the tongue in the middle of the production of /s/, during the English word 'set' (the tongue tip is on the right in the midsagittal image). It is possible to view much of the tongue's length in the sagittal plane (Figure 12.4a). This figure shows the characteristic bright white line of the tongue, which is the reflection caused by the ultrasound waves from the probe under the chin hitting the air at the tongue surface. The dark area underneath the bright white line is the tongue body. In the sagittal image the mandible and hyoid bone create a shadow (black region) at both edges of the image, obscuring parts of the tongue tip and root. Figure 12.4b is an ultrasound image in the coronal plane, and shows the raised lateral edges of the tongue as well as medial compression.

The figure shows that ultrasound images provide only a partial view; it is often impossible to see the tongue tip and root because the tip is obscured by the air beneath it and the root is obscured by the hyoid bone shadow. Another limitation is that the white line of the tongue surface becomes murky or disappears when there is no air above it, which happens when the tongue makes contact with the hard or soft palate. This factor makes ultrasound more suited to recording aspects of tongue articulation that do not involve complete constriction. A further limitation is that ultrasound does not give images of the vocal tract structures beyond the surface of the tongue, making it difficult to know the tongue's position in relation to the hard and soft palates or the pharynx.

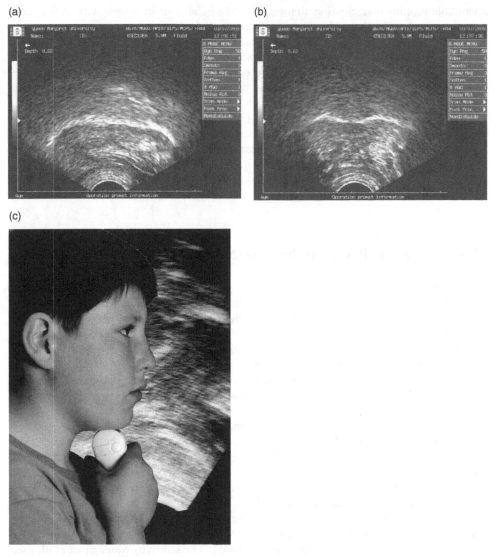

Figure 12.4 An example of a sagittal ultrasound image of the tongue is shown in (a), with the anterior tongue towards the right side of the image. An example of a coronal section is shown in (b). The images are from the middle of the consonant /s/ of the word 'set'. The images are taken by a probe placed below the chin as shown in (c) (Photo courtesy of Sara Howard).

The number of studies using ultrasound for investigating tongue behaviour in adult speech is growing, although there are a limited number reporting its application to the cleft palate population. One exception is a study by Gibbon and Wolters (2005) which used ultrasound to investigate the speech an adult with repaired cleft palate. Although reporting just a single case, this study showed that ultrasound has potential to become a valuable tool for investigating abnormal tongue behaviour in people with cleft palate. An attractive feature that is likely to promote its clinical application in the area of cleft palate is that ultrasound, like EPG, has a facility to provide visual feedback of tongue shape and movement. Ultrasound can display dynamic images of the tongue that are not only relatively intuitive and therefore easy to interpret but are also in real time. These features mean that the technique can be used for visual feedback of tongue shape and position with children and adults with speech disorders (Bernhardt *et al.*, 2005; Shawker and Sonies, 1985). Bernhardt *et al.* (2005) have developed ultrasound treatment guidelines for English lingual stops, vowels, sibilants and liquids based on a series of studies with adolescents and adults with hearing impairment or residual speech impairments. Although a promising new approach, there is a need for adequately controlled studies to determine whether it is beneficial for individuals with articulation disorders associated with cleft palate.

12.3.3   Magnetic Resonance Imaging (MRI)

MRI is another biologically safe, non-invasive technique that gives high quality images of the hard and soft tissues of the full length of the vocal tract, from lips to larynx (Baer *et al.*, 1991; Stone, 1991). MRI uses radiofrequency waves with scanners consisting of electromagnets that surround the body to create a magnetic field. MRI scanning detects the presence of hydrogen atoms with the images highlighting differences in the water content and distribution in body tissues. The result is that tissue with fewer hydrogen atoms, such as bones and air, is dark, whereas tissue with many hydrogen atoms, such as muscle, is lighter. Like ultrasound, MRI scans generate two-dimensional images, which can be combined to produce three-dimensional images. Although MRI is now used increasingly to investigate tongue movement in speech, it has been used primarily to identify abnormal mass (Wein *et al.*, 1991). In the past, the technique's slow temporal resolution made it unsuitable for investigating dynamic aspects of speech. However, recent advances mean that it is now possible to record the dynamics of speech, including segment durations, articulator positions, vocal tract constrictions and inter-articulator timing (Narayanan *et al.*, 2004).

Recent studies of adults with cleft palate have reported dynamic MRI images, which have proved valuable in revealing abnormal features of articulation (Sato-Wakabayashi *et al.*, 2008; Shinagawa *et al.*, 2005). The study by Shinagawa *et al.* used so-called 'MRI movies' to investigate vocal tract constrictions and inter-articulator coordination in an adult with repaired cleft palate and mildly hypernasal speech. These researchers recorded an MRI movie of the sound sequences /pa/, /ta/ and /ka/, which revealed abnormal movements of the tongue, soft palate and posterior pharyngeal wall. Furthermore, velopharyngeal closure was observed during /pa/, /ta/ and /ka/ articulation in the control speaker. A larger study by Sato-Wakabayashi *et al.* (2008) used the same technique of MRI movie. They observed complete velopharyngeal closure in 12 individuals with normal speech during the production of /pa/ and /ka/. In contrast, a speaker with repaired unilateral cleft lip and palate showed reduced movement of the lips, tongue and velum during articulation (Figure 12.5). In summarizing the clinical application of MRI, Shinagawa *et al.* (2005, p.225) state that the dynamic movies are 'a promising

(a)

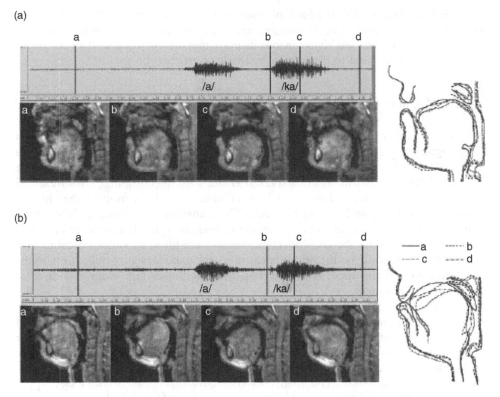

(b)

Figure 12.5 Movement of articulators captured by a magnetic resonance imaging movie during the production of /aka/ by a speaker with bilateral cleft lip and palate (a) and a speaker with normal craniofacial structures (b). (Adapted from Sato-Wakabayashi *et al.*, 2008, p. 314).

tool for evaluating speech function in patients with (cleft lip and palate) because of their non-invasive and non-radiation nature'.

12.4 Motion Tracking

Two varieties of instruments – magnetic and optoelectronic systems – are discussed in this section. They are biologically safe but collectively more invasive and, therefore, more disruptive potentially to natural speech compared to the techniques described in the previous section. The so-called 'point tracking' systems can measure movement of discrete flesh points at high sampling rates. Their capability to measure articulatory kinematics, such as displacement, velocity, acceleration, duration and amplitude, makes them instruments of choice for measuring speech motor control in normal and disordered speech. Despite a growing literature on their use with adults and typical children, only a few report their application to cleft palate speech. The data recorded by these instruments are displayed in the form of traces that are less immediately intuitive, and more difficult to interpret, than the images produced by the techniques already discussed in previous sections. The less than obvious displays may be one reason why these techniques have not been used to provide biofeedback of articulation yet.

12.4.1   Magnetic Systems

The most frequently used magnetic motion capture system used in speech research is electromagnetic articulography (EMA) or electromagnetic midsagittal articulography (EMMA). The two most widely used systems have been developed in Europe (Schönle et al., 1987) and the North America (Perkell et al., 1992). Transmitter coils mounted on a specially constructed helmet form an equilateral triangle in front of the chin, in front of the forehead, and behind the neck. The transmitters produce an alternating magnetic field at different frequencies, making it possible to track movement at points in the vocal tract during speech production. Sensors are glued to various locations on the vocal tract – typically on the bridge of the nose, the maxillary gum ridge (to monitor head movement) on the upper and lower lips, the mandibular gum ridge and three or four points on the tongue.

Few studies report EMA data for cleft palate speech. An exception is one by van Lieshout, Rutjens and Spauwen (2002), which recorded lip kinematics for bilabial sounds in adolescents and young adults with repaired unilateral cleft lip. The results showed that, compared to typical speakers, individuals with cleft lip had reduced range of movement of the upper lip and a more variable spatiotemporal pattern for upper lip movement cycles and inter-lip coupling. They concluded that speakers with a cleft upper lip may have difficulty producing stable movement patterns for bilabials due to reduced movement range or speed for the upper lip. They go on to say 'the fact that bilabials are not affected in a perceptually salient way suggests that the speech production system has a relatively high tolerance for dealing with movement variability' (van Lieshout, Rutjens and Spauwen, 2002, p. 16).

12.4.2   Optoelectronic Systems

An ordinary cine or video camera can be used to investigate the coordinated actions of visually accessible articulators, namely the lips and jaw. More sophisticated optical motion systems, such as Optotrak (Guiard-Marigny and Ostry, 1997), Selspot (Kelso et al., 1985) and VICON (Gibert et al., 2005), can record movement at discrete points located on the lips and jaw in three dimensions. These systems collect movement data with a video camera by attaching small infrared, light emitting diodes or reflective markers to the articulators. The camera tracks the markers attached to the jaw and lips, and using several cameras together makes it possible to measure the movements of each marker. Although the markers used in systems such as VICON may interfere with natural speech to some extent, an important advantage of this technique is that it is one of the few that can record orofacial movements in young children, infants and even new born babies. An obvious limitation of this technique, however, is that it records externally visible structures only and cannot investigate the major articulators situated within the vocal tract. This technique has not been used to study articulation in individuals with cleft palate so far, but future studies could adopt a similar approach to that of Green, Moore and Reilly (2002) to investigate the development of speech in young children with atypical lip and jaw structures associated with craniofacial anomalies.

12.5   Conclusion

The past decade has seen an increase in the variety of instruments available, as well as their technical sophistication and user friendliness. Although generally underused to measure articulation, some of the instruments described in this chapter are becoming more widely available now and research on their application in cleft palate speech is expanding. A reason for the increased interest in some instruments, such as EPG and ultrasound, is their facility to provide visual feedback, which can be used in speech therapy to modify abnormal articulations. The development of new technologies that offer the prospect of more effective diagnosis and treatments is highly desirable in order to improve health care provision and quality of life for individuals with speech disorders associated with cleft palate.

Although the value of instrumental data is high, there is a price to pay and there are challenges to overcome to obtain the data. Many instruments are expensive and have high maintenance and operational costs. The procedural demands of using many techniques make them unsuitable for use with some populations, such as young children or those in poor health. The analysis of instrumental data can be a technically complex and time consuming task and often involves processing large quantities of data. Some techniques are invasive or uncomfortable for the speaker and so are not well suited for gathering naturalistic speech samples or large data sets. Taken together, these factors restrict the use of many instruments to research conducted in specialized laboratories or medical facilities. Overcoming these challenges and translating the results into routine practice requires strong collaborative links between researchers in the academic setting, clinical professionals in the health services, and people who experience articulation disorders in their everyday lives. These links ensure that research is relevant, practical and effectively disseminated.

Acknowledgement

We thank Dr Natasha Zharkova for providing the ultrasound images shown in Figure 12.4.

References

Articulate Instruments Ltd (2008) *Articulate Assistant User Guide (version 1.17) and WinEPG Installation and Users Manual (revision 1.15)*. Articulate Instruments Ltd, Edinburgh, UK.

Baer, T., Gore, J.C., Gracco, L.C. and Nye, P.W. (1991) Analysis of vocal tract shape and dimensions using magnetic resonance imaging: vowels. *Journal of the Acoustical Society of America*, 90, 799–828.

Baken, R.J. and Orlikoff, R.F. (2000) *Clinical Measurement of Speech and Voice*, 2nd edn. Singular, San Diego.

Bernhardt, B., Gick, B., Bacsfalvi, P. and Adler-Bock, M. (2005) Ultrasound in speech therapy with adolescents and adults. *Clinical Linguistics & Phonetics*, 19, 605–617.

Brooks, A.R., Shelton, R.L. and Youngstrom, K.A. (1965) Compensatory tongue-palate-posterior pharyngeal wall relationships in cleft palate. *Journal of Speech and Hearing Disorders*, 30, 166–173.

Cheng, H.Y., Murdoch, B.E., Goozée, J.V. and Scott, D. (2007) Electropalatographic assessment of tongue-to-palate contact patterns and variability in children, adolescents, and adults. *Journal of Speech, Language, and Hearing Research*, 50, 375–392.

Chi-Fishman, G. (2005) Quantitative lingual, pharyngeal and laryngeal ultrasonography in swallowing research: a technical review. *Clinical Linguistics & Phonetics*, 19, 589–604.

Fletcher, S. (1983) New prospects for speech by the hearing impaired, in *Speech and Language: Advances in Basic Research and Practice* (ed. N. Lass), Academic Press, New York, pp. 1–42.

Fujimura, O., Tatsumi, I.F. and Kagaya, R. (1973) Computational processing of palatographic patterns. *Journal of Phonetics*, 1, 47–54.

Fujiwara, Y. (2007) Electropalatography home training using a portable training unit for Japanese children with cleft palate. *Advances in Speech-Language Pathology*, 9, 65–72.

Gibbon, F.E. (2004) Abnormal patterns of tongue-palate contact in the speech of individuals with cleft palate. *Clinical Linguistics & Phonetics*, 18, 285–311.

Gibbon, F.E. and Crampin, L. (2001) An electropalatographic investigation of middorsum palatal stops in an adult with repaired cleft palate. *Cleft Palate-Craniofacial Journal*, 38, 96–105.

Gibbon, F.E. and Crampin, L. (2002) Labial-lingual double articulations in cleft palate speech. *Cleft Palate-Craniofacial Journal*, 39, 40–49.

Gibbon, F.E. and Lee, A. (2010) Producing turbulent speech sounds in the context of cleft palate, in *Turbulent Sounds: An Interdisciplinary Guide* (eds S. Fuchs, M. Zygis, C. Shadle and M. Toda), DeGruyter, Germany, pp. 303–341.

Gibbon, F.E., Ellis, L. and Crampin, L. (2004) Articulatory placement for /t/, /d/, /k/ and /g/ targets in school age children with speech disorders associated with cleft palate. *Clinical Linguistics & Phonetics*, 18, 391–404.

Gibbon, F.E. and Wolters, M. (2005) A new application of ultrasound to image tongue behaviour in cleft palate speech. Poster presentation at the Craniofacial Society of Great Britain and Ireland Annual Scientific Conference, Swansea, UK (13–15 April 2005).

Gibbon, F.E. and Wood, S. (2010) Visual feedback therapy with electropalatography (EPG) for speech sound disorders in children, in *Interventions in Speech Sound Disorders* (eds L. Williams, S. McLeod and R. McCauley), Brookes, Baltimore, pp. 509–536.

Gibbon, F.E., Smeaton-Ewins, P. and Crampin, L. (2005) Tongue-palate contact during selected vowels in children with cleft palate. *Folia Phoniatrica and Logopaedica*, 4, 181–192.

Gibbon, F.E., Lee, A., Yuen, I. and Crampin, L. (2008) Clicks produced as compensatory articulations in two adolescents with velocardiofacial syndrome. *Cleft Palate-Craniofacial Journal*, 45, 381–392.

Gibert, G., Bailly, G., Beautemps, D. *et al.* (2005) Analysis and synthesis of the three-dimensional movements of the head, face and hand of a speaker using cued speech. *Journal of the Acoustical Society of America*, 118, 1144–1153.

Green, J.R., Moore, C.A. and Reilly, K.J. (2002) The sequential development of jaw and lip control for speech. *Journal of Speech, Language, and Hearing Research*, 45, 66–79.

Guiard-Marigny, T. and Ostry, D.J. (1997) A system for three-dimensional visualization of human jaw motion in speech. *Journal of Speech, Language, and Hearing Research*, 40, 1118–1121.

Hardcastle, W.J. and Gibbon, F.E. (1997) Electropalatography and its clinical applications, in *Instrumental Clinical Phonetics* (eds M.J. Ball and C. Code), Whurr Publishers, London, pp. 149–193.

Hardcastle, W., Morgan Barry, R. and Nunn, M. (1989) Instrumental articulatory phonetics in assessment and remediation: case studies with the electropalatograph, in *Cleft Palate: The Nature and Remediation of Communication Problems* (ed. J. Stengelhofen), Churchill Livingstone, Edinburgh, pp. 136–164.

Hiiemae, K.M. and Palmer, J.B. (2003) Tongue movements in feeding and speech. *Critical Reviews in Oral Biology and Medicine*, **14**, 413–429.

Honjo, I. and Isshiki, N. (1971) Pharyngeal stop in cleft palate speech. *Folia Phoniatrica*, **23**, 347–354.

Howard, S. (2004) Compensatory articulatory behaviours in adolescents with cleft palate: comparing the perceptual and instrumental evidence. *Clinical Linguistics & Phonetics*, **18**, 313–340.

Howard, S. and Pickstone, C. (1995) Cleft palate: perceptual and instrumental analysis of a phonological system, in *Case Studies in Clinical Linguistics* (eds M. Perkins and S. Howard), Whurr Publishers, London, pp. 65–90.

Kawano, M., Isshiki, N., Honjo, I. *et al.* (1997) Recent progress in treating patients with cleft palate. *Folia Phoniatrica et Logopaedica*, **49**, 117–138.

Kelso, J.A.S., Vatikiotis-Bateson, E., Saltzman, E.L. and Kay, B. (1985) A qualitative dynamic analysis of reiterant speech production: phase portraits, kinematics, and dynamic modeling. *Journal of the Acoustical Society of America*, **77**, 266–280.

Lee, A., Law, J. and Gibbon, F.E. (2009) Electropalatography for Articulation Disorders Associated with Cleft Palate. *Cochrane Database of Systematic Reviews* 3 (Art. No.: CD006854). doi: 10.1002/14651858.CD006854.pub2.

Lundberg, A. and Stone, M. (1999) Three-dimensional tongue surface reconstruction: practical considerations for ultrasound data. *Journal of the Acoustical Society of America*, **106**, 2858–2867.

McLeod, S. and Searl, J. (2006) Adaptation to an electropalatography palate: acoustic, impressionistic, and perceptual data. *American Journal of Speech-Language Pathology*, **15**, 192–206.

McLeod, S. and Singh, S. (2009) *Speech Sounds: A Pictorial Guide to Typical and Atypical Speech*, Plural Publishing, San Diego.

Michi, K., Suzuki, N., Yamashita, Y. and Imai, S. (1986) Visual training and correction of articulation disorders by use of dynamic palatography: serial observation in a case of cleft palate. *Journal of Speech and Hearing Disorders*, **51**, 226–238.

Michi, K., Yamashita, Y., Imai, S. *et al.* (1993) Role of visual feedback treatment for defective /s/ sounds in patients with cleft palate. *Journal of Speech and Hearing Research*, **36**, 277–285.

Narayanan, S., Nayak, K., Lee, S. *et al.* (2004) An approach to real-time magnetic resonance imaging for speech production. *Journal of the Acoustical Society of America*, **115**, 1771–1776.

Perkell, J.S., Cohen, M.H., Svirsky, M.A. *et al.* (1992) Electromagnetic midsagittal articulometer systems for transducing speech articulatory movements. *Journal of the Acoustical Society of America*, **92**, 3078–3096.

Powers, G.R. (1962) Cinefluorographic investigation of articulatory movements of selected individuals with cleft palates. *Journal of Speech and Hearing Research*, **5**, 59–69.

Sato-Wakabayashi, M., Inoue-Arai, M.S., Ono, T. *et al.* (2008) Combined fMRI ad MRI movie in the evaluation of articulation in subjects with and without cleft lip and palate. *Cleft Palate-Craniofacial Journal*, **45**, 309–314.

Schmidt, A.M. (2007) Evaluating a new clinical palatometry system. *Advances in Speech-Language Pathology*, **9**, 73–81.

Schönle, P.W., Gräbe, K., Wenig, P. *et al.* (1987) Electromagnetic articulography: use of alternating magnetic fields for tracking movements of multiple points inside and outside the vocal tract. *Brain and Language*, **31**, 26–35.

Shawker, T.H. and Sonies, B.C. (1985) Ultrasound biofeedback for speech training: instrumentation and preliminary results. *Investigative Radiology*, **20**, 90–93.

Shinagawa, H., Ono, T., Honda, E. *et al.* (2005) Dynamic analysis of articulatory movement using magnetic resonance imaging movies: methods and implications in cleft lip and palate. *Cleft Palate-Craniofacial Journal*, **42**, 225–230.

Stone, M. (1991) Towards a model of three-dimensional tongue movement. *Journal of Phonetics*, **19**, 309–320.

Stone, M. (1997) Laboratory techniques for investigating speech articulation, in *The Handbook of Phonetic Sciences* (eds W.J. Hardcastle and J. Laver), Blackwell Publishers, Oxford, pp. 11–32.

Stone, M. (2005) A guide to analysing tongue motion from ultrasound images. *Clinical Linguistics & Phonetics*, **19**, 455–501.

Stone, M. and Lundberg, A. (1996) Three-dimensional tongue surface shapes of English consonants and vowels. *Journal of the Acoustical Society of America*, **99**, 3728–3737.

Suzuki, N. (1989) Clinical applications of EPG to Japanese cleft palate and glossectomy patients. *Clinical Linguistics & Phonetics*, **3**, 127–136.

Tanimoto, K., Henningsson, G., Isberg, A. and Ren, Y.F. (1994) Comparison of tongue position during speech before and after pharyngeal flap surgery in hypernasal speakers. *Cleft Palate-Craniofacial Journal*, **31**, 280–286.

Thompson-Ward, E.C. and Murdoch, B.E. (1998) Instrumental assessment of the speech mechanism, in *Dysarthria: A Physiological Approach* (ed. B.E. Murdoch), Stanley Thornes, Cheltenham, pp. 68–101.

Trost, J.E. (1981) Articulatory additions to the classical description of the speech of persons with cleft palate. *Cleft Palate Journal*, **18**, 193–203.

van Lieshout, P.H., Rutjens, C.A. and Spauwen, P.H. (2002) The dynamics of interlip coupling in speakers with a repaired unilateral cleft-lip history. *Journal of Speech, Language, and Hearing Research*, **45**, 5–19.

Wein, B.B., Drobnitzky, M., Klajman, S. and Angerstein, W. (1991) Evaluation of functional positions of tongue and soft palate with MR imaging: initial clinical results. *Journal of Magnetic Resonance Imaging*, **1**, 381–383.

Whitehill, T.L., Stokes, S.F. and Man, Y.H.Y. (1996) Electropalatography treatment in an adult with late repair of cleft palate. *Cleft Palate-Craniofacial Journal*, **33**, 160–168.

Wood, S. and Hardcastle, W.J. (2000) Instrumentation in the assessment and therapy of motor-speech disorders: a survey of techniques and case studies with EPG, in *Acquired Neurogenic Communication Disorders: A Clinical Perspective* (ed. I. Papathanasiou), Whurr Publishers, London, pp. 203–248.

Wrench, A.A. (2007) Advances in EPG palate design. *Advances in Speech-Language Pathology*, **9**, 3–12.

Yamashita, Y. and Michi, K. (1991) Misarticulation caused by abnormal lingual-palatal contact in patients with cleft palate with adequate velopharyngeal function. *Cleft Palate-Craniofacial Journal*, **28**, 360–366.

Yamashita, Y., Michi, K., Imai, S. *et al.* (1992) Electropalatographic investigation of abnormal lingual-palatal contact patterns in cleft palate patients. *Clinical Linguistics & Phonetics*, **6**, 201–217.

13

Psycholinguistic Assessment and Intervention

Joy Stackhouse

University of Sheffield, Department of Human Communication Sciences, Sheffield, S10 2TA, UK

13.1   Introduction

This chapter aims to introduce a psycholinguistic approach to readers with a particular interest in cleft lip and palate and associated conditions. It is divided into four parts:

- What is a Psycholinguistic Approach?

- A Psycholinguistic Assessment Framework

- Intervention from a Psycholinguistic Perspective

- Literacy: Phonological Awareness and Spelling

The chapter focuses mainly on school-age children and so the term 'child' is used throughout. However, the psycholinguistic approach has been adopted across the

Cleft Palate Speech: Assessment and Intervention, First Edition. Edited by Sara Howard, Anette Lohmander.
© 2011 John Wiley & Sons, Ltd. Published 2011 by John Wiley & Sons, Ltd.

life span from toddlers and pre-school children through to adolescence and adulthood. SLT represents speech and language therapist specifically but the terms 'adult' or 'user' are used generally to denote that psycholinguistic activities are often carried out by parents or teaching staff. CLP is used as an abbreviation to refer to children with cleft lip and palate, velopharyngeal incompetence and associated conditions/syndromes

13.2   What is a Psycholinguistic Approach?

A psycholinguistic approach is just one of the approaches that it is necessary to include when working with children with speech difficulties arising from CLP; it does not stand alone or replace any other. The other approaches include medical, linguistic, developmental, educational and psychosocial. To understand the contribution a psycholinguistic approach makes, it helps to compare it with these and examine how each might influence our assessment and management of a child with CLP.

13.2.1   Medical Approach

The medical approach looks for 'aetiology' and a 'diagnosis' as a basis for intervention. This results in classification models based on possible causes, for example speech difficulties arising from CLP, or hearing loss, or dyspraxia (Shriberg *et al.*, 1997). It is particularly important when working with children with CLP as medical intervention may be part of their management, for example surgery. However, there is not necessarily a one to one match between a diagnostic label and how that condition manifests itself in a child's speech, language and literacy performance. Further, children with CLP form heterogeneous groups with regards to their speech and language development (Morris and Ozanne, 2003). It is therefore important to take on board other perspectives, even when there appears to be an obvious medical 'cause' for a child's communication difficulty.

13.2.2   Linguistic Approach

A linguistic approach describes a child's speech difficulties through phonetic, phonological and prosodic analyses. It allows us to establish if a child has a limited phonetic inventory for the language(s) they speak and if this is affecting their phonological performance, that is how they contrast sounds to convey meaning. This description can be particularly challenging when working with children with CLP and may involve advanced phonetic skills on the part of the transcriber (Chapter 7). A linguistic approach also allows a description of a child's language performance in terms of their morphology, syntax, semantics and pragmatics. Carrying out a linguistic assessment is not dependant on knowing what has caused a child's speech difficulties. Its aim is to have sufficient information to plan appropriate speech targets for intervention.

13.2.3   A Developmental Approach

This is important when working with children who, regardless of any special needs, are constantly changing. By combining the linguistic approach with a developmental one, it can be established if a child's speech performance is delayed for their age and if it is following a typical or atypical pathway. Children with CLP may have atypical speech characteristics; for example, 'backing' (e.g. /t/ → [k]), a common speech characteristic of children with cleft palate, is the opposite of 'fronting', a 'normal simplifying process' evident in the speech of typically developing young children (Ingram, 1976). However, a child with CLP may also have features of speech delay as well as age appropriate utterances. A unique role of an SLT is to understand this mix and establish what speech aspects are directly related to the structural capabilities of the child, what are compensatory productions and what, if any, fall into the category of developmental immaturities. Each of these may be targeted differently in an intervention programme.

13.2.4   Psycholinguistic Approach

A psycholinguistic approach attempts to bridge the gap between the medical and linguistic approaches while maintaining a developmental perspective. It addresses what might be causing a child's speech difficulties in terms of their underlying speech processing skills. This is done with reference to theoretical models of speech processing that attempt to describe how we process speech input, programme speech output and keep a store of information about speech and language that we can use as needed (Baker *et al.*, 2001). This can be represented in the simple speech processing model presented in Figure 13.1.

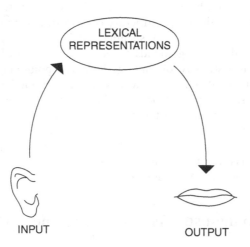

Figure 13.1   A simple speech processing model (from Stackhouse and Wells, 1997, p. 9). Reproduced with permission of John Wiley & Sons, Ltd.

The basic premise of a psycholinguistic approach is that children's speech difficulties arise at one or more points around this speech processing model. A child born with CLP has a difficulty at the bottom right of the model, that is, in the mouth. However, this does not preclude processing difficulties elsewhere in the model at either the input or output sides, or both. A fundamental principle of a psycholinguistic approach is to ignore any diagnostic labels initially (e.g. CLP, dyspraxia, stammer, dyslexia) and to establish an unbiased view of a child's speech processing skills. A psycholinguistic assessment therefore checks a child's speech input and output skills, and the precision of their lexical representations, that is, how well information about a word has been stored. This information includes:

- meaning (semantics);

- morphology (e.g. plural marking) and grammatical use (e.g. in a sentence);

- phonological information sufficient to distinguish between similar sounding words for example 'key' vs 'tea';

- a motor programme for accuracy and efficiency of production;

- the written form to allow automatic recognition of a word in print and ease of spelling.

Integral to the psycholinguistic approach presented here is that literacy development is also dependant on an intact speech processing system. For example, difficulty discriminating between similar sounding words will lead to 'fuzzy' representations being stored, which will not only impact on speech performance but also on spelling, since the child is not sure what letters to use to represent these imprecise 'sounds' (Stackhouse, 2006). Difficulties with speech production, particularly if inconsistent, can interfere with a child's ability to reflect on the sound structure of a word and to decide what it begins or ends with, another necessary skill for spelling. Similarly, motor programming difficulties can prevent a child blending sounds together to form words, which inhibits the development of a phonics strategy for reading; there is no point in learning how to sound out letters in order to read unfamiliar words if they cannot be blended together to produce the word. In short, speech processing difficulties can interfere with the development of 'phonological awareness' – the ability to reflect on the sound structure of a word as opposed to its meaning, a necessary skill for literacy to develop in alphabetic languages. Given literacy is essential for accessing the school curriculum and fulfilling academic potential, it is important to maintain an educational perspective when working with children with speech and language difficulties.

13.3   A Psycholinguistic Assessment Framework

The Psycholinguistic Framework developed by Stackhouse and Wells (1997) for practice and research comprises three key components:

1. Speech Processing Profile – a means of collating assessment results as a basis for intervention.

2. Box and Arrow Model – to allow further theoretical interpretation of a child's performance.

3. Developmental Phase Model – to chart the relationship between a child's speech and literacy development.

This chapter focuses on the first component: the Speech Processing Profile (Figure 13.2).

This profile drives an assessment as well as records its findings. It is based on the simple speech processing model illustrated in Figure 13.1. Input skills are represented on the left of the profile and output skills on the right. Bottom left (A) is at the level of the ear and bottom right (K) is at the level of the mouth. The higher the question on the profile the nearer it is to the stored representations at the top of the model. Assessments at this level require the child to access information stored in their lexical representations, for example naming pictures is at top right: Level G. A child's speech processing profile of strengths and weaknesses is constructed by providing answers to at least some of the questions posed in A–L. The 'answers' may be derived from observations of speech behaviour, informal tasks or spontaneous play, a child's own reflections of their speech processing skills, or more formal assessment procedures and standardized tests. In short, the psycholinguistic approach is a very flexible one, since it is 'an approach carried in the head of the user and not in a case of tests' (Stackhouse and Wells, 1997, p. 49), that is, it is a way of thinking about a child's skills and can take as little or as much time as is wished.

Not every question needs to be answered in order to plan therapy in everyday practice. A typical way of completing this profile is to place a tick in boxes where the child is performing within normal limits for their age and put a cross where they are not. Sometimes these ticks and crosses are based on the adult's knowledge of what is typical performance, or are used to mark relative difficulties within the child; for example, although the child is struggling with many speech processing tasks they struggle less with some (marked by one X) than others (marked by two XX). On other occasions normative data are available and a child's difficulties in terms of distance from the mean in standard deviations (sds) can be recorded more objectively, for example X = –1 sd, XX = –2 sd, XXX = –3 sd (examples of completed profiles are given in Pascoe, Stackhouse and Wells, 2006, and Stackhouse and Wells 2001).

13.3.1   Principles of a Psycholinguistic Assessment

To carry the approach in your head, the following three key questions need to be asked about an assessment task in order to understand 'What do Tests Really Test?' in psycholinguistic terms:

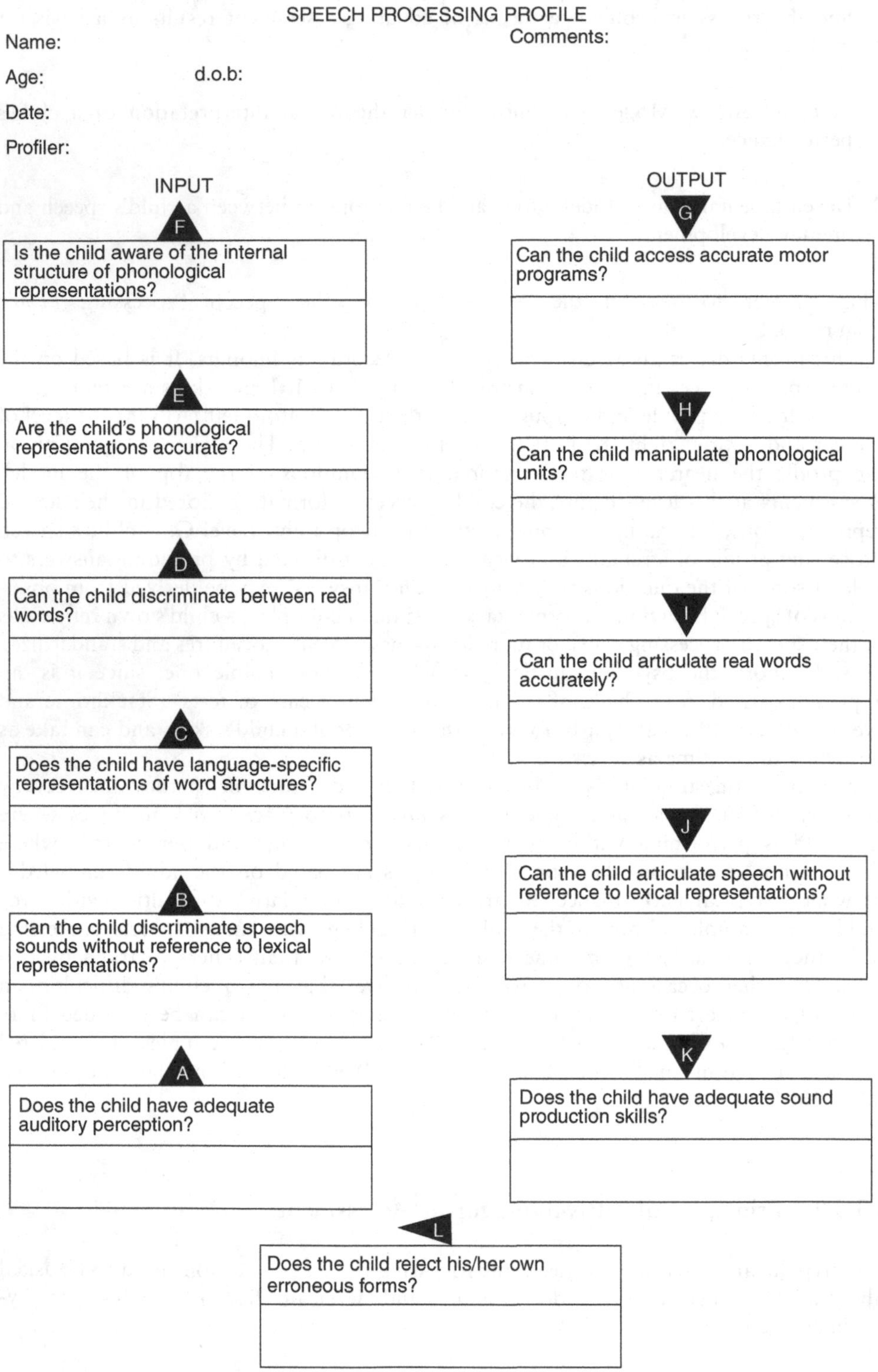

SPEECH PROCESSING PROFILE

Name: Comments:

Age: d.o.b:

Date:

Profiler:

INPUT

F
Is the child aware of the internal structure of phonological representations?

E
Are the child's phonological representations accurate?

D
Can the child discriminate between real words?

C
Does the child have language-specific representations of word structures?

B
Can the child discriminate speech sounds without reference to lexical representations?

A
Does the child have adequate auditory perception?

OUTPUT

G
Can the child access accurate motor programs?

H
Can the child manipulate phonological units?

I
Can the child articulate real words accurately?

J
Can the child articulate speech without reference to lexical representations?

K
Does the child have adequate sound production skills?

L
Does the child reject his/her own erroneous forms?

Figure 13.2 The speech processing profile (from Stackhouse and Wells, 1997). Reproduced with permission of John Wiley & Sons, Ltd.

1. *'Does the task tap input or output skills?'* An output task requires more from the child than saying 'yes' or 'no'. It should generate different answers for each item, for example producing a string of rhyming words.

2. *'Does the child have lexical representations for the stimuli used in the task?'* If the answer to this question is 'Yes', then the task is tapping a higher level on the profile. However, just because a child 'knows' the stimuli (e.g. if a familiar word) it does not follow that they *do* access their representations fully in order to complete the task. For example, it is possible to decide if two spoken words sound the same or different without accessing all stored information about the word. A third question is therefore required.

3. *Does the child **have to** access their lexical representations to successfully complete the task?* Tasks involving pictures where the adult does not name the stimuli require the child to access their own representations of the stimuli. For example, if asked to look at three pictures and decide which two rhyme the child has to access the words from their own representations and then reflect on what these sound like without any help being provided by the adult.

To help users of the assessment framework, this analysis has been carried out on a range of speech input and output tasks designed to answer the questions on the profile (Stackhouse and Wells, 1997) and a compendium of speech processing tasks with a CD-ROM of the stimuli has been produced (Stackhouse *et al.*, 2007). These tasks include auditory discrimination of simple and complex real and non-words; mispronunciation detection tasks to check precision of the representations and word-finding skill; naming and repetition tasks to compare a child's performance based on their own representations with that following the adult model; connected speech tasks; stimulability; and consistency and diadochokinetic tasks. However, as the essence of a psycholinguistic approach is that it is 'within the head of the user', assessment procedures designed for individual children are encouraged. For example, if on a naming test a child produces 'car' for 'tar', it is important to know if that speech error is derived from a speech output difficulty alone or compounded by speech input problems. It is necessary, therefore, to carry out a simple input task, for example auditory discrimination of minimal pair words which involve the child's speech target and error (e.g. tar ~ car; tea ~ key).

Using the Speech Processing Profile allows a range of assessment findings to be collated systematically on one sheet and for progress to be monitored over time. It has been used in research to predict children at risk for persisting speech and literacy problems (Nathan, *et al.*, 2004a; Stackhouse *et al.*, 2007), to investigate stored representations (Claessen, Leitao and Barrett, 2010) and to uncover hidden speech processing difficulties (Nathan and Simpson, 2001). Most of all, however, it is a basis for planning and evaluating intervention and has been used specifically with children with CLP (Patrick, 2005).

13.4   Intervention from a Psycholinguistic Perspective

A basic principle when planning intervention within a psycholinguistic framework is that a child's speech processing strengths can be used to support any weaknesses.

Another is that there are no specific 'psycholinguistic' resources for this. All familiar therapy activities can be used in a psycholinguistic way if the user thinks in that way. The *Nuffield Centre Dyspraxia Programme* (Williams and Stephens, 2004) is a good example of how a programme originally designed to improve articulatory production can be reinterpreted to deliver a psycholinguistic approach (see Stackhouse and Pascoe, 2010, for a DVD illustrating this). However, as stated at the beginning of this chapter, a psycholinguistic approach is not used in isolation. It is important to have the information derived from other approaches to develop the hypotheses on which the intervention will be based.

13.4.1   Interaction between Psycholinguistic and Medical Intervention

If a child with a CLP is producing speech as well as they can given their atypical structure and is awaiting corrective surgery, there is little point in targeting articulation directly. Indeed, such children may not be seen by an SLT during this time. A child with intact speech processing skills (ticks all round the profile presented in Figure 13.2) who is developing literacy normally should not be disadvantaged by this wait. However, a child with speech input difficulties, who is also having trouble developing phonological awareness and literacy could benefit from intervention which targets these areas and sharpens up their lexical representations as a foundation for speech production intervention post-surgery. The adoption of 'input modelling' with young children with CLP serves a similar purpose (Calladine, 2009; Chapter 15).

13.4.2   Interaction between Psycholinguistic and Linguistic Intervention

The data derived from phonetic and phonological analyses indicate *what* needs to be worked on in therapy; for example, what 'sounds' or 'utterances' to target. It helps us to decide if a child needs articulation therapy to improve sound production; or phonological therapy to use segments contrastively to convey meaning; or, as is more likely with persisting and complex speech difficulties associated with CLP or Childhood Apraxia of Speech, articulation practice for some aspects of speech production and phonological therapy for others (Stackhouse, Pascoe and Gardner, 2006).

   The data derived from a psycholinguistic assessment indicate *how* to work on the chosen targets; for example, can auditory discrimination be used as a strength in therapy to support output? (Waters, Hawkes and Burnett, 1998; Waters, 2001); are phonological awareness skills or written words a target for intervention or support for speech production? Although a psycholinguistic approach is typically based on individual profiles it does not necessarily follow that intervention is given on a one-to-one basis. Successful intervention can be carried out in groups and, as long as directed by a trained user (normally the SLT), activities can be delivered by parents, teachers/teaching assistant or peers. Whatever the format, intervention tasks are likely to incorporate the following: auditory discrimination; articulatory ease as a prerequisite to phonological therapy; mispronunciation detection to sharpen the representations; phonological awareness to heighten generalization of sound production and support literacy development; self-monitoring to ensure independence from the adult; and, depending on the age of the child, reading and spelling activities to develop the lexical representations further and to support speech production.

13.4.3   Task Design

This is a key feature of a psycholinguistic approach. Having addressed 'What Do Tests Really Test?' at the assessment phase, intervention can now be asked about ' What Do Tasks Really Tap?'

A 'task' includes any materials used for intervention, the procedure followed (including any instructions), the feedback given to the child (verbal or visual) and any technique used to support speech processing, (e.g. cueing through signs or symbols). This is summarized by Rees (2001, p67) as follows:

TASK = Materials + Procedure + Feedback +/– Technique

Learning to use a psycholinguistic approach involves working through the following three levels, level 3 being the most advanced:

1. Design intervention tasks based on the above equation.

2. Understand why altering any one of the four components, even minimally, can change the psycholinguistic demands made on the child.

3. Use this knowledge to manipulate tasks at the time of delivery to meet the needs of the child, that is, how to make a task easier or more challenging depending on the child's response.

To help achieve these levels, Rees (2001) lists seven key questions that need to be addressed when designing tasks. Question 4 of these has four parts and is related to phonological awareness specifically:

Q4a. Does the child have to reflect on his/ her speech production?

Q4b. Does the child have to show awareness of the internal structure of phonological representations or of spoken stimuli?

Q4c. If so, what kind of segmentation is required?

Q4d. Does the child have to manipulate phonological units?

Consider these questions in the following two tasks designed for Martin, a five-year-old boy with speech difficulties associated with CLP. Martin is backing alveolar sounds and the aim is to target front and back sounds to ensure that (i) he can discriminate between them, (ii) his phonological representations for front versus back sounds are specified well enough for speech and literacy to develop smoothly and (iii) he is making some contrast between them in his speech production.

Task A

Materials and Procedure: Three pairs of words beginning with /t/ and /k/ (e.g. tea and key) are represented twice on 12 cards and placed face down in front of Martin. The adult has one copy of each picture card face up in front of them. A small table top screen is between the adult and the child so they cannot see each other's cards. Martin turns over one of his cards without showing it to the adult and names it. The adult selects the picture from their cards that represents what they heard Martin say.

Feedback: When Martin names his picture correctly the adult holds up the appropriate card and Martin's speech production is rewarded as the adult's picture matches what he thought he had said. If Martin's production of 'tea' sounded more like 'key' the adult selects the picture of key and says 'It sounded like this but I'm not sure. Can you try again'. The visual feedback for Martin via the adult's card is that his production did not convey what he meant. If Martin's second response is not closer to the target then the adult offers more direct help for his speech production.

Task B

Materials and Procedure: Eight picture cards of simple familiar words are shuffled and placed face downwards in front of Martin. Four of these begin with /t/ and four with /k/. Two posting boxes are on the table, one marked with the letter 't' and one with 'k'. Martin picks up each picture in turn, names it, decides whether it starts with /t/ or /k/, matches his decision to the label on one of the boxes and posts the card in the appropriate box.

Feedback: If Martin chooses the correct box the adult rewards him verbally. If he is not sure which box to choose, the adult says the word for him and asks him to look and listen to what sound the word starts with. If Martin is unable to respond, the adult presents a written form of the target word, repeats the onset (t or k) and points to the corresponding letter on the written word card – he can then match that letter visually to one on the posting box at the same time as listening to its production. If helpful, an accompanying *Cued Articulation* gesture can be added (Passy, 1993).

Check your answers to Questions 4a–d against the key at the end of this chapter.

Both tasks require Martin to reflect on his speech production, but to different degrees. Explicit sound segmentation is not necessary to complete Task A successfully (e.g. Martin does not have to decide what each target begins with). Rather, it encourages tacit awareness of differences between onsets because when Martin pronounces 'tea' more like 'key', the adult does not pick up the picture Martin is focusing on, thus making Martin aware that something is not right.

In contrast, to carry out Task B successfully, explicit sound segmentation and knowledge is required. Martin has to segment and identify the first consonant from the rest of the word. It is impossible to do this without having onset/rime segmentation knowledge and skill, as Martin has to match the segmented consonant to a symbol on the posting box. However, not even Task B requires him to manipulate phonological units (question 4d). If we want to challenge Martin further by adding this, we could ask him to produce syllables (e.g. 'oo') with a /k/ or /t/ at the beginning; this involves him blending the unit onset/rime. If we asked him to take the onset off one syllable and put it on another (e.g. take the 't' off 'tea' and put it at the beginning of 'ie' or 'ay'), this would involve both segmentation and blending. If we want him to make connections in his lexical representations, we can also ask him to decide if what he has produced is a real word or not (i.e. 'tie' vs 'tay'). Psycholinguistic intervention is therefore about manipulating the components of a task in order to hit the target as planned.

13.4.4   Monitoring and Evaluation

Measuring success of intervention is an important aspect of evidence based practice. The psycholinguistic approach has built in mechanisms for this (Pascoe, Stackhouse and Wells, 2006). For example, the Speech Processing Profile can be used to chart a child's progress over time (e.g. case study of Zoe whose progress was summarized at three points in time between the ages of three, five and nine years of age, Stackhouse and Wells, 1997) and has been used in longitudinal studies of speech and literacy development (Nathan *et al.*, 2004b; Stackhouse *et al.*, 2007). However, standardized tests can be too blunt an instrument to measure change over shorter periods, and more qualitative measures are required. Level L on the profile (at the bottom centre between level A, the ear and level K, the mouth) is particularly useful for this. Its focus is on how a child monitors their own speech output performance, that is the feedback loop between their mouth (K) and their ear (A). There is no test for L. Rather, the adult needs to observe how the child manages their speech output difficulties and the interaction with the listener (the scoring procedure for this is given in Stackhouse *et al.*, 2007). For example, when first meeting a child the following can be noted:

1. Is there spontaneous speech correction indicating not only self-monitoring skills but also an ability to change speech production?

2. Are there spontaneous attempts at speech correction but these are not always successful because of difficulties elsewhere (e.g. articulatory production or programming)?

3. Does the child only change their speech output when the listener misunderstands what they have said?

4. Does the child only change their speech output when directed to do so by an adult, for example when required to modify their production as part of an intervention task?

5. If there is a mixture of response to Question L, are these related to specific phonetic structures, lexical items, environmental contexts, or conversational partners?

A further key area for evaluating the success of the intervention is how far it has been generalized (Pascoe, Stackhouse and Wells, 2006). This generalization includes within and across domains, as follows:

a) from speech segments targeted in therapy (e.g. ['f']) to others which were not (e.g. ['s'], ['sh']);

b) from targeted production of a segment in initial position in a word (e.g. <u>s</u>un) to non-targeted final position in a word (e.g. hor<u>s</u>e).

c) from a specific set of practised words to words that were not used in therapy;

d) from sounds practised in words to connected speech;

e) from speech input work (e.g. auditory discrimination) to speech output;

f) from speech production to spelling.

In children with persisting speech difficulties this generalization may not happen without specific training, for example transfer from single words to connected speech (Pascoe, Stackhouse and Wells, 2005). However, generalization can be facilitated if the child can use phonological awareness skills to reflect on their speech production. In turn, this can also contribute to the development of their literacy skills if the intervention for speech makes sound-letter linkage explicit (Hatcher, 2006).

13.5   Literacy: Phonological Awareness and Spelling

Children whose speech difficulties persist beyond five years of age are at risk for literacy problems (Bishop and Adams, 1990; Nathan *et al.*, 2004a; Leitao and Fletcher, 2004). However, this is more likely to be the case when there are associated language problems and when there is no obvious cause of the speech difficulties. For example, children described as having 'verbal dyspraxia' or 'phonological impairments' are more at risk of literacy difficulties than those with CLP (Stackhouse, 1982).

However, although CLP in itself does not directly 'cause' *specific* literacy problems in children, children with CLP are vulnerable in terms of keeping up with learning about literacy at school. They may miss lessons because of hospitalization, frequent appointments and illnesses; they may have hearing difficulties which can impact on transcribing written language; or they may have resonance issues which may affect perception and coding of vowels. For some, the CLP may be associated with more general learning difficulties. This heterogeneity of the group of children with CLP may account for why there have been mixed reports in the literature about the level and nature of reading performance in children with CLP (Richman and Ryan, 2003).

Table 13.1 Examples of reading and spelling errors made by children with Cleft Palate and Verbal Dyspraxia (Reproduced from Stackhouse, 1982, with permission from the Royal College of Speech & Language Therapists) (Key: Target → Response).

	Cleft palate	Verbal dyspraxia
Reading	choir → chore	canary → competition
	sabre → sabrey	dream → under
	ceiling → kelin	think → teacher
Spelling	sooner → soona	yet → ygt
	headache → headache	year → andere
	boat → bot	slippery → greid

In the study by Stackhouse (1982) the reading and spelling performance of three groups of children in the age range from 7 to 11 years were compared: (i) children with speech difficulties associated with CLP; (ii) children described as having 'verbal dyspraxia'; and (iii) typically developing peers with no speech difficulties. Table 13.1 presents examples of the reading and spelling skills of the children with CLP and verbal dyspraxia.

The errors of the children with CLP appear more logical. For example, when reading unfamiliar words they translated the letters into sounds and blended them together, that is they have cracked the alphabetic code of English. In contrast, the children with dyspraxia are guessing what the word might be. When spelling, the children with CLP have letter-sound correspondence skills; they have listened to the word, segmented it into its components and written appropriate letters for these. Thus, as a group, the children with CLP have more systematic spellings and are ready to learn about the conventions of English spelling. The children with CLP performed no differently from the typically developing group. However, the children with verbal dyspraxia were both quantitatively poorer (in terms of their performance on standardized tests) and qualitatively different (in the types of errors they produced) from both the group with CLP and the typically developing children. They had not moved into an alphabetic stage of literacy development, which requires an understanding of sound-to-letter correspondencies (Frith, 1985).

A recent study by Collett, Leroux and Speltz (2010) compared the language and early reading skills at ages five and seven years of children with isolated cleft lip and palate, cleft palate only and typically developing non-cleft controls. The outcome that children with clefts performed better than the controls on early reading tests supports the view that children with CLP are not at risk for literacy difficulties. More important factors for language and reading outcomes are demographic, mother–child interaction and early cognitive scores. Therefore, if presented with a child with CLP who also has literacy problems which cannot be explained by other factors (e.g. hearing loss, general learning difficulties, absence from school, socio-economic status), these may indicate in psycholinguistic terms that the speech difficulties could be arising at any point(s) on the speech processing profile, and not only at Level K, that is in the mouth.

This was the case for Tim, an 11-year-old boy with a repaired CLP and persisting speech difficulties. Although communicative, his speech was hypernasal and often unintelligible to the listener. Now that he was attending secondary school, questions were being asked about his poor literacy performance. Although reading for pleasure, he chose books typically read by younger children and his writing contained spelling and grammatical errors. A sample of 14 single word spellings contained eight errors. Three of these were immature for his age and suggested he needed help to understand the conventions of English spelling:

storm → stom;

cream → crem;

puppy → pupey.

The remaining five indicated more significant speech processing difficulties:

crab → caprt;

cloud → clim;

pound → pang;

ladder → ladiger;

marble → mloered.

The aim of Tim's psycholinguistic assessment was to try and establish in one short session if he had specific speech processing difficulties and, if so, how these might be affecting his spoken and written language. The following is a summary of this session (he should be 100% accurate on these tasks at his age).

1. **Letter-sound knowledge**

Unclear and unconfident. Does not know all letter-sound correspondences.

2. **Non-word reading** (e.g. mosp; prab)

Scored 0. Unable to read 'new' words.

3. **Auditory Discrimination of pairs of non-words (with and without clusters)**

16/20 correct. He accepted the following different non-word pairs as the 'same': bleis ~ bleit; bleist ~ bleits, as well as other non-word pairs beginning with sk ~ st.

4. **Rhyme detection**

9/13 correct. When correct he was still slow at responding indicating that he needed more processing time than peers to make a correct decision.

5. **Half Spoonerisms** (e.g. say 'cat' without /k/)

   8/10 attempted; 4/10 correct.

6. **Blending**

   Unable to read/blend clusters written on cards (e.g br; spl).

Transferring these results onto a Speech Processing Profile shows that Tim has difficulties at both input and output sides. Given his age, his significant difficulties with phonological awareness activities (e.g. rhyme and blending) and poor letter-sound knowledge alerts us to the fact that he may have specific literacy difficulties that are unlikely to be explained by his CLP. This hypothesis can be investigated further by examining his spelling data. Spelling is well worth including in a speech processing assessment as like speech it develops in a predictable way and is another output from a child's stored representations. However, unlike speech it is not distorted by articulatory difficulties associated with CLP which can be difficult to transcribe. The following hypotheses are suggested for Tim's spellings of single words produced at chronological age 11;05 (key: target -> spelling response):

1. 'Fuzzy' representations of plosives (e.g. p ~ t; t ~ k; d ~ g):

   do<u>t</u> → dor<u>p</u>; wee<u>k</u> → we<u>t</u>r; min<u>d</u> → min<u>g</u>er; <u>sk</u>ate → <u>st</u>ore

   and plosive vs homorganic nasal, (e.g. d ~ n):

   staye<u>d</u> → sta<u>n</u>e

2. Confusion at word ends, for example when to mark 'er' and when not. This may be arising from exaggerated pronunciation of the last part of the word as he tries to spell it:

   sooner → son<u>e</u>; dream → demy<u>er</u>; sight → siy<u>er</u>; might → mitr<u>er</u>; mouth → moll<u>er</u>

3. Marking the beginning and end of a two-syllable words but not the 'middle':

   <u>m</u>ista<u>k</u>e → <u>m</u>e<u>k</u>ra

4. Not sure how to transcribe vowels:

   h<u>ay</u> → h<u>ey</u>; b<u>oa</u>t → b<u>ao</u>t; c<u>u</u>t → c<u>o</u>t

5. Letter order confusion:

   help → hlep; large → lrangh

6. Transcribing a related word to the target:

while → wiuth; pair → pear; been → be; brought → buyer

This examination of spelling errors contributes valuable information for an educational approach to planning Tim's intervention in collaboration with the teaching staff at his school. His literacy difficulties had not been picked up fully at primary school as they were attributed to him having a CLP. However, given the evidence that children with CLP are no more at risk for specific literacy problems that their peers, there must be some further explanation of Tim's atypical performance. Indeed, there was a history of dyslexia in Tim's family and his sister was receiving help at school for her specific literacy difficulties. The conclusion is that Tim has dyslexic difficulties in addition to his CLP. Although much of his unintelligibility can be attributed to his oral structural and functional difficulties, he also has pervasive speech processing difficulties which compound his articulatory difficulties, interfere with his ability to develop phonological awareness and thus impact on his literacy development.

13.6 Summary

This chapter presents a range of approaches to the assessment and management of children with CLP. The contribution of a psycholinguistic approach is to:

- investigate a child's speech processing strengths and weaknesses;

- ensure systematic assessment which goes beyond the obvious presenting condition;

- develop a better understanding of the relationship between speech, language and literacy difficulties;

- identify children at risk of literacy difficulties;

- use medical and linguistic information;

- maintain developmental, educational and psychosocial perspectives;

- integrate speech and literacy goals;

- set realistic intervention targets;

- design activities which can be manipulated and interpreted;

- incorporate evaluation;

- facilitate communication between users;

- provide training and learning opportunities.

However, the focus on the psycholinguistic approach is not at the expense of any other; each has an important role to play.

Key to Tasks for Martin

Q4a. Does the child have to reflect on his/her speech production?
Task A: Yes   Task B: Yes

Q4b. Does the child have to show awareness of the internal structure of phonological representations/spoken stimuli?
Task A: No   Task B: Yes

Q4c. If yes, what kind of segmentation is required?
Task A: —   Task B: onset/rime

Q4d. Does the child have to manipulate phonological units?
Task A: No   Task B: No

Bibliography

The following book series presents the psycholinguistic approach with training activities and assessment materials:

Stackhouse, J. and Wells, B. (1997) *Children's Speech and Literacy Difficulties 1: A Psycholinguistic Framework*, Whurr Publishers, London.

Stackhouse, J. and Wells, B. (2001) *Children's Speech and Literacy Difficulties 2: Identification and Intervention*, Whurr Publishers, London.

Pascoe, M., Stackhouse, J. and Wells, B. (2006) *Children with Persisting Speech Difficulties. Children's Speech and Literacy Difficulties 3*, John Wiley & Sons Ltd, Chichester.

Stackhouse, J., Vance, M., Pascoe, M. and Wells, B. (2007) *A Compendium of Speech and Auditory Procedures. Children's Speech and Literacy Difficulties 4*, John Wiley & Sons Ltd, Chichester.

References

Baker, E., Croot, K., Mcleod, S. and Paul, R. (2001) Psycholinguistic models of speech development and their application to clinical practice. *Journal of Speech, Language and Hearing Research*, 44, 685–702.

Bishop, D. and Adams, C. (1990) A prospective study of the relationship between specific language impairment, phonological disorders and reading retardation. *Journal of Child Psychology and Psychiatry*, 31, 1027–1050.

Calladine, S. (2009) Multi-sensory input modelling therapy: intervention for young children with cleft palate. MSc Dissertation, University of Sheffield, UK.

Claessen, M., Leitao, S. and Barrett, N. (2010) Investigating children's ability to reflect on stored phonological representations: the Silent Deletion of Phonemes Task. *International Journal of Language and Communication Disorders*, 45, 411–423.

Collett, B.R., Leroux, B..L. and Speltz, M.L. (2010) Language and early reading among children with orofacial clefts. *Cleft Palate–Craniofacial Journal*, 47, 284–292.

Frith, U. (1985) Beneath the surface of developmental dyslexia, in *Surface Dyslexia* (eds K.E. Patterson, J.C. Marshall and M. Coltheart), Routledge & Kegan Paul, London, pp. 301–330.

Hatcher, P. (2006) Phonological awareness and reading intervention, *Dyslexia Speech and Language: A Practitioner's Handbook*, 2nd edn (eds M. Snowling and J. Stackhouse), Whurr, London, pp. 167–197.

Ingram, D. (1976) *Phonological Disability in Children*, Elsevier, New York.

Leitao, S. and Fletcher, J. (2004) Literacy outcomes for students with speech impairment: long term follow up. *International Journal of Language and Communication Disorders*, 39, 245–256.

Morris, H. and Ozanne, A. (2003) Phonetic, phonological, and language skills of children with a cleft palate. *Cleft Palate–Craniofacial Journal*, 40, 460–470.

Nathan, L. and Simpson, S. (2001) Designing a literacy programme for a child with a history of speech difficulties, in *Children's Speech and Literacy Difficulties, 2: Identification and Intervention* (eds J. Stackhouse and B. Wells), Whurr Publishers, London, pp. 249–298.

Nathan, L., Stackhouse, J., Goulandris, N. and Snowling, M. (2004a) The development of early literacy skills among children with speech difficulties: a test of the 'critical age hypothesis.'. *Journal of Speech, Language, and Hearing Research*, 47, 377–391.

Nathan, L., Stackhouse, J., Goulandris, N. and Snowling, M. (2004b) Educational consequences of developmental speech disorder: key stage I national curriculum assessment results in English and mathematics. *British Journal of Educational Psychology*, 74, 173–186.

Pascoe, M., B. (2005) Phonological therapy within a psycholinguistic framework: promoting change in a child with persisting speech difficulties. *International Journal of Language and Communication Disorders*, 39, 1–32.

Pascoe, M., Stackhouse, J. and Wells, B. (2006) *Children with Persisting Speech Difficulties. Children's Speech and Literacy Difficulties 3*, John Wiley & Sons Ltd, Chichester.

Passy, J. (1993) *Cued Articulation*, STASS Publications, Ponteland, Northumberland, UK.

Patrick, K. (2005) A psycholinguistic based approach to the assessment and treatment of cleft palate speech: a pilot therapy outcome study. MSc Dissertation, Leicester: De Montfort University.

Rees, R. (2001) What do tasks really tap? in *Children's Speech and Literacy Difficulties, 2: Identification and Intervention* (eds J. Stackhouse and B. Wells), Whurr, London., pp. 66–95.

Richman, L.C. and Ryan, S.M. (2003) Do the reading disabilities of children with cleft fit into current models of developmental dyslexia? *Cleft Palate-Craniofacial Journal*, 40, 154–157.

Shriberg, L.D., Austin, D., Lewis, B.A. *et al.* (1997) The Speech Disorders Classification System (SDCS). *Journal of Speech, Language and Hearing Research*, 40, 723–740.

Stackhouse, J. (1982) An investigation of reading and spelling performance in speech disordered children. *British Journal of Disorders of Communication*, 17, 53–60.

Stackhouse, J. (2006) Speech and spelling difficulties: what to look for, *Dyslexia, Speech and Language: A Practitioner's Handbook*, 2nd edn (eds M. Snowling and J. Stackhouse), Whurr Publishers, London., pp. 15–35.

Stackhouse, J. and Pascoe, M. (2010) Psycholinguistic intervention, in *Interventions in Speech Sound Disorders in Children* (eds A.L. Williams, S. McLeod and R.J. McCauley), Paul H. Brookes Publishing Co, Baltimore., pp. 219–246.

Stackhouse, J. and Wells, B. (1997) *Children's Speech and Literacy Difficulties, 1: A Psycholinguistic Framework*, Whurr Publishers, London.

Stackhouse, J., Pascoe, M. and Gardner, H. (2006) Intervention for a child with persisting speech and literacy difficulties: a psycholinguistic approach. *Advances in Speech-Language Pathology*, 8, 231–244.

Stackhouse, J., Vance, M., Pascoe, M. and Wells, B. (2007) *A Compendium of Speech and Auditory Procedures. Children's Speech and Literacy Difficulties, 4*, John Wiley & Sons Ltd, Chichester.

Waters, D. (2001) Using input processing strengths to overcome speech output difficulties, in *Children's Speech and Literacy Difficulties, 2: Identification and Intervention* (eds J. Stackhouse and B. Wells), Whurr, London., pp. 164–203.

Waters, D., Hawkes, C. and Burnett, E. (1998) Targeting speech processing strengths to facilitate pronunciation change. *International Journal of Language and Communication Disorders*, **33** (Suppl.):469–474.

Williams, P. and Stephens, H. (2004) *Nuffield Centre Dyspraxia Programme*, 3rd edn. Miracle Factory, Windsor, UK.

14

Early Communication Assessment and Intervention

Nancy Scherer and Brenda Louw

East Tennessee State University, Department of Audiology and Speech-Language Pathology, Johnson City, TN 37614, USA

14.1 Introduction

This chapter focuses on early assessment and intervention for children with cleft palate from a transdisciplinary approach. It is felt that this approach provides a comprehensive framework for viewing early treatment that is beneficial for the continuum of disabilities that may occur in the population of children with craniofacial disorders and clefts. Children with cleft palate are often assessed only for their speech production, while other developmental and family issues that may impact success of early intervention are not addressed. This chapter provides guidelines for early assessment and intervention with a focus on identifying the child's strengths and weaknesses in order to optimize early intervention. While some children may not require the full complement of assessment if seen by a speech–language pathologist with craniofacial experience, this chapter provides guidelines for children seen in other settings where speech–language pathologists have limited craniofacial experience. There is a growing body of literature on the progression of early communicative skills in children with clefts and the impact of

Cleft Palate Speech: Assessment and Intervention, First Edition. Edited by Sara Howard, Anette Lohmander.
© 2011 John Wiley & Sons, Ltd. Published 2011 by John Wiley & Sons, Ltd.

some early intervention programmes for this population. This chapter also describes early intervention for children with clefts from a data driven and evidenced based perspective.

14.2   Assessment

Early communication assessment of children with cleft palate and multi-anomaly disorders is aimed at identifying communication and developmental delays in order to minimize the impact of clefting on the young child and the family through early intervention (D'Antonio and Scherer, 1995). The assessment of a child with cleft lip and palate is a continuing, dynamic process, starting from early infancy (ACPA: American Cleft Palate-Craniofacial Association, 2007). Early assessment involves a chronological process of describing a young child's communication behaviour, identifying strengths and needs in the child and family, and planning intervention. Best practice requires that a family centred, multidisciplinary approach be followed.

In children with CLP without additional anomalies the focus is traditionally centred on the assessment of speech, resonance, voice quality and language based on the evidence described in studies of early communicative development (Chapman, Hardin-Jones and Halter, 2003; Scherer, Williams and Proctor-Williams, 2008). These studies indicate deficits in the onset and composition of their babbling, onset of first words and early expressive vocabulary development. However, palatal clefting is often associated with syndromes in which the communication impairment is one feature of multi-anomaly disorders requiring a more comprehensive assessment (D'Antonio and Scherer, 2009).

The heterogeneity of the cleft population and the wide range of communication skills necessitate a broad framework for assessment and intervention which can be adapted according to the child's and family's needs and the context in which the assessment takes place. Furthermore, assessment over time also needs to follow a developmental approach to address the important milestones at each stage of development (D'Antonio and Scherer, 1995) and to allow for the outcomes of other interventions.

While comprehensive standardized tests of early communicative development are available, they are not particularly sensitive until 18 months of age. Conducting systematic, but less formal, observations of young children using checklists and parental report measures tends to be more ecologically valid as these occur in naturalistic contexts and are individualized. Specific domains known to be problematic for children with clefts (e.g. babbling, consonant inventories and expressive vocabulary) can be targeted while broader developmental domains are screened.

14.2.1   Model of Assessment

A four-level assessment framework for a comprehensive assessment of young children with CLP and multi-anomaly disorders is presented in Figure 14.1 (Kritzinger and Louw, 2000, 2002; Louw and Kritzinger, 2008). Information gathering from the family is followed by assessing the child and family on four levels, namely: level one, which assesses physical features and sensory integrity and processing of the child; level two, which

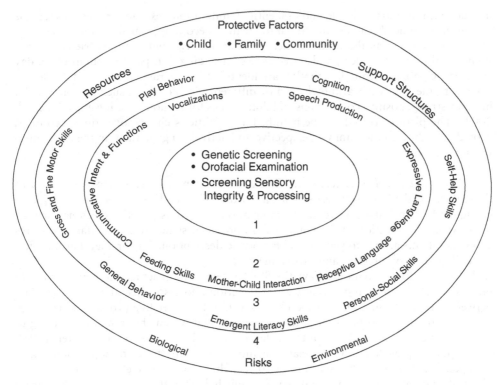

Figure 14.1 Four level assessment framework. (Based on Louw, 1986; Kritzinger and Louw, 2002; Louw and Kritzinger, 2008.)

focuses on communicative and feeding skills; level three, which targets general developmental skills; and level four, which identifies risk and protective factors to determine child and family resilience (Louw and Kritzinger, 2008).

The framework guides a comprehensive first evaluation for children with CLP. The first assessment should include all levels and domains and, during subsequent follow up assessments, the speech–language pathologist (SLP) selects the level and areas according to each individual child's and family's needs. Based on the data collected and analyses of the behaviours, the SLP will be able to identify areas of normality, strength and concern and make recommendations. The SLP is often the first person to recognize the possibility of a multi-anomaly disorder in young children with cleft lip and palate. Evaluation is a multidisciplinary effort and recommendations may include referrals to other team members based on the findings on each of the four assessment levels.

Assessment needs to start with the family before focusing on the child. In addition to routine case history information, a family assessment also requires a family conversation, rather than a traditional interview format, to share the many factors they deem important to their family dynamics and the elements that they deal with from day to day (Billeaud, 2003). During such a conversation team members such as the SLP, social worker or psychologist may guide the family to create a visual representation of their family structure, interaction, functions and life cycle through an eco-map of how they interact with the outside world and to identify family resources, support networks, areas of concern and need. Circles are drawn to create an eco-map, starting with the family's identified members as the centre circle. Associations (e.g. with family, friends, neighbours, health care providers) and activities (e.g. attending cleft palate team meeting, day care, participating in church activities) are identified in separate circles and the connections with the family are acknowledged by different kinds of lines, such as double solid lines for strong, positive connections and dotted lines for tenuous relationships (Billeaud, 2003). The picture created can be modified as conditions change over time. Eco-maps provide insight into the family's perspective and actively engage them in the early intervention process.

14.2.1.1 *First Level of Assessment*

The assessment process can then be directed to the child using the four level assessment framework. The first level of assessment depicted in Figure 14.1 includes an orofacial examination as well as genetic screening through direct visual observation of the young child's orofacial structures, craniofacial features and general appearance to generate a phenotypic description. The first level also targets the child's sensory integrity and processing.

An orofacial examination allows the SLP to determine whether there are structural factors which could be interfering with articulation and resonance and to differentiate between structural versus motor speech causes. In infants, feeding provides a means for assessing structure and function of the mechanism and, when children are beginning to talk, both non-speech and speech tasks should be used (D'Antonio and Scherer, 1995). The reported prevalence of associated malformations in the cleft population varies (Chapter 3). Peterson-Falzone *et al.* (2010) conclude that the likelihood of associated physical anomalies and functional issues is much higher than indicted in the earlier literature. Associated anomalies, like clefts themselves, may vary in severity of expression and some significant findings may be minute and easy to miss (Peterson-Falzone, Hardin-Jones and Karnell, 2010). Clinicians therefore need a systematic approach for recognizing and identifying normal and abnormal variations in structure.

It is important to remember that speech abnormalities in young children with clefts may be related not only to anatomic abnormalities due directly to the cleft but also to a global communication impairment associated with the underlying cause of the cleft. By following these guidelines the SLP will be able to compile a detailed phenotypic description. Although SLPs are not qualified to make a diagnosis of a syndrome based on their observations, such a description is an important first step in identifying syndromic characteristics. These observations need to be discussed with the surgeon and paediatrician and a genetic evaluation may be suggested. Identification of associated anomalies at an early age is critical for the child, family and care providers (Coston *et al.*, 1992).

Level one also includes the screening assessment of the child's sensory integrity and sensory processing. The auditory, visual, tactile, proprioceptive, olfactory and gustatory senses, vestibular mechanism, muscle tone, coordination, self-regulation are included in level one of the assessment.

Hearing screening is essential, as ear disease and hearing loss constitute a major potential threat to children with cleft palate and multi-anomaly disorders (Peterson-Falzone, Hardin-Jones and Karnell, 2010). These children are at risk for recurrent otitis media and associated conductive hearing loss and remain at risk in the pre-school years and beyond. Routine referrals to an audiologist for hearing screening, diagnostic testing if indicated, and regular and continued monitoring of hearing status is recommended by the ACPA: American Cleft Palate-Craniofacial Association (2007). A pediatric hearing test battery for infants and toddlers, depending on their age, should include otoscopy, auditory brainstem response (ABR) testing, otoacoustic emissions (OAE), acoustic immitance assessment, visual reinforcement audiometry (VRA) and functional assessment of auditory skill development performed by an audiologist (ASHA: American Speech-Language-Hearing Association, 2004). Any sign of ear disease or hearing loss should be cause for referral to an otolaryngologist for examination and treatment (Peterson-Falzone, Hardin-Jones and Karnell, 2010).

Poor sensory integration affects social, cognitive and sensorimotor development, and early identification is important as a preventative measure. Vulnerable children are more likely to have extreme patterns of sensory processing that interfere with everyday life (Dunn and Westman, 1997; Dunn, 2007). Identifying and describing the child's sensory processing helps the SLP to understand the child's behavior and to explain it to parents. Such knowledge is important for further referrals to an occupational therapist and for planning interventions to support children to participate better in everyday activities (Dunn, 2007).

The child's responses to sensory input (auditory, visual, tactile, proprioceptive, olfactory and gustatory) and vestibular sensations can be categorized according to patterns of sensory processing as described by Dunn and Westman (1997) and Dunn (2007). Transdisciplinary play based assessment (Linder, 1993) is particularly useful in assessing young children's sensory integrity. Based on the observations, referrals for a formal assessment of sensory integration and processing by an occupational therapist or physical therapist may be necessary. Assessment results obtained from level one may be used to identify contributing factors, indicate the need for and justify further diagnostic testing and referrals, and to make treatment recommendations.

14.2.1.2 The Second Level of Assessment This level, as illustrated in Figure 14.1, addresses feeding and communication skills. Commonly the feeding problems experienced reflect the type, severity of the cleft or presence of other physical or developmental disorders (Peterson-Falzone, Hardin-Jones and Karnell, 2010). While most children with non-syndromic clefts do not experience significant feeding difficulties, factors such as prematurity, low birth weight, cardiac or pulmonary disease, functional or structural abnormalities of the oro-pharynx or gastrointestinal tract may contribute to the feeding difficulties (Reid, Kilpatrick and Reilly, 2006).

Screening of feeding skills through observation, use of checklists, feeding scales such as the Oral-Motor/Feeding Rating Scale (Jelm, 1990) and parent interviews will indicate the need for a team evaluation and further referral by the team for objective measures such as Fibre-optic Endoscopic Evaluation of Swallowing (FEES) and Videofluoroscopic Swallowing Study (VSS). Based on observations of the infant's feeding patterns informed choices of feeding modifications can be made by the SLP, nurse practitioner and other team members.

Several speech and language assessment protocols for young children with cleft palate have been described (Peterson-Falzone, Hardin-Jones and Karnell, 2010). A wide range of early communication screening and assessment tools is commercially available in English, such as the Denver Developmental Screening Test-II, Early Language Milestone

Scale, MacArthur Bates Communicative Development Inventories: Words and Sentences (CDI:WS) (Fenson *et al.*, 2007), Rossetti Infant–Toddler Language Scale (Rossetti, 1990), Preschool Language Scale-4, and the Receptive-Emergent Language Scale (REEL-3) (Anderson & Teilly, 2002; Berglund and Eriksson, 2000; Bleses *et al.*, 2008; Hamilton, Plunkett and Schafer, 2000; Jackson-Maldanado *et al.*, 1993; Kern, 2007; Rossetti, 1990; Tardif *et al.*, 2009). The Communicative Development Inventories have been normed in a number of languages and provide a resource for early vocabulary assessment. Informal observational screening forms exist such as the pre-linguistic and linguistic screening forms for infants and toddlers with cleft palate by D'Antonio and Scherer (1995) and Peterson-Falzone, Hardin-Jones and Karnell (2010). These assessment tools and many more are listed and described by a number of authors (Billeaud, 2003; D'Antonio and Scherer, 2009; Tiegerman-Farber and Radziewicz, 2008).

The focus of the infant pre-linguistic communication assessment is to identify early precursors of receptive and expressive language and speech function. A sample of infant vocal behaviour needs to be collected and video-or audiotaped by the parents if possible or by the SLP. The child's consonant vowel inventory, level of vocal development (reflexive, cooing, vocal play, canonical babble) and syllable structure (e.g. V, CV, VC, CVCV) should be described. The presence of any maladaptive articulations should be noted (D'Antonio and Scherer, 1995).

Describing the emergence of communicative intent in the pre-linguistic stage is important to identify readiness for emergence of words. Observation of caregiver child interaction allows for description of the adult's sensitivity and responsiveness within the caregiver child dyad as well as the child's responses, joint attention and turn taking within social exchanges (D'Antonio and Scherer, 1995).

Once the child begins to use words, speech production is assessed by analysing his/her consonant inventory to identify the number, manner and place of articulation features. Atypical sound substitutions such as glottal stops and nasal substitutions need to be identified. Information about positional constraints, word shape and complexity of consonants also assist in planning intervention. The resonance type and the severity of hyper or hyponasality needs to be noted, as well as audible nasal emission and the frequency thereof. The methodology most suited to screening and assessment of children on a linguistic level is a spontaneous language sample and speech and language questionnaires collected by parents and video-or audiotaped by the parents if possible or by the SLP. The language sample needs to be analysed to determine the number of different words, word combinations, Mean Length of Utterance (MLU) as well as the child's conversational skills. Informal observations of the toddler's receptive and expressive language again supplement the information on the toddler's communication development.

Based on the assessment results the infant and toddler's individual profile of speech and language development can be determined; this will identify the need for further referrals and inform treatment decisions, such as monitoring of speech, language and hearing, providing language intervention and targeting speech production. Children with limited consonant inventories as toddlers demonstrate delays in phonological development (Chapman, Hardin-Jones and Halter, 2003). While randomized studies exploring the impact of early intervention are just now being conducted, experts recommend early intervention for toddlers with limited consonant inventories (Peterson-Falzone *et al.*, 2006).

14.2.1.3   The Third of Assessment   The third level of assessment provides information on the general functioning of the young child with CLP (Figure 14.1). Children with CLP and multi-anomaly disorders exhibit both biologic and environmental risk factors that interact and place them at risk for developmental disorders (Neiman and Savage, 1997). Researchers do concur that children with CLP, particularly those with multi-anomaly disorders, have an elevated risk for developmental delay (Neiman and Savage, 1997; Strauss and Broder, 1993) Assessment of motor skills, cognitive skills, play behavior and social emotional behaviour is therefore necessitated.

Motor milestones are an indicator of general development and relate to speech and language acquisition. Delayed motor milestones may be an indicator of a multi-anomaly condition or an indication of a specific motor impairment. Parental report, behavioural observation and developmental screening tests, such as the Bayley Scales of Infant Development-2 (BSID-2) (Bayley, 1993), may be applied to determine the level of functioning and identity of a motor delay (D'Antonio and Scherer, 1995). A developmental motor delay may be an indication of a specific motor impairment or predictive of later speech and language delay or impairment and may require referrals to a paediatrician and a physical therapist for further assessment.

Early play behaviours may assist in the identification of children with clefts who are at risk for later language development. Play assessment provides an estimate of the child's developmental level and correlates highly with language skills (Snyder and Scherer, 2004). The Symbolic Play Scale Checklist (Westby, 2000) and the Communication and Symbolic Behaviour Scales (CSBS) (Wetherby and Prizant, 1998) are clinically useful tools to assess the developmental relationship between cognitive development, language and play. When play behaviours are of concern, they need to be addressed in early intervention with cognitive and language skills and, depending on the concern, referrals should be made to early education specialists, occupational therapists and mental health professionals.

Research supports the long held belief that children with CLP are at risk for socio-emotional problems (Bzoch, 2004; Collett and Speltz, 2006). Early identification of social and emotional problems in young children is critical for improving developmental outcomes (Squires, 2000). Screening of social and emotional development needs to take place within the context of the child's and family's life through the observation of play, parental report and by using tools such as, for example, The Ages and Stages Questionnaires: Social-Emotional (ASQ-SE) (Squires, Bricker and Twombly, 2000), which provides information on self-regulation, compliance, communication, adaptive functioning, autonomy, affective functioning and interaction with others. If the child is identified as having a potential social-emotional difficulty, referral to mental health services is called for. If the child appears to be developing typically but the family is still concerned, the SLP should help the family to access community resources such as parent support groups and parenting classes (Squires, 2000).

The third level of assessment allows the SLP to identify areas of normality, strengths and to detect and identify additional areas of concern as well as subtle problems. Appropriate referrals and intervention recommendations can then be made. Video recording all or portions of the assessment through levels one to three is recommended. It frees up the SLP from documentation notes during the evaluation and provides a baseline reference for later comparisons. It also allows for later viewing by other team members not present during the assessment.

14.2.1.4 The Fourth Level of Assessment The final assessment level in Figure 14.1 aims to identify protective mechanisms and risk factors to determine child and family resilience. Risk factors associated with children with communication delays and CLP have been well documented (Billeaud, 2003; Rossetti, 2001; Peterson-Falzone, Hardin-Jones and Karnell, 2010). In children with clefts and multi-anomaly disorders risk factors within the child, such as low birth weight, the number of surgeries undergone and hospitalizations, high susceptibility to middle ear disease, and challenging family and community issues, such as teenage motherhood, low literacy levels of parents, substance abuse, family instability, incarceration and poverty, are cause for concern. The combination and interaction of risk factors need to be determined for each child and family.

Documented research based on longitudinal studies of infants and young children who grew up in adverse conditions, has identified protective factors and mechanisms in the child, the family and the community that buffer a child's reaction to a stressful situation or chronic adversity, so that his or her adaptation is more successful than would be the case if protective factors were not present. Protective factors relating to at-risk children in infancy include such factors as alertness and high vigour, sociability and engaging temperament (Werner, 2000). Within a strengths based approach to early intervention with children with cleft palate and their families, an assessment needs to focus not only risk factors in the children and families, but also on the protective factors. A favourable balance between risk and protective factors allows for successful adaptation. Intervention needs to shift the balance from vulnerability to resilience, either by decreasing the exposure to risk factors or by increasing the number of available protective factors (Werner, 2000).

Conversations with families and parental report can be used to guide them to identify protective factors such as competencies and informal sources of support that already exist. Categories of biological and environmental risks (Rossetti, 2001) and lists of protective factors within the child, the family and the community (Werner, 2000) may be used to understand and address the balance between the risks and protective factors to foster the child's and family's resilience. This strengths based approach helps parents to reframe their child and his or her diagnosis more positively, which may impact their relationship with their child, and their approach to intervention.

In conclusion, the four level assessment framework allows the SLP to identify strengths and concerns and to distinguish between infants and toddlers who are developing appropriately for their age, have a developmental delay and those with multi-anomaly disorders. Based on the assessment results, recommendations regarding future management can be made. Children who are functioning on an age-appropriate level need to be followed up annually. Some children with age-appropriate development, who are more vulnerable due to a combination of biological and environmental risk factors and poor resilience, require regular monitoring on a three to six monthly basis. Such children are often missed during the first assessment, as the range of normality is so broad but through regular monitoring early identification is possible.

Children identified with significant issues and delays on assessment levels one and two of the assessment framework, but function well and develop appropriately on level three of the assessment, require early intervention to address both speech and language development. Children identified with developmental delay and associated impairments on assessment level three, require referrals to other team members and professionals and comprehensive multidisciplinary early intervention.

14.3   Intervention

Early intervention for children with CLP could take several different forms as a result of the assessment. Some children may require monitoring of development while others need specific interventions that focus on one or more developmental areas. This chapter discusses the specific interventions that have data available on the effectiveness with a focus on speech and language interventions.

14.3.1   Early Speech Intervention Programmes

Early intervention for children with clefts has focused on three general approaches: speech intervention that emphasizes expansion of speech sound inventories and phonological intervention: programmes that simultaneously intervene in speech and language areas; and parent training or education programmes. Programmes that focus on sound production exclusively have been the mainstay of speech therapy for children of pre-school age and above. However, children under the age of three do not respond consistently to conventional clinician directed articulation or phonological approaches (Paul, 2001). Cognition and attentional demands of traditional programmes present difficulties for children under three. For intervention that focuses on speech sounds, treatment often takes the form of sound stimulation activities that incorporate vocal play with nasal and oral consonants, modelling place of articulation and oral airflow for sounds, and modelling vocabulary (Peterson-Falzone *et al.*, 2006). While these sound stimulation activities have anecdotal evidence, their effectiveness has not been investigated in a systematic way.

14.3.2   Programmes that Simultaneously Treat Language and Speech Production

14.3.2.1   Focused Stimulation   The Focused Stimulation (FS) model is a naturalistic intervention that emphasizes modelling and responsive interaction with little direct prompting of the child's language production (Girolametto, Pearce and Weitzman, 1996, 1997). Target vocabulary is selected and the clinician or parent provides high density of models of the target words in a meaningful context, usually play. This approach has been successful with children who demonstrate communicative intent and joint attention (Fey *et al.*, 2006). The approach manipulates the environment to provide opportunities for target vocabulary use. Most studies suggest that at least 10 vocabulary words be targeted in a session (Girolametto, Pearce and Weitzman, 1996). An adaptation of the model includes adding emphasis or stress to the target words or by positioning the target word at the beginning or end of a carrier phrase to call attention to the targets. This approach does not require a response from the children but spontaneous imitation of the target words is desired.

The effectiveness of FS was investigated in a study of 10 children with CLP (Scherer, D'Antonio and McGahey, 2008). Parents were trained to implement the FS treatment for a set of target words containing stop consonants. These parents learned the FS procedures readily and their children acquired the target words. Production of stop consonants in the target words was acquired for most target words.

14.3.2.2   Enhanced Milieu Teaching with Phonological Emphasis (EMT/PE)   This intervention consists of seven strategies to facilitate language and speech (*Scherer and Kaiser, 2010*).

14.3.2.2.1   Environmental Arrangement   The component of environmental arrangement is designed to increase the child's engagement with the physical setting, which then can provide more frequent opportunities for the parent to communicate with the child, to elicit communicative responses, to model appropriate language forms and to respond contingently to the child's verbal and non-verbal communication attempts. Parents are taught to select toys and materials that are of interest to the child, to engage in play with the child with the toys and materials, and to match and elaborate the child's play schemes as a means of promoting and enhancing the child's engagement with the environment.

Environmental strategies have been shown to increase the likelihood that children will show interest in the environment and make communicative attempts. The goal of these strategies is to engage the child in activities that promote vocalizations and word attempts. These strategies provide a context for prompting vocabulary, as well as facilitating spontaneous production attempts that can be recast by the adult to include phonologically correct models. Table 14.1 provides a description of environmental strategies to select, arrange and manage materials to that will increase the likelihood that the child will initiate and maintain communicative interaction.

14.3.2.2.2   Responsive Interaction   In the responsive interaction component of EMT, emphasis is placed on developing a conversational style of interaction that promotes balanced turn taking between adult and child while providing models of appropriate language. The basic responsive interaction strategies include the interactional components of responsiveness (e.g. responding to every child communication attempt, responding to the meaning of child utterances with related comments or questions), following the child's lead in play and conversation, facilitating turn taking, matching and extending the child's topic. Language modelling strategies include matching the child's linguistic level, imitating or mirroring the child's words and actions and systematically expanding child utterances while maintaining child meanings.

14.3.2.2.3   Modelling   Elicited modelling may be considered the most fundamental Milieu Teaching strategy. Following the establishment of joint attention, the adult presents a verbal model of target language that is related to the child's immediate interest. The adult prompts the child's production of the model with 'Say X'. If the child imitates the model correctly, it receives immediate positive feedback (which includes an expansion of the child's response) and the material of interest is given. If the child does not respond to the initial model or responds with a partial, incorrect or unrelated response, the adult establishes joint attention again and presents the model a second time (a corrective model). If the child responds with an unintelligible response, a speech

Table 14.1 Environmental arrangement principles.

Selecting materials

1. Select toys/materials that are high preference and interesting to the child.
2. Select toys with multiple parts (e.g. Lego, Mr Potato Head) or add-ons (e.g. add the barnyard animals to water play).
3. Select toys that require assistance opening (e.g. play dough) or putting together (e.g. a train track).
4. Select toys/tasks that require turn taking with the child (e.g. throwing and catching a ball, hiding and finding an object). Non-verbal turn taking provides a foundation for verbal turn taking (balanced conversation).

Arranging materials

1. Limit the number of materials/toys available to the child at any one time. Limiting materials helps your child attend to the toys you are playing with rather than being overwhelmed by too many toys. It also may provide an opportunity for your child to request additional materials.
2. Have some toys in your child's view but out of reach (e.g. on a high shelf or in plastic containers up on a counter).
3. Keep toys in containers that your child will need assistance opening.

Managing materials

1. Be a gatekeeper. Place yourself between your child and the materials or keep some portion of the materials in your control.
2. Seat the child in a highchair or in a location that limits their easy access to toys.
3. When the child seems to start losing interest, add in materials to keep the play going. Be creative as you mix toys and materials that may not generally go together. For example, add food colouring to water play or have the barnyard animals go through the car wash made for the Matchbox cars.
4. When the child does not receive all of the toys or materials at once, there is an opportunity to request more. For example, give him or her two Lego blocks instead of the whole container of Lego.
5. Provide incomplete toy sets. You can also provide an opportunity for the child to communicate with you by not providing all the materials he or she might need for an activity. For example, you could give the child a jar of bubbles without a wand, so he or she will need to ask for the material.
6. Provide opportunities for unexpected events. For example, if you put Mr Potato Head's arm where his eye goes, your child may use language to tell you that it is wrong or to move it to the right location.

---

recast is provided (discussed below). If the child does respond to the corrective model, the adult simply models desired verbal response and then gives the material to the child.

14.3.2.2.4 Mand-Model The mand-model procedure begins with a verbal prompt in the form of a real question (e.g. 'What do you want?') or a choice (e.g. 'Would you like the car or ball?') or a mand to verbalize (e.g. 'Tell me what you want.'). If the child responds with a target vocabulary word, the adult acknowledges the child's response and provides the requested material. If the child does not respond or gives an incorrect response, the adult models the desired target vocabulary. By arranging the environment and presenting choices among interesting materials, toys or activities, the adult makes the child's language immediately functional. Model and mand-model procedures provide a means of structuring child responses to facilitate the use of target vocabulary. However, it is also important to provide opportunities for the child to initiate conversation in order to foster spontaneous use of the target vocabulary. The time delay procedure was developed to establish child initiation instead of relying on models and mands as cues for vocabulary.

14.3.2.2.5   Time Delay   Once joint attention has been established, the adult waits for the child to initiate communication. If the child initiates but does not use his specific targets, other strategies (mands, models) can be used as follow up prompts to elicit specific vocabulary forms. Time delay can be an important bridging strategy for helping children who rely on prompts to move toward more independent and spontaneous use of language.

14.3.2.2.6   Incidental Teaching   Incidental teaching was developed to encourage children to use elaborated language in conversational interaction. The environment is arranged to promote requesting objects and assistance; ideally, the environmental arrangement includes contrasting features that make use of specific vocabulary necessary for adequate communication and for improving conversational skills. For children with CLP, these strategies provide opportunities for generalization of vocabulary and speech production targets into conversational use; when the child makes a request, the adult responds by modelling, making another request or waiting for a more elaborated response or for a targeted vocabulary response. Child attempts to produce targeted vocabulary can then be recast to model the correct phonology and to facilitate child acquisition of speech sound targets. Ability to request verbally or non-verbally and ability to imitate target forms are the only prerequisite child skills for incidental teaching.

A comparison of FS and Enhanced Milieu Teaching (EMT), which does emphasize a verbal response, showed that three toddlers with cleft lip and/or palate responded faster to the EMT procedures than to the FS procedures (Scherer, 1999). These children acquired new vocabulary faster with the EMT approach, even though both approaches did facilitate vocabulary learning. While FS was not intended to modify phonology, Girolametto, Pearce and Weitzman (1997) report that changes in consonant inventories were observed for late-talkers receiving treatment. Phonological change can be optimized through selection of treatment target vocabulary incorporating target sounds.

14.3.2.2.7   Speech Recasts   This strategy provides a cue to the child to modify substitution or omission errors within naturalistic interaction. Recasting is the repetition of the child's utterance using correct grammar and/or phonological forms. Speech recasts are those recasts that provide correct phonological information in response to a child's incorrect production. For example, the child may say 'ba' for 'ball' and the adult would provide a speech recast by responding with 'Ball. You want the ball?' The effectiveness of speech recasts has been described within naturalistic conversational intervention for pre-school children with speech and language impairments. Scherer and Kaiser (2010) have applied speech recasts to children with organic speech disorders under three years of age by embedding speech recasts into the EMT model.

14.3.3   Parent Training Programmes

Training parents to facilitate speech and language requires skills different from those used to teach children. Traditionally, parent training programmes for children with clefts include a review of speech and language milestones and a description of specific speech and language and other issues commonly observed in children with cleft palate, such as feeding, timing of palate repair and identification of compensatory articulation errors (Russell, 1989; Lynch, Brookshire and Fox, 1993). Most early intervention programmes do not address the professional skills that are important when working with adults. Clinician's often include parents in the intervention process by having them observe the session and/or giving them handouts or assignments to complete at home. While these strategies appear to have face validity, their impact on children's speech and language development has not been documented. Anecdotally, these strategies often result in limited carryover in the home or, in some cases, inappropriate application of the strategies. The Hanen Centre in Canada has developed a series of parent training programmes to facilitate speech and language development (http://www.hanen.org/web/Home/tabid/36/Default.aspx). The Hanen programmes, based on Focused Stimulation, combine group parent classes with home visits to provide parents with the skills to facilitate their child's speech and language progress. While these programmes are not specifically designed for children with cleft palate, they have been shown to benefit those children (Scherer, D'Antonio and McGahey, 2008). Kaiser and her colleagues have developed and tested the efficacy of training parents to use Enhanced Milieu Teaching to facilitate speech and language development in children with cleft palate and other developmental disabilities (Scherer and Kaiser, 2010). A typical hour parent training session includes a 15–20 minute segment to present facilitation strategies to parents. Strategies are presented through handouts, demonstration, role play and video. During a second 20 minute segment, the clinician demonstrates the strategies with the child while the parent observes, then the parent practices the strategies with their child for another 20 minutes while the clinician coaches the parent during the activities. Coaching provides supportive feedback regarding implementation of the strategies, environmental arrangement and behavioural management (Kaiser and Hancock, 2003). The parent training typically continues for 15–24 sessions. This approach combines parent training with direct intervention for the child in a way the results in the parents' ability to deliver the intervention in the home.

14.3.4   Oral Motor Programmes

Oral motor programmes have become widely used with young children with cleft lip and/or palate despite the lack of evidence to support their use. It has been difficult to justify the use of these programmes given the absence of neuromotor deficits in non-syndromic children with clefts and the general lack of treatment efficacy for oral motor programmes (Peterson-Falzone *et al.*, 2006). There is no evidence to support the association between oral motor programmes and improved articulation or velopharyngeal function for children with cleft lip and/or palate (Peterson-Falzone, Hardin-Jones and Karnell, 2010). The concern is that oral motor programs are replacing more traditional articulation and language based programs and, thereby, reducing the time devoted to articulation and language goals.

In conclusion, the evidence suggests that early intervention for children with clefts can be effective if it uses naturalistic conversational procedures, treats both early vocabulary and speech sounds simultaneously, and includes parents as intervention agents. Research into outcomes of early intervention should continue to explore the effectiveness of different timing of intervention, dosage and adaptation for rural and developing countries.

References

ACPA: American Cleft Palate-Craniofacial Association (2007) Parameters for evaluation and treatment of patients with cleft lip/palate or other craniofacial anomalies. http://www.acpa-cpf.org (accessed 23 March 2011).

Anderson, D. and Teilly, J. (2002) The MacArthur communicative developmental inventory: normative data for American sign language. *Journal of Deaf Studies and Deaf Education*, 7, 83–106.

ASHA: American Speech-Language-Hearing Association (2004) Guidelines for the audiologic assessment of children from birth to 5 years of age (guidelines). http://www.asha.org/docs/html/GL2004-00002.html (accessed 23 March 2011).

Bayley, N. (1993) *Bayley Scales of Infant Development*, Psychological Corporation, San Antonio, TX.

Berglund, E. and Eriksson, M. (2000) Communicative development in Swedish children 16–28 months old: the Swedish early communicative development inventory-words and sentences. *Scandinavian Journal of Psychology*, 41, 133–144.

Billeaud, F.P. (2003) *Communication Disorders in Infants and Toddlers: Assessment and Intervention*, Elsevier, New York.

Bleses, D., Vach, W., Slott, M. et al. (2008) Early vocabulary development in Danish and other languages: a CDI-based comparison. *Journal of Child Language*, 35, 619–650.

Bzoch, K. (2004) *Communicative disorders related to cleft lip and palate*, 5th edn, Pro-Ed, Austin, TX.

Chapman, K.L., Hardin-Jones, M.A. and Halter, K.L. (2003) The relationship between early speech and later speech and language performance for children with cleft lip and palate. *Clinical Linguistics & Phonetics*, 17, 173–197.

Collett, B.R. and Speltz, M.L. (2006) Social-emotional development of infants and young children with orofacial clefts. *Infants & Young Children*, 19 (4), 262–291.

Coston, G.N., Sayetta, R.B., Friedman, H.I. et al. (1992) Craniofacial screening profile: quick screening for congenital malformations. *Cleft Palate-Craniofacial Journal*, 291, 87–91.

D'Antonio, L.L. and Scherer, N.J. (1995) The evaluation of speech disorders associated with clefting, in *Cleft Palate Speech Managament: A Multidisciplinary Approach* (eds R. Shprintzen and J. Bardach), Mosby, St Louis, Missouri, pp. 176–220.

D'Antonio, L.L. and Scherer, N.J. (2009) Communication disorders associated with cleft palate, in *Comprehensive Cleft Care* (eds J.E. Losee and R.E. Kirschner), McGraw-Hill Medical, New York, Chapter 35.

Dunn, W. (2007) Supporting children to participate successfully in everyday life by using sensory processing knowledge. *Infants & Young Children*, 20, 84–101.

Dunn, W. and Westman, K. (1997) The sensory profile: the performance of a national sample of children without disabilities. *American Journal of Occupational Therapy*, 51, 25–34.

Fenson, L., Marchman, V.A., Thal, D. *et al.* (2007) *The MacArthur-Bates Communicative Development Inventories*, 2nd edn. Brookes, Baltimore.

Fey, M.E., Warren, S.F., Brady, N. *et al.* (2006 Early effects of responsivity education/prelinguistic milieu teaching for children with developmental delays and their parents. *Journal of Speech, Language, and Hearing Research*, **49** (3), 526–548.

Girolametto, L., Pearce, P. and Weitzman, E. (1996) Interactive focused-stimulation for toddlers with expressive vocabulary delays. *Journal of Speech and Hearing Research*, **39**, 1274–1283.

Girolametto, L., Pearce, P. and Weitzman, E. (1997) Effects of lexical intervention on the phonology of late-talkers. *Journal of Speech, Language, Hearing Research*, **40**, 338–348.

Hamilton, A., Plunkett, K. and Schafer, G. (2000) Infant vocabulary assessed with British communicative development inventory. *Journal of Child Language*, **27**, 689–705.

Jackson-Maldanado, D., Thal, D., Marchman, V. *et al.* (1993) Early lexical development in Spanish-speaking infants and toddlers. *Journal of Child Language*, **20**, 523–549.

Jelm, J.M. (1990) *Oral-Motor/Feeding Rating Scale*, Therapy Skill Builders, Tucson.

Kaiser, A. and Hancock, T. (2003) Teaching parents how to shift and support their young children's development. *Infants and Young Children*, **16**, 9–12.

Kern, S. (2007) Lexicon development in French-speaking infants. *First Language*, **27**, 227–250.

Kritzinger, A. and Louw, B. (2000) A comprehensive assessment protocol for infants and toddlers at risk for communication disorders. Part I: case history. CLINICA: applications in clinical practice of communication pathology. Monograph 5. University of Pretoria, South Africs.

Kritzinger, A. and Louw, B. (2002) A comprehensive assessment protocol for infants and toddlers at risk for communication disorders. Part II: assessment protocol. CLINICA: applications in clinical practice of communication pathology. Monograph 6. University of Pretoria, South Africa.

Linder, T.W. (1993) *Transdisciplinary Play Based Assessment*, Brookes, Baltimore, MD.

Louw, B. (1986) Black Infants with Cleft Lip and Plate: A Morpho-Functional Study. Doctoral Dissertation, University of Pretoria, South Africa.

Louw, B. and Kritzinger, A. (2008) Early communication intervention: a bright future. Paper presented at the Centenary conference: fast forward over a century. University of Pretoria, South Africa (September 2008).

Lynch, J.I., Brookshire, B.B. and Fox, D.R. (1993) *A Curriculum for Infants and Toddlers with Cleft Palate: Developing Speech and Language*, Pro Ed, Austin, TX.

Neiman, G.S. and Savage, H.E. (1997) Development of infants and toddlers with clefts from birth to three years of age. *Cleft Palate-Craniofacial Journal*, **34**, 218–225.

Paul, R. (2001) *Language Disorders from Infancy through Adolescence*, 2nd edn. Mosby, St. Louis, MO.

Peterson-Falzone, S.J., Trost-Cardamone, J., Karnell, M. and Hardin-Jones, M. (2006) *The Clinician's Guide to Treating Cleft Palate Speech*, Mosby, St Louis, MO.

Peterson-Falzone, S.J., Hardin-Jones, J. and Karnell, M. (2010) *Cleft Palate Speech*, 4th edn. Mosby, St Louis, MO.

Reid, J., Kilpatrick, N. and Reilly, S. (2006) A prospective, longitudinal study of feeding skills in a cohort of babies with cleft conditions. *Cleft Palate-Craniofacial Journal*, **43**, 702–709.

Rossetti, L.M. (1990) *The Rossetti Infant Toddler Language Scale: A Measure of Communication and Interaction*, Lingui Systems, East Moline, IL.Rossetti, L.M. (2001) *Communication Intervention. Birth to Three*, 2nd edn, Singular Thomson Learning, San Diego, CA.

Russell, J. (1989) Early intervention, in *Cleft Palate: The Nature and Remediation of Communication Problems* (ed. J. Stengelhofen), Churchill Livingstone, London, pp. 31–63.

Scherer, N.J. (1999) The speech and language status of toddlers with cleft lip and/or palate following early vocabulary intervention. *American Journal of Speech-Language Pathology*, **8**, 81–93.

Scherer, N.J. and Kaiser, A. (2010) Enhanced Milieu teaching with phonological emphasis: application for children with cleft lip and palate, in *Treatment of Speech Sound Disorders in Children* (eds A.L. Williams, S. McLeod and R. McCauley), Brookes Publishing, New York, pp. 427–452.

Scherer, N.J., D'Antonio, L.L. and McGahey, H. (2008) Early intervention for speech impairment in children with cleft palate. *Cleft Palate-Craniofacial Journal*, **45**, 18–31.

Scherer, N.J., Williams, A.L. and Proctor-Williams, K. (2008) Early and later vocalization skills in children with and without cleft palate. *International Journal of Pediatric Otorhinolaryngology*, **72**, 827–840.

Snyder, L.E. and Scherer, N.J. (2004) The development of play and language in toddlers with cleft palate. *American Journal of Speech-Language Pathology*, **13**, 1366–1380.

Squires, J.K. (2000) Identifying social/emotional and behavioural problems in infants and toddlers. *Infant-Toddler Intervention: The Transdisciplinary Journal*, **10**, 107–119.

Squires, J.K., Bricker, D. and Twombly, L. (2000) *The Ages and Stages Questionnaires: Social-Emotional (ASQ-SE)*, Brookes, Baltimore, MD.

Strauss, R.P. and Broder, H. (1993) Children with cleft lip/palate and mental retardation: a subpopulation of cleft-craniofacial team patients. *Cleft Palate-Craniofacial Journal*, **30**, 548–556.

Tardif, T., Fletcher, P., Liange, W. and Karirote, N. (2009) Early vocabulary development in Mandarin (Putonghua) and Cantonese. *Journal of Child Language*, **36**, 1115–1144.

Tiegerman-Farber, E. and Radziewicz, C. (2008) *Language Disorders in Children: Real Families, Real Issues, and Real Interventions*, Pearson, New Jersey.

Werner, E.E. (2000) Protective factors and individual resilience, in *Handbook of Early Childhood Intervention* (eds J.P. Shonkoff and S.M. Meisels), Cambridge University Press, New York City, NY, pp. 115–132.

Westby, C.E. (2000) A scale for assessing development of children's play, in *Play Diagnosis and Assessment* (eds K. Gitlin-Weiner, A. Sandgund and C. Schaefer), John Wiley & Sons, Inc., New York, pp. 15–57.

Wetherby, A. and Prizant, B.M. (1998) *Communication and Symbolic Behavior Play Scales*, Brookes, Baltimore, MD.

15

Phonological Approaches to Speech Difficulties Associated with Cleft Palate

Anne Harding-Bell[1] and Sara Howard[2]

[1] Cambridge University Hospitals NHS Foundation Trust, East of England Cleft Lip and Palate Network, Addenbrookes Hospital, Cambridge, CB2 0QQ, UK
[2] University of Sheffield, Department of Human Communication Sciences, Sheffield, S10 2TA, UK

15.1   Introduction

While speech production difficulties associated with cleft palate have traditionally been categorized as 'articulation disorders' (Morley, 1945; McWilliams and Musgrave, 1971), more recent research has recognized that the articulatory and perceptual constraints presented by a cleft palate can influence phonological development and the child's capacity to signal the phonological contrasts essential to meaningful speech. The 1980s and 1990s saw the first significant body of work on phonological approaches to speech assessment and intervention for cleft palate. Case studies by Hodson *et al.* (1983) and Lynch, Fox and Brookshire (1983), for example, used a phonological approach to identify a range of processes in the children's speech, some of which could be related directly to the effects of the cleft, whereas others resembled speech patterns found in typical phonological development. This notion of the combination of atypical and typical developmental patterns in the speech of children with a history of cleft, and of the clinical importance of trying to differentiate between the two in an individual speaker, was

Cleft Palate Speech: Assessment and Intervention, First Edition. Edited by Sara Howard, Anette Lohmander.
© 2011 John Wiley & Sons, Ltd. Published 2011 by John Wiley & Sons, Ltd.

further developed by Grunwell and Russell (1988) in a detailed study of two children with repaired cleft palate. The longitudinal nature of the study also permitted the authors to explore the relationship between early babble and pre-speech and later phonological development, and to speculate on the impact a delay in phonetic development could have on phonological development. Chapman and Hardin (1992) and Chapman (1993), in the first larger group investigations of phonological processes in the speech of children with a cleft palate, identified a considerable number of phonological processes in their data. Significantly, however, although several processes were unique to speakers with a cleft, many of the processes found were also characteristic of typical speech development. A key difference in the phonological development of the children with a repaired cleft palate seemed to be that these typical processes tend to persist for longer than in children without a cleft.

Further issues complicate the presentation of cleft-related speech difficulties. Thus, for example, over 90% of children with a cleft palate under the age of two will experience some degree of fluctuating hearing loss, which may affect their speech development (Broen et al., 1996; Shriberg et al., 2003). In addition, a link between phonological problems and language impairment in children with cleft palate has also been noted (Pamplona et al., 2000) and Morris and Ozanne (2003) emphasize the need to incorporate both phonological and language measures into assessment protocols for children with cleft palate. The picture is thus not a simple one, and Harding and Grunwell (1998) stress the importance, in speech analysis for cleft palate, of differentiating carefully between those processes which are to be expected in typical phonological development, those which may characterize non-cleft speech delay or disorder, and those which can be directly related to the history of cleft and associated hearing problems. This chapter explores the phonological perspective on assessment and intervention for cleft-related speech impairment, drawing on examples from clinical data to demonstrate the impact of articulatory and perceptual constraints on phonology in individuals with a cleft palate.

A phonological approach to speech related to cleft palate shifts the focus away from the articulation of individual sound segments, to the consideration of patterns of sound use. At the heart of phonological analysis lies the premise that individual sound segments do not operate in isolation. Sounds group together to form sound classes (e.g. nasals; plosives; voiceless plosives; sibilant fricatives etc.) which are likely to behave in the same ways in a particular child's speech production (for example, all fricatives may be subject to the process of stopping, or all word-final consonants may be subject to deletion). Furthermore, the realization of particular sounds and sound classes may be significantly influenced by their position within a particular syllable, word or even phrase (Grunwell, 1982; Sosa and Bybee, 2008). It is important, therefore, to reflect on both the systemic and distributional properties of the child's phonological system: that is to say, on the set of sounds which the child is using contrastively and on their distribution within syllables and words (and perhaps larger contexts). Phonological process analysis has proved a popular and effective framework for working with speech related to cleft palate, and it is particularly useful because it provides direct comparisons with the immature speech production patterns found in typical speech development, and with atypical patterns characteristic of other types of developmental speech disorder (Grunwell, 1982; Miccio and Scarpino, 2008).

15.2   Variability, Variation and Compensation

Although consistent speech output patterns can be expected in speech data associated with cleft palate, this is not to say that individual speakers will be entirely consistent across all contexts and situations, and nor can consistency be expected across different speakers. Rather, the literature reports considerable intra- and inter-speaker variation (Lynch, Fox and Brookshire, 1983; Grunwell and Russell, 1988; Estrem and Broen, 1989; Chapman, 1993). Intra-speaker variability may be characteristic of typical speech development in very young children (McLeod and Hewett, 2008) and could suggest that normal developmental simplifications are gradually resolving, therefore being seen as a positive sign in a child's speech production, or, where more severe, may be indicative of a phonological impairment (Grunwell, 1982; Dodd, 1995) or specifically related to the influence of a cleft (Harding and Grunwell, 1996).

Inter-speaker variation may have significant clinical implications for diagnosis and intervention. Thus, for example, Grunwell and Russell (1988) and Estrem and Broen (1989) both illustrate contrasting cases, where the speech output of one child can be explained largely by the impact of the cleft, whereas the speech patterns of the second child are better understood with reference to typical phonological developmental processes. Inter-speaker variation also, of course, illustrates the diverse and creative responses of individual speakers to the articulatory and perceptual constraints presented by the cleft. Hutters and Brønsted (1987) and Harding and Grunwell (1998) discuss the consequences for speech output of a speaker adopting either a passive or active approach to the problems presented by cleft-related speech production difficulties. Thus, for some speakers, consciously or subconsciously, maintaining accurate place and manner of articulation for consonant segments may be paramount, but at the cost of accompanying hypernasal resonance and nasal emission. Where control of resonance and airflow takes precedence, however, this may be achieved by significant changes in the place, manner and voicing characteristics of target consonants. Broen, Doyle and Bacon (1993) and Howard (1993) stress the creative and sometimes rather subtle ways in which children with a cleft signal phonological distinctions. Although the patterns identified for an individual speaker may be unusual and unpredictable, they nevertheless represent a reasonable response to the challenge of signalling phonological and lexical contrasts in the face of articulatory and/or perceptual constraints. In some cases, consistent patterns of production may not be detectable by human eye or ear, even though they are clearly demonstrable by instrumental analysis (Howard, 1993; Gibbon, 2004): in this case, even though the child appears to be intending to signal phonological contrasts, these are not apparent to the listener and thus intelligibility is reduced even in the presence of consistent phonological behaviour.

A further response to speech production constraints for some children with a cleft palate, in the very early stages of phonological development, is that of lexical selectivity, or an avoidance of words containing challenging sounds (Estrem and Broen, 1989; Scherer, 1999). This phenomenon is also found in typical speech development, and in other kinds of speech impairment (Stoel-Gammon, 2011), and may serve to partially explain the finding of Chapman and Hardin (1992) that the two-year-olds in their study produced very few compensatory articulations.

15.3   Classification of Speech Difficulties Related to Cleft Palate

Speech production related to a cleft palate, whilst demonstrating characteristic patterns and behaviours, also displays rich variety when individual speakers are compared. For each child, a complex set of structural, perceptual, cognitive and developmental circumstances, and the child's responses to these circumstances, produces a unique profile of speech production. Where differential diagnosis of the nature of the child's speech difficulties is necessary, phonological analysis can contribute to this process. Harding and Sell (2001) provide an extensive list of 'speech diagnostic categories' associated with cleft palate. Amongst these categories are 'Articulatory disorder related to structural constraints' and 'Phonological disorder', but also 'Articulatory disorder with phonological consequences'.

This last is worth a little further comment here. In a phonological disorder, it may be expected that the systemic and/or distributional limitations present in a child's phonological system will, in turn, create difficulties for the listener: the speaker's intelligibility is reduced by lack of ability to signal phonological contrasts appropriately. Significantly, however, what constitutes a phonological problem from the *listener's* perspective may have different explanations when speech production is examined from the perspective of the *speaker*. Thus some children will have cognitive problems related to the mental representation and organization of the phonological system, and their speech production will reflect these difficulties: this would be categorized as a true 'phonological disorder' in Harding and Sell's classificatory system. For other children, however, cognitive organization and mental representation is normal, but cannot be successfully expressed in speech output due to physical constraints: an 'articulatory disorder' from the point of view of the speaker, which has 'phonological consequences' for intelligibility from the perspective of the listener (Hewlett, 1985, and Grundy and Harding, 1995, provide further discussion of this issue). It is important to distinguish between these two possibilities, because they have significant implications for planning appropriate intervention.

15.4   Phonological Assessment of Speech Data Related to Cleft Palate

To assess the phonological dimensions of the speech production difficulties of a child with cleft palate, it is imperative that this analysis should (i) be based on good quality phonetic data, using narrow phonetic transcription (Chapter 7) and (ii) be systematic and replicable. In the United Kingdom the standard assessment for speech related to cleft palate (the GOS.SP.ASS; Sell, Harding and Grunwell, 1994, 1999) contains sections which capture phonological information. In Scandinavia standardized procedures for the assessment of speech related to cleft palate have also been developed. The Swedish Articulation and Nasality test (SVANTE) provides an opportunity to perform analysis of both articulation and phonology (Lohmander et al., 2005). In addition, a restricted part of the test may be used for the purposes of cross-linguistic comparison (www.clispi.org). The test will soon be available in Norwegian (SVANTE-N). Where a more detailed phonological analysis is deemed necessary, the DEAP (Diagnostic Evaluation of Articulation and Phonology; Dodd *et al.*, 2002) and PACSTOYS (Grunwell and Harding-Bell, 2005) are useful tools for English speaking children; helpful resources for use in a number of other languages are shown at the clispi website (www.clispi.se).

The 'Consonant Production' section of the GOSS.SP.ASS, displays English consonant targets in tabular form along a horizontal axis, grouped by place of articulation. This horizontal arrangement reflects the organization of the IPA chart (itself designed to reflect the spatial relationships of the vocal organs), thus facilitating rapid identification of any patterns in the phonological system that might be directly related to articulatory constraints. Consonant realizations are documented for two different contexts, Syllable Initial Word Initial (SIWI) and Syllable Final Word Final (SFWF), thus allowing for identification of at least some contextual influences on segmental productions. The authors also stress the importance of including transcriptions of different realizations of the same target in the same context in order to capture information on speaker variability, and suggest that phonetic transcription of spontaneous speech should also be included, as this 'may reveal phonological information not available from the sentence imitation data' (Sell, Harding and Grunwell, 1994, p. 7). This is an important point, as for some children there are important differences between speech production data collected using formal assessments and that which occurs in spontaneous connected speech (Howard, 2007; Speake, Howard and Vance, in press). The DEAP and PACSTOYS, meanwhile, provide a tool for more extensive exploration of a child's phonological organization, which can be very useful in differentiating patterns associated with typical development and non-cleft developmental speech delay and disorders from those associated with cleft-related difficulties.

15.5   Phonological Consequences of Speech Production Related to Cleft Palate

In this section, some real clinical data from the speech production of three young children with a cleft palate are used to illustrate and exemplify phonological patterns found in speech associated with cleft palate and to explore their consequences for intelligible speech. The table from the 'Consonant Production' section of the GOS.SP.ASS is used to present the data, but it should be noted that this only provides a partial phonological analysis. Importantly, however, the tables clearly demonstrate the relevance of including a phonological perspective in routine speech assessment for speech related to a cleft, in order to demonstrate the extent to which meaningful contrasts are constrained by the limitations of the child's systemic and distributional use of sounds.

15.5.1   Taylor: The Phonological Consequences of Backing

Examined in this first example are speech production data from Taylor, a two-year-old child who realises almost all oral consonants in word-initial position as the voiced velar plosive [g] and does not realize consonant targets in word final position. Table 15.1a

Table 15.1a Taylor's speech production: Sample single word data at age 2;0.

fish	/fɪʃ/	[gɪ]	dish	/dɪʃ/	[gɪ]
pig	/pɪg/	[gɪ]	biscuit	/'bɪskɪt/	['gɪgɪ]
doggy	/'dɒgi/	['gɒgi]	ship	/ʃɪp/	[gɪ]
shop	/ʃɒp/	[gɒ]	dog	/dɒg/	[gɒ]

Table 15.1b Taylor's consonant realizations at age 2;0.

		Labial				Alveolar						Postalveolar			Velar			Gl.
Target	m	p	b	f	v	n	l	t	d	s	z	ʃ	tʃ	dʒ	ŋ	k	g	h
SIWI	m, ŋ	g	g	g	g	-	ŋ	j	g	g	g	g	g	g	-	g	g	-
SFWF	ø	ø	ø	ø	-	ø	-	ø	ø	ø	-	ø	ø	-	-	ø	ø	-

shows a small sample of single word data and Table 15.1b plots his consonant realizations in SIWI and SFWF contexts.

The considerable restrictions in phonological contrastivity in Taylor's speech output can best be explained as the product of a combination of typical developmental processes and cleft related processes. Thus, realizations of /f, s, ʃ/ as [g] are affected by both a pervasive cleft-related backing process and also the typical developmental process of stopping. The word final deletion pattern is developmentally typical at age 2.0, but in addition might be related to cleft-related hearing problems. The backing pattern in these data is particularly pervasive, affecting not only the coronal consonant targets /t, d, n, s, z, ʃ, tʃ, dʒ/ but also the labials /p, b, f, v/. It is not usual to define velar realization of bilabial consonant targets as 'backing' because the process involves a shift from one set of articulators (the lips) to another (the tongue), so we may just want to describe this pattern as velar realization of bilabial and alveolar targets. Backing patterns are not exclusive to the speech of individuals with a cleft palate, but they are less commonly reported in non-cleft speech difficulties and it would certainly be unusual to find labial /p, b, f, v/ realised as [g] in children without a cleft palate. In speech production associated with cleft palate, the process of backing is generally interpreted as the consequence of an active strategy of retraction which preserves the manner of articulation of anterior plosive targets, but with the consequent sacrifice of anterior place of articulation for an entire class of consonants (Harding and Grunwell, 1998). Such realizations have frequently been associated with the presence of a residual cleft or a fistula (Lohmander, Persson and Owman-Moll, 2002), although Trost-Cardamone and Bernthal (1993) remind us that retracted articulations may also be linked to an early history of hearing loss consequent on otitis media. In Taylor's case, despite a history of bilateral cleft, no anterior fistula could be identified. He was, however, diagnosed with bilateral hearing loss.

15.5.2 Joe: The Phonological Consequences of Glottal Articulation

The data in Tables 15.2a–15.2d present speech data from Joe, a boy with speech production affected by a cleft, at age 2;0, 3;0 and 4;6, illustrating how a predominantly

Table 15.2a   Joe's speech production: sample single word data at age 2;0.

chair	/tʃɛə/	[ʔɛə]	teddy	/'tɛdi/	['ʔɛʔi]
shoe	/ʃu/	[ʔu]	fish	/fɪʃ/	[ʔɪʔ]
book	/bʊk/	[(b͡)ʔʊʔ]	two	/tu/	[ʔu]
zoo	/zu/	[ʔu]	baby	/'beɪbi/	['(b͡)ʔeɪ(b͡)ʔɪ]

Table 15.2b   Joe's consonant realizations at age 2;0.

	Labial					Alveolar						Postalveolar			Velar			Gl.
Target	**m**	p	b	f	v	**n**	l	t	d	s	z	ʃ	tʃ	dʒ	ŋ	k	g	h
SIWI		?	(b͡)ʔ	?	-		-	-	?	-	?	-	?	?		-	?	
SFWF		-	-	ø	-		-	?	ø	ø	ø	?	ø	ø		?	-	

Items in bold were accurately realised in both SIWI and SFWF positions.

Table 15.2c   Joe's consonant realizations at age 3;0.

	Labial					Alveolar						Postalveolar			Velar			Gl.
Target	**m**	p	b	f	v	**n**	l	t	d	s	z	ʃ	tʃ	dʒ	ŋ	k	g	h
SIWI		h	b͡ʔ	-	-		j	h	?	h	?	h	?	?		h	?	
SFWF		?	?	?	-		-	?	?	?	?	?	?	?		?	?	

Items in bold were accurately realised in both SIWI and SFWF positions.

Table 15.2d   Joe's consonant realizations at age 4;6.

	Labial					Alveolar						Postalveolar			Velar			Gl.
Target	**m**	**p**	**b**	**f**	**v**	**n**	**l**	**t**	**d**	**s**	**z**	**ʃ**	**tʃ**	**dʒ**	**ŋ**	**d**	**k**	**h**
SIWI																		
SFWF										ɦ	ɦ	ɦ						

Items in bold were accurately realised in both SIWI and SFWF positions.

glottal pattern of articulation at age 2;0 evolved, with a gradual expansion of both systemic and distributional possibilities.

As with Taylor's speech data, above, when Joe is 2;0 we can see evidence of the typical developmental phonological processes of stopping and, variably, of final consonant deletion. However, the most pervasive pattern in Joe's phonological system, and one which is greatly detrimental to his intelligibility, is his glottal realization of all obstruent consonants. For the listener, this results in a massive collapse of phonological contrastivity.

By age 3;0 the speech data reveal that Joe has begun to distinguish between voiced and voiceless plosives in word initial position, realising the former as a glottal stop [ʔ], and the latter as a voiceless glottal fricative [h]. It might be hypothesized from these data that the salient contrastive feature which Joe has settled on to distinguish between these two sound classes is the aspiration component typical of initial, pre-vocalic realizations of /p, t, k/ in his accent of British English, where /p, t, k/ are realised as [pʰ, tʰ, kʰ]. At age 4;6 a context-sensitive pattern is now identifiable for fricatives and affricates, whereby Joe continues to realize them as glottal stops in word-initial position, but realises them as voiceless pharyngeal fricatives in word-final position. Hence Joe's speech data at this point show that he is highly systematic in his phonological behaviour, but that as he has attempted to expand his repertoire of phonological contrasts, he has introduced more compensatory strategies into his sound system.

In both Taylor and Joe's cases, aspects of their speech data could not be definitively or exclusively attributed to their cleft palate: some patterns might also have been related to their histories of conductive hearing loss, or to a co-occurring developmental phonological disorder. The common occurrence of fluctuating conductive hearing loss in children with a cleft palate is likely to affect speech perception and production and speech problems associated with hearing loss, including initial and final consonant deletion, glottalization of initial consonants the voicing of voiceless consonants, vowel distortions and backing of anterior fricatives and stops are all reported consequences of hearing impairment (Oller and Kelly, 1974; Shriberg *et al.*, 2003). In the clinical context, uncertain attribution of individual speech characteristics indicates the need to gather more evidence in order to facilitate accurate differential diagnosis and to plan effective intervention.

15.5.3 Jamie: The Phonological Consequences of Nasal Realization of Plosives and Fricatives

Tables 15.3a and 15.3b show data from Jamie, a two-year-old boy who has a pattern of nasal realization of oral consonants in his speech production. This is a pervasive

Table 15.3a Jamie's speech production: Sample single word data at age 2;0.

cup	/kʌp/	[nʌʔ]	book	/bʊk/	[mʊʔ]
shoe	/ʃu/	[nu]	pen	/pɛn/	[mɛn]
bed	/bɛd/	[mɛ]	teddy	/'tɛdi/	['nɛni]
dolly	/'dɒli/	['nɒni]	cat	/kæt/	[næʔ]

Table 15.3b Jamie's consonant realizations at age 2;0.

	Labial					Alveolar							Postalveolar		Velar			Gl.
Target	**m**	p	b	f	v	n	l	t	d	s	z	ʃ	tʃ	dʒ	ŋ	k	g	**h**
SIWI		m	m	m	m	n	n	n	n	n	n		n	n		n	n	
SFWF		?		(f)	(v)	ø	?	ø	?	ø	?		?	ø		?	ø	

Items in bold were accurately realised in both SIWI and SFWF positions.

pattern affecting all obstruent consonants in SIWI position. In SFWF almost all consonants, whether oral or nasal, are omitted or realised as a glottal stop. The negative consequences for Jamie's ability to signal phonological contrasts and for the intelligibility of his speech output are severe. Such a prevalence of nasal realizations is strong evidence of velopharyngeal dysfunction (VPD), but it could also relate to hearing loss (Donahue, 1993).

In Jamie's speech output the conflation of the set of consonants in SIWI position into a single contrast, [m] versus [n], can be interpreted as a passive process (Harding and Grunwell, 1998) in the face of suspected velopharyngeal dysfunction. Nasal realization of plosive targets combines with the typical developmental processes of context-sensitive voicing (all pre-vocalic consonant realizations are voiced, regardless of the voicing status of the target); stopping (fricative and affricate targets are realised as stops), and fronting of velar plosives.

15.6   Intervention

15.6.1   Aims of Intervention

Phonologically-based therapy for children with developmental speech disorders (including those with a cleft palate) aims to change a child's speech output by bringing it closer to an age-appropriate and sociophonetically-appropriate system. In achieving this, improvements in speech intelligibility and acceptability should follow. As Tyler (2005, p. 127) notes, 'children with phonological disorders may encounter difficulties at peripheral auditory or articulatory levels, as well as at a higher organizational level': thus phonological therapy will aim to tackle potential problems at any or all of these levels. For children with phonological difficulties who have a repaired cleft palate, where both articulatory and auditory constraints are likely to contribute to their speech problems, it may be particularly important to combine phonological principles with more traditionally-based articulatory intervention techniques (Grunwell and Dive, 1988; Russell, 2010).

15.6.2   Phonological Principles in Intervention Change,
Expansion and Generalization

Grunwell (1992, p. 101) notes that, 'The essence of speech therapy is to facilitate change in a person's communication abilities: change furthermore that is progressive' and describes a sequence of four processes required to bring about positive phonological change: destablization, innovation, stabilization and generalization. To facilitate the introduction of new speech output patterns, the child's current, stable and inaccurate output patterns need to be destabilized. This then allows for innovation: the introduction of new (and preferred) patterns into the child's speech output, which should in turn expand the phonological system. As the new patterns are introduced there is likely to be a period of variable speech output, but the aim should be the gradual stabilization of the new patterns and the consequent gradual disappearance of the old patterns.

Generalization of the patterns to new contexts (whether these be phonological, lexical, linguistic or socio-environmental) will also be a gradual process, involving variability and progressive stabilization. Generalization of a specific contrast could include work on phonetically selected syllable and word contexts, as well as on phrase contexts (Pascoe, Stackhouse and Wells, 2005) and ultimately, if necessary, on spontaneous connected speech (Howard, 2007).

15.6.3   The Child's Perspective

It is quite possible that a child's perception of their own speech may be quite different from that of other listeners and they may have quite different attributions for their lack of intelligibility and consequent breakdowns in communication (Howard, 2004; Holliday, Harrison and McLeod, 2009). It may help parents to understand that young children with a speech impairment often attribute their communication difficulties to the inattention or auditory difficulties of the listener, and therefore no assumptions can be made that children are motivated to change or improve their speech. This was the case for two of the children discussed above: both Joe and Taylor perceived their own speech output as normal. Divergent opinions exist in the literature about the need for children to understand the nature of their inaccurate speech and for them to be motivated to change before therapy can be effective. For some children, however, it may be important to explore their recognition of their difficulties and the extent of their motivation to change their speech (Havstam, Sandberg and Lohmander, 2010).

15.6.4   Phonologically Based Therapies

In the same way that non-cleft phonological disorders are most effectively addressed through targeting phonological patterns, rather than individual sounds (Stoel-Gammon, Stone-Goldman and Glaspey, 2002), phonological approaches can also be fruitfully applied to therapy for cleft palate speech disorders. The aim, as stated earlier, is to improve intelligibility by expanding the child's sound system and the syllabic and lexical contexts in which target sounds may occur. Various current approaches have been used in intervention with children with cleft palate, or have been noted for their potential in cleft intervention. These include the Cycles approach (Hodson and Paden, 1991), Stimulability Intervention (Miccio and Elbert, 1996), Multiple Exemplar Training (Bowen and Cupples, 1999) and Multiple Opposition intervention (Williams, 2000). Detailed accounts of these and other phonological interventions have been provided by Williams, McLeod and McCauley (2010); Howard (2010) supplies a summary of current approaches.

The greater emphasis in recent literature on specifically addressing speech output in phonological interventions (in addition to the more traditional phonological emphasis on perception, discrimination and organization) is helpful in planning intervention for children with a cleft palate, who are likely to benefit most from an approach which combines articulatory and cognitive principles to changing speech output. In an early account of such a combined approach to intervention, Grunwell and Dive (1988) describe a programme where the initial emphasis is on auditory work, drawing the child's attention to the phonological properties of sounds and sounds classes, with production of sounds only targeted at a relatively late stage in the intervention as a whole. More recently, Pamplona, Ysunza and Espinosa (1999) have reported that intervention which combines articulation and phonology is more effective than a purely articulatory approach.

15.6.5   Combining Phonological and Articulatory Approaches

Whilst intervention approaches for non-cleft speech disorders are frequently designed to reflect the course of typical phonological development, goal setting in the presence of structural and articulatory constraints can only be guided, but not exclusively driven, by typical developmental patterns. Attention must be paid to the child's articulatory capacities in the light of their individual cleft history and their individual speech output profile. Harding and Grunwell (1998) provide explicit advice on principled target selection and therapy planning, based on the phonetic features of place, manner and voicing, and on the ways in which these features, and their contrastive function, might be specifically challenged by a cleft palate.

They identify four principles to assist the decision making process for target selection. Three of these processes are systemic: (i) fricative targets (especially in word-final position) may be stimulable in advance of plosives because of differences in air pressure requirements between the two sound classes; (ii) a focus on alveolar sounds may be necessary because, unlike in typical speech development, velar segments commonly emerge before alveolars in the cleft population; and (iii) voiceless pressure consonants (plosives, fricatives and affricates) may be more achievable than their voiced counterparts, because the open glottis in voiceless segments facilitates airflow from the lungs. The fourth principle relates to phonological structure: (iv) Harding and Grunwell observe that word-final pressure consonants might be more achievable than word-initial pressure consonants. These phonetic–phonological considerations might discourage use of a typical developmental perspective in selecting the order in which consonant classes are targeted in intervention.

Planning appropriate intervention entails detailed knowledge of the phonetics of speech production, of normal phonological development and of the recognized phonological patterns associated with cleft palate. By working on sound classes, on features which are common to groups of sounds, rather than on individual sound segments, and on specific phonological contexts, widespread change through the child's phonological system can be facilitated. Harding and Grunwell (1998) emphasize the need to pay attention to the visual, as well as auditory, aspects of speech production in working on input with children. They also recommend that all models are presented with minimum effort: in contrast to Golding-Kushner's recommendation (2001) of exaggerated articulatory models, Russell and Harding (2001) suggest that effortful models may encourage or perpetuate effortful compensatory articulation. Avoidance of exaggeration in modelling consonant patterns is also more likely to produce models which more closely reflect the phonetics of real connected speech.

15.6.6   Intervention Principles in Action

For each of the children whose assessment data were discussed earlier, decisions regarding intervention were subsequently necessary. The analysis of Jamie's pattern of nasal realizations suggested that they were the passive consequence of velopharyngeal dysfunction, a hypothesis which was confirmed with videofluoroscopy (Chapter 8) and treated with secondary surgery (Chapter 5). Speech patterns normalized rapidly following surgery and no further speech therapy was needed. In contrast, Taylor and Joe's speech output, dominated by the active processes of backing and glottal realization respectively, indicated that therapy would be beneficial in both cases. Here a brief summary is presented of the ways in which phonological and articulatory principles were combined to address their speech output problems.

15.6.6.1   Selecting the Therapy Approach: Output Versus Input Based Therapy   Both boys were very young when the phonological consequences of cleft palate were identified and each presented with a history of hearing loss. They were both reluctant to engage with output activities, but it was felt that urgent active intervention was needed in order to facilitate effective spoken communication by the time of school entry, so input based approaches were adopted. Principles from pattern based therapy (Stoel-Gammon, Stone-Goldman and Glaspey, 2002), multiple exemplar training (Bowen and Cupples, 1999) and multisensory input therapy (Harding and Bryan, 2000; Calladine, 2009) were used in combination to produce a hierarchically-ordered programme aimed to intensify the boys awareness of specific contrastive features, without the requirement for them to produce speech targets.

15.6.6.2   Phonological Goals   The primary phonological goal in both cases was to introduce place of articulation contrasts, with a focus on classes of sounds, rather than on individual segments. Conventional phonological therapy would have focussed solely on auditory processing but these boys, in common with many children with cleft palate, had a history of hearing problems, so emphasis was also placed on highlighting the visual information available in speech production. Activities which combined visual and auditory bombardment were carried out, with a particular focus on maximizing opportunities to *see* (as well as hear) the difference between articulatory gestures for bilabials, alveolars and velars. Activities designed to increase the salience of the place of articulation included visual discrimination, visual recognition, deliberate error activities in the context of conventional scaffolding activities (sound in isolation, sound sequences, whole word, phrases), all without any requirement for output practice. This emphasis on awareness of place of articulation through visual models was designed to supplement auditory representations which might have been affected by early conductive hearing loss. Given that both boys were using place-related processes which affected whole classes of consonants, a horizontal intervention approach was adopted (Bowen and Cupples, 1999), in which all alveolar targets were presented over a period of weeks, thus emphasizing the shared feature of place of articulation.

In each case, principles taken from maximal opposition therapy (Gierut, 2001; Williams, 2000) informed the development of activities demonstrating place of articulation contrasts with an identifiable visual component, in this case between bilabial sounds (e.g. [p] and [b]) and posterior sounds produced with open lips (e.g. [k, h]). Unlike conventional articulation therapy the emphasis was initially on the visual, rather than auditory, characteristics of the sound classes being contrasted, and the modelled sounds were identified as 'sound-shapes' rather than sounds. Activities followed a hierarchy from shapes in isolation to contrasting sound shapes in word, phrase and sentence level. Neither boy was asked for, and neither spontaneously offered, speech output during this phase of intervention.

Manner of articulation was also addressed in therapy by working on the contrast between plosives and fricatives: once again the focus was on contrasting sound classes, rather than individual pairs of sounds. This contrast was presented in word-final position, based on the observation by Harding and Grunwell (1998) that pressure consonants tend to emerge first in this context. Care was taken not to produce exaggerated models of either fricative or plosive segments, so as to better match their auditory properties in real connected speech.

The voiced–voiceless contrast was targeted by modelling plosive contrasts, where the voiceless models were weakly articulated, with prolonged aspiration [$p^{h:}$, $t^{h:}$, $k^{h:}$], in order to maximize the contrasting input. A conventional, developmental approach would have suggested a specific focus on voiced targets, but the particular problems associated with voiced plosives in terms of the control of sub- and supra-glottal pressure and air flow (Isshiki and Ringel, 1964) suggested that the class of voiceless plosives would provide a better starting point for intervention.

15.6.7 Intervention Summary

Two principles underpinned intervention for both Taylor and Joe. The first was the focus on input activities combining visual and auditory components, to inform and change their mental phonological representations without requiring them to produce sounds themselves. The second was the focus on classes of sounds, rather than on individual sounds or contrasts between individual segments, and on phonological structure and word and syllable contexts, in order to maximize change throughout the system.

15.7 Summary

Phonological processes and patterns in speech related to cleft palate develop from the consonant repertoire available in early speech, which itself is influenced by the presence of both structural and perceptual constraints. Phonological assessment identifies phonological processes or patterns operating across classes of sounds and occurring in specific contexts. The information derived from a rudimentary phonological analysis in a routine clinical assessment, such as GOSSPASS (Sell, Harding and Grunwell, 1999) and SVANTE (Lohmander et al., 2005), contributes to differential diagnosis and may help to identify velopharyngeal problems, the presence of a fistula and/or hearing-related speech difficulties.

Intervention planning can be based on articulatory–phonological principles by selecting classes of consonants based on the phonetic requirements of specific consonants in relation to articulatory constraints. Activities incorporate auditory and visual input work as well as production with an emphasis on visual attention to the articulatory pattern, in order to supplement variable auditory perception. Targets for therapy include classes of sounds in specific phonological contexts in order to expand and normalize the phonological system. Passive processes, as illustrated by Jamie's data, are likely to be improved by surgery, but active processes, such as Joe's prevalent glottal pattern and Taylor's backing pattern, require speech interventions based on phonological principles in order to destabilize atypical phonological processes, and to introduce and stabilize new, preferred patterns.

Partnership with parents and children enhances the effectiveness of therapy and early intervention, with focussed parental input from infancy, should optimize listening skills and stimulate articulatory and phonological awareness so as to normalize early phonological behaviours and discourage the establishment of compensatory strategies and active processes.

References

Bowen, C. and Cupples, L. (1999) Parents and Children Together (PACT): a collaborative approach to phonological therapy. *International Journal of Language and Communication Disorders*, 34 (1), 35–35.

Broen, P.A., Doyle, S. and Bacon, C.K. (1993) The velopharyngeally inadequate child: phonologic change with intervention. *Cleft Palate-Craniofacial Journal*, 30 (5), 500–507.

Broen, P.A., Moller, K., Carlstrom, J. *et al.* (1996) Comparison of the hearing histories of children with and without cleft palate. *Cleft Palate-Craniofacial Journal*, 33 (2), 127–133.

Calladine, S. (2009) Multi-sensory input modelling with children with cleft palate. MSc dissertation. University of Sheffield, UK.

Chapman, K.L. (1993) Phonologic processes in children with cleft palate. *Cleft Palate-Craniofacial Journal*, 30 (1), 64–72.

Chapman, K.L. and Hardin, M.A. (1992) Phonetic and phonological skills of two-year-olds with cleft palate. *Cleft Palate-Craniofacial Journal*, 29 (5), 435–443.

Dodd, B. (1995) *Differential Diagnosis and Treatment of Children with Speech Disorder*, Whurr, London.

Dodd, B., Zhu, H., Crosbie, S. *et al.* (2002) *Diagnostic Evaluation of Articulation and Phonology*, Psychological Press, London.

Donahue, M.L. (1993) Early phonological and lexical development in otitis media: a diary study. *Journal of Child Language*, 20 (3), 489–501.

Estrem, T. and Broen, P.A. (1989) Early speech production of children with cleft palate. *Journal of Speech and Hearing Research*, 32 (1), 12–23.

Gibbon, F.E. (2004) Abnormal patterns of tongue-palate contact in the speech of individuals with cleft palate. *Clinical Linguistics & Phonetics*, 18 (4/5), 285–311.

Gierut, J. (2001) Complexity in phonological treatment: clinical factors. *Language, Speech and Hearing Services in Schools*, 32, 229–241.

Golding-Kushner, K.J. (2001) *Therapy Techniques for Cleft Palate Speech and Related Disorders*, Singular, San Diego.

Grundy, K. and Harding, A. (1995) Disorders of speech production, *Linguistics in Clinical Practice*, 2nd edn (ed. K. Grundy), Whurr, London, pp. 329–357.

Grunwell, P. (1982) *Clinical Phonology*, Croom Helm, London.

Grunwell, P. (1992) Processes of phonological change in developmental speech disorders. *Clinical Linguistics & Phonetics*, 6 (1&2), 101–122.

Grunwell, P. and Dive, D. (1988) Treating 'cleft palate speech': combining phonological techniques with articulation therapy. *Child Language Teaching and Therapy*, **4** (2), 193–210.

Grunwell, P. and Harding-Bell, A. (2005) *PACSTOYS*, STASS Publications, Ponteland.

Grunwell, P. and Russell, J. (1988) Phonological development in children with cleft lip and palate. *Clinical Linguistics & Phonetics*, **2** (2), 75–95.

Harding, A. and Bryan, A. (2000) Multi-sensory input modelling. Video available from Cleft.Net. East Box 46 Addenbrookes Hospital, Cambridge University Hospitals, NHS Foundation Trust, Hills Road Cambridge CB2 0QQ.

Harding, A. and Grunwell, P. (1996) Characteristics of cleft palate speech. *European Journal of Disorders of Communication*, **31** (4): 331–358.

Harding, A. and Grunwell, P. (1998) Active versus passive cleft-type speech characteristics. *International Journal of Language and Communication Disorders*, **33** (3), 329–352.

Harding, A. and Sell, D. (2001) Cleft palate and velopharyngeal anomalies, in *Speech and Language Therapy: The Decision-Making Process When Working with Children* (eds M. Kersner and J. Wright), David Fulton, London, pp. 215–230.

Havstam, C., Sandberg, A. and Lohmander, A. (2010) Communication attitude and speech in 10-year-old children with cleft (lip and) palate in an ICF perspective. *International Journal of Speech-Language Pathology*, **13** (2), E-publication ahead of print.

Hewlett, N. (1985) Phonological versus phonetic disorders: some suggested modifications to the current use of the distinction. *British Journal of Disorders of Communication*, **20** (2), 155–164.

Hodson, B. and Paden, E. (1991) *Targetting Intelligible Speech: A Phonological Approach to Remediation*, 2nd edn. Pro-Ed, Austin, Texas.

Hodson, B.W., Chin, L., Redmond, B. and Simpson, R. (1983) Phonological evaluation and remediation of a child with a repaired cleft palate. *Journal of Speech & Hearing Disorders*, **48** (1), 93–98.

Holliday, E.L., Harrison, L.J. and McLeod, S. (2009) Listening to children with communication impairment talking through their drawings. *Journal of Early Childhood Research*, **7** (3), 244–263.

Howard, S.J. (1993) Articulatory constraints on a phonological system: a case study of cleft palate speech. *Clinical Linguistics & Phonetics*, **7** (4), 299–317.

Howard, S.J. (2004) Compensatory articulatory behaviours in adolescents with cleft palate: comparing the perceptual and instrumental evidence. *Clinical Linguistics & Phonetics*, **18** (4–5), 313–340.

Howard, S.J. (2007) The interplay between articulation and prosody in children with impaired speech: observations from electropalatography and perceptual analysis. *International Journal of Speech-Language Pathology*, **9** (1), 20–35.

Howard, S. (2010) Children's speech disorders, in *The Handbook of Language and Speech Disorders* (eds J. Damico, N. Müller and M. Ball), Wiley-Blackwell, Oxford, pp. 337–361.

Hutters, B. and Brønsted, K. (1987) Strategies in cleft palate speech – with special reference to Danish. *Cleft Palate-Craniofacial Journal*, **24** (2), 126–136.

Isshiki, N. and Ringel, R. (1964) Airflow during the production of selected consonants. *Journal of Speech and Hearing Research*, **7**, 233–244.

Lohmander, A., Persson, C. and Owman-Moll, P. (2002) Unrepaired clefts in the hard palate: speech deficits at the ages of 5 and 7 years and their relationship to size of the cleft. *Scandinavian Journal of Plastic and Reconstructive Surgery and Hand Surgery*, **36**, 332–339.

Lohmander, A., Borell, E., Henningsson, G. *et al.* (2005) SVANTE – SVenskt Artikulations- och NasalitetsTEst [English: Swedish Articulation and NAsality test], Lund, Studentlitteratur.

Lynch, J.I., Fox, D.R. and Brookshire, B.L. (1983) Phonological proficiency of two cleft palate toddlers with school-age follow-up. *Journal of Speech and Hearing Disorders*, **48** (2), 274–285.

McLeod, S. and Hewett, S.R. (2008) Variability in the production of words containing consonant clusters by typically-developing 2- and 3-year-old children. *Folia Phoniatrica et Logopaedica*, 60 (4), 163–172.

McWilliams, B.J. and Musgrave, R.H. (1971) Diagnosis of speech problems in patients with cleft palate. *British Journal of Disorders of Communication*, 6 (1), 26–32.

Miccio, A.W. and Elbert, M. (1996) Enhancing stimulability: a treatment program. *Journal of Communication Disorders*, 29, 335–351.

Miccio, A.W. and Scarpino, S.E. (2008) Phonological analysis, phonological processes, in *The Handbook of Clinical Linguistics* (eds M.J. Ball, M.R. Perkins, N. Müller and S. Howard), Blackwell, Oxford, pp. 412–422.

Morley, M.E. (1945) *Cleft Palate and Speech*, Churchill Livingstone, Edinburgh.

Morris, H. and Ozanne, A. (2003) Phonetic, phonological and language skills of children with a cleft palate. *The Cleft Palate – Craniofacial Journal*, 40 (5), 460–470.

Oller, D. and Kelly, C. (1974) Phonological substitutions of a hard-of-hearing child. *Journal of Speech and Hearing Disorders*, 39, 65–74.

Pamplona, M.C., Ysunza, A. and Espinosa, J. (1999) A comparative trial of two modalities of speech intervention for compensatory articulation in cleft palate children, phonologic approach versus articulatory approach. *International Journal of Pediatric Otolaryngology*, 49 (1), 21–26.

Pamplona, M.C., Ysunza, A., Gonzalez, M. *et al.* (2000) Linguistic development ini cleft palate patients with and without compensatory articulation disorder. *International Journal of Pediatric Otolaryngology*, 54 (2), 81–91.

Pascoe, M., Stackhouse, J. and Wells, B. (2005) Phonological therapy within a psycholinguistic framework: promoting change within a child with persisting speech difficulties. *International Journal of Language and Communication Disorders*, 40 (2), 189–220.

Russell, J. (2010) Orofacial anomalies, in *The Handbook of Language and Speech Disorders* (eds J. Damico, N. Müller and M. Ball), Wiley-Blackwell, Oxford, pp. 474–496.

Russell, J. and Harding, A. (2001) Speech development and early intervention, in *Management of Cleft Lip and Palate* (eds A.C.H. Watson, D. Sell and P. Grunwell), Whurr, London, pp. 191–209.

Scherer, N.J. (1999) Speech language status of toddlers with cleft lip and/or palate following early vocabulary intervention. *American Journal of Speech-Language Pathology*, 8 (1), 81–93.

Sell, D., Harding, A. and Grunwell, P. (1994) A screening assessment for cleft palate speech (Great Ormond Street Speech Assessment). *European Journal of Disorders of Communication*, 29 (1), 1–16.

Sell, D., Harding, A. and Grunwell, P. (1999) GOS.SP.ASS.'98: an assessment for speech disorders associated with cleft palate and/or velopharyngeal dysfunction. *International Journal of Language & Communication Disorders*, 34 (1), 17–33.

Shriberg, L.D., Kent, R.D., Karlsson, H.B. *et al.* (2003) A diagnostic marker for speech delay associated with otitis media with effusion: backing of obstruents. *Clinical Linguistics & Phonetics*, 17 (7), 529–547.

Sosa, A.V. and Bybee, J.L. (2008) A cognitive approach to clinical phonology, in *The Handbook of Clinical Linguistics* (eds M.J. Ball, M.R. Perkins, N. Müller and S. Howard), Blackwell Publishing Ltd, Oxford, pp. 480–490.

Speake, J., Howard, S. and Vance, M. (in press) Intelligibility in children with persisting speech disorders: a case study. *Journal of Interactional Research in Communication Disorders*.

Stoel-Gammon, C. (2011) Relationships between lexical and phonological development in young children. *Journal of Child Language*, 38 (1), 1–34.

Stoel-Gammon, C., Stone-Goldman, J. and Glaspey, A. (2002) Pattern-based approaches to phonological therapy. *Seminars in Speech and Language*, 23, 3–13.

Trost-Cardamone, J.E. and Bernthal, J.E. (1993) Articulation assessment procedures and treatment decisions, in *Cleft Palate: Interdisciplinary Issues and Treatment* (eds K.T. Moller and C.D. Starr), Pro-Ed, Austin, TX, pp. 307–336.

Tyler, A. (2005) Planning and monitoring intervention programmes, in *Phonological Disorders in Children* (eds A. Kamhi and K. Pollock), Brookes, Baltimore, pp. 123–137.

Williams, A.L. (2000) Multiple oppositions: case studies of variables in phonological intervention. *American Journal of Speech-Language Pathology*, **9** (4), 289–299.

Williams, A.L., McLeod, S. and McCauley, R.J. (2010) *Interventions for Speech Sound Disorders in Children*, Brookes, Baltimore.

16

Speech Intelligibility

Tara L. Whitehill[1], Carrie L. Gotzke[2] and Megan Hodge[2]

[1]University of Hong Kong, Faculty of Education, Division of Speech and Hearing Sciences, Hong Kong
[2]University of Alberta, Department of Speech Pathology and Audiology, Edmonton, Alberta, Canada T6G 2G4

16.1 Introduction

One of the primary goals for the cleft palate–craniofacial team is to ensure that the speech of individuals born with cleft palate is understandable to others. Speech intelligibility is an outcome measure for determining how successful the team has been at reaching this goal. Individuals born with cleft palate are at an increased risk for demonstrating speech, language and hearing problems, when compared to peers without cleft palate. These problems include phonological/articulation delay or disorder, resonance disorders (e.g. hypernasality, hyponasality), voice disorders (e.g. harsh voice or reduced vocal intensity), expressive language delay or disorder and hearing impairment (Kuehn and Moller, 2000). Phonological/articulation disorders that result in the loss of identity of phonemic contrasts are considered the primary contributor to reduced intelligibility (Kent et al., 1989). However, problems with voice, hearing and expressive language may further compromise speech intelligibility. In this chapter, speech intelligibility is defined, issues involved in its measurement are outlined, key findings for intelligibility in individuals with cleft palate are reviewed, and current and emerging directions for research on speech intelligibility for this population are highlighted.

Cleft Palate Speech: Assessment and Intervention, First Edition. Edited by Sara Howard, Anette Lohmander.
© 2011 John Wiley & Sons, Ltd. Published 2011 by John Wiley & Sons, Ltd.

16.2   Definition of Intelligibility and Related Concepts

Speech intelligibility has been defined as 'the accuracy with which a speaker transmits verbally the set of symbols he/she intends to utter' (Fletcher, 1978, p. 173) and also as 'how well a listener understands [speech]' (Witzel, 1995, p. 173). Operationally, intelligibility scores have been described as the percentage of words identified correctly by listeners (Hodge and Gotzke, 2007). In a critical review of 57 studies involving the evaluation of intelligibility in individuals with cleft palate, Whitehill (2002) found that intelligibility was rarely defined. Furthermore, several terms related to intelligibility appeared to be used interchangeably. For example, the term intelligibility was frequently (and probably incorrectly) used to refer to global judgements of speech severity.

Acceptability, naturalness and understandability are other global measures of speech outcome that are closely associated but not synonymous with intelligibility. Witzel (1995) defined acceptability as 'the subjective impression of the pleasingness of speech' (p. 147). Naturalness has been defined (for speakers with dysarthria) as the overall prosodic adequacy of speech (Southwood and Weismer, 1993). A recent recommendation for 'universal parameters' for reporting speech outcomes in individuals born with cleft palate included two global outcome measures: acceptability and understandability (Henningsson et al., 2008). Speech understandability was defined as 'the degree to which the speaker's message can be understood by the listener' and acceptability as 'the degree to which speech calls attention to itself apart from the content of the spoken message' (p. 9). It is likely that the term naturalness is closely related to acceptability and the term understandability is closely related to intelligibility. The relationships among these measures have not been systematically examined for individuals with cleft palate (but see Southwood and Weismer, 1993, for a study of these relationships in individuals with dysarthria).

The relationship between acceptability and intelligibility has been investigated for individuals born with cleft palate. For example, Whitehill and Chun (2002) found a positive correlation (0.61) between intelligibility (as measured by a multiple-choice task employing phonetic contrasts) and acceptability (measured using a seven-point equal-appearing interval (EAI) scale); Moller and Starr (1984) also found a positive correlation (0.79) between these two measures, using an eight-point rating scale for acceptability and percentage estimation for intelligibility. However, these two variables have different relationships with other speech variables. For example, Whitehill and Chun found that intelligibility had a high correlation with articulation (as measured by percentage of single words transcribed as correct, 0.77) and no significant correlation with ratings of nasality (as measured using a seven-point EAI scale). In contrast, acceptability had a higher correlation with nasality (0.78) than with articulation (0.56).

16.3   Measurement Issues

Intelligibility is not an absolute quantity, as an individual's intelligibility score may vary depending on how it is measured. The speech stimuli chosen, speaker and listener characteristics, and how the stimuli are recorded, presented to listeners and judged, all influence intelligibility scores. Therefore, these variables must be selected thoughtfully and specified carefully when undertaking intelligibility measurement and interpreting the results. These issues are detailed in Hodge and Whitehill (2010), but summarized here.

The *judgement tasks* that have been used to measure intelligibility can be broadly separated into rating scales and identification tasks. Rating scales are the most commonly used method for assessing the intelligibility of individuals born with cleft palate (Kuehn and Moller, 2000; Peterson-Falzone, Hardin-Jones and Karnell, 2001; Whitehill, 2002). While EAI scales (Konst *et al.*, 2003) are used most commonly, categorical or descriptive scales (Sell *et al.*, 2001) and visual analogue scales (Keuning, Wieneke and Dejonckere, 1999) have also been used. Another scaling method, direct magnitude estimation, has been used to rate intelligibility in speakers with dysarthria and other speech disorders (Weismer and Laures, 2002).

Seven-point scales are used most frequently in EAI scaling (Konst *et al.*, 2003). However, the number of points on EAI scales used to rate intelligibility varies widely; there has been little systematic investigation of this variable. There is some concern regarding the appropriateness of using an EAI scale for rating intelligibility. Using speech samples from individuals with hearing impairment, Schiavetti, Metz and Sitler (1981) demonstrated that listeners do not treat each point on an EAI scale as equally distant from the next and subdivide the ends of the scale differently from the middle points of the scale. This finding has been replicated for other clinical populations (e.g. dysarthria) and suggests that intelligibility should not be assessed using an EAI scale. An additional limitation of using rating scales for assessing intelligibility is that other aspects of the speech signal (e.g. resonance, voice quality, speaking rate) may make it difficult to focus on only intelligibility (Samar and Metz, 1988; Witzel, 1995; Konst *et al.*, 2000). This issue can be minimized through the use of identification tasks.

Both multiple choice (i.e. closed-set) and transcription (i.e. open-set) identification tasks have been used to obtain intelligibility scores. In closed-set tasks, the listener is asked to select which item from a list of choices most closely matches what was heard. In open-set tasks, the listener is asked to transcribe (usually orthographically) what he or she has heard. For both open-set and closed-set tasks, the percentage of words identified correctly serves as the intelligibility score. While identification tasks appear to have greater face validity than rating scales, they are generally more time consuming (Konst *et al.*, 2000).

Single words, sentences, reading passages and spontaneous speech have all been used as *speech stimuli* in intelligibility measurement for individuals born with cleft palate. While spontaneous speech may best represent the individual's everyday speech (and thus have the highest face validity), examiners may have difficulty eliciting a sufficient sample of speech and, in the case of severely impaired speech, glossing the sample in preparation for listener judgement. When choosing a speech sample, it is important that the speaking task(s) be appropriate for the abilities of the speaker. Consideration must be given, for example, to expressive language abilities in a sentence repetition task, literacy abilities in an oral reading task, or speech severity in tasks involving more than single word utterances. Details of the speech stimuli used in intelligibility assessment need to be described when reporting results.

There are a number of *listener characteristics* that may influence the outcome of intelligibility measurement. One listener variable that has been investigated in research with individuals with cleft palate is the amount of experience raters have had in listening to and rating the speech of individuals with cleft palate. For example, speech–language pathologists (SLPs) with experience judging the speech of individuals with cleft palate were slightly more consistent in rating intelligibility than SLPs without such experience (Keuning, Wieneke and Dejonckere, 1999). Pannbacker (1975) also found that raters with experience with cleft palate were more reliable than inexperienced raters in judging intelligibility; the experienced listeners also had a tendency to rate the speech of individuals with cleft palate as poorer than did the less experienced listeners. There is a recent trend towards involving individuals with cleft palate, their family members and/or lay listeners in measuring the intelligibility of individuals with cleft palate, in an effort to improve the validity of evaluations (Bagnall and David, 1988; Purcell, 2006; Witt et al., 1996). However, there has been little systematic comparison of the effect of lay versus professional listeners on intelligibility scores (but see Tonz et al. (2002) for a recent study of this issue).

The use of a panel of listeners, versus a single listener, has been recommended to increase the stability of intelligibility judgements (McWilliams, Morris and Shelton, 1984; Peterson-Falzone, Hardin-Jones and Karnell, 2001). However, this can prove challenging in the clinical setting. When intelligibility judgements are made for research or clinical audit purposes, it is recommended that listeners should be experienced in judging the speech of individuals with cleft palate, but not directly involved in the management of the particular speaker or group of speakers (such as the surgeon or team speech–language pathologist), so as to avoid potential bias; blind evaluation of randomized recordings is recommended (Sell, 2005; Lohmander et al., 2009). *Listening conditions* may also influence intelligibility measurements. Moller and Starr (1984) examined the effect of live audio, live audiovisual or recorded audio only presentation of speech stimuli on trained listeners' ratings of intelligibility for individuals born with cleft palate. Intelligibility ratings were not affected by the listening condition. Other studies have found that visual information does have an effect on ratings of other speech dimensions in individuals with cleft palate (Podol and Salvia, 1976). Although this particular issue may require further study, it is strongly recommended that the speech samples used in evaluating intelligibility be audio and/or audiovisually recorded (as opposed to rated 'live'), so as to permit determination of inter-listener and intra-listener reliability and to allow for future possibility of audit or review (Sell, 2005).

16.4   Studies of Intelligibility in Speakers with Cleft Palate

This section provides an overview of the variety of purposes for which intelligibility has been studied in individuals with cleft palate and key findings in each area.

A number of descriptive studies have sought to *compare individuals with cleft palate with their non-cleft peers*. Not surprisingly, a consistent finding has been that children born with cleft palate have significantly lower intelligibility scores when compared with typically developing children, using a variety of evaluation methods including rating scales (Van Lierde et al., 2002; Van Lierde et al., 2004), word identification (Hodge and Gotzke, 2007; Pannbacker, 1975) and automatic speech recognition (Schuster et al., 2006). Adults with cleft palate have also been shown to have significantly lower intelligibility than matched adults without a cleft (Pannbacker, 1975; Van Lierde et al., 2004). However, it is important to note that the range of intelligibility scores for speakers with cleft palate is usually wide, with some individuals clearly achieving age-appropriate intelligibility scores. In addition, several studies have shown significant *age differences* in intelligibility in individuals with cleft palate. Sell *et al.* (2001) found that 19% of five-year olds with cleft palate were rated as 'impossible to understand' or 'only just intelligible to strangers', while only 4% of 12-year olds were assigned these ratings. Similarly, in a longitudinal study of 26 children who had undergone two-stage palatal repair, at age three years, 13 of the children had intelligibility that was rated by expert listeners as 'moderately or severely reduced' (using a three-point scale, based on a spontaneous speech sample) whereas at age 10, none of the 26 children had speech intelligibility rated in that category (i.e. all had intelligibility that was rated as 'everything intelligible' or 'mildly reduced') (Lohmander *et al.*, 2006).

Studies comparing the intelligibility of *speakers with different types of cleft palate* have reported conflicting results. Using intelligibility scores obtained from an open-set single word identification task, Leeper, Pannbacker and Roginski (1980) found that individuals with cleft palate only (CPO) had the lowest intelligibility score, followed by speakers with bilateral cleft lip and palate (BCLP) and then speakers with unilateral cleft lip and palate (UCLP). Conversely, Van Lierde *et al.* (2004), using a four-point rating scale and connected speech samples, found no significant difference in intelligibility between individuals with unilateral cleft lip and palate and those with bilateral cleft lip and palate. The variability in results may be due to differing methods for evaluating intelligibility, differences in surgical technique and timing, equivalency of subjects and other factors.

Speech intelligibility is frequently used as an *outcome measure for surgery* in individuals with cleft palate. For example, using a four-point scale where 0 = normal and 3 = grossly impaired, Rohrich *et al.* (1996) compared the intelligibility of a group of individuals born with cleft palate whose hard palate was closed early (average 10.8 months) and a group whose hard palate was closed late (average 48.6 months). A significantly greater percentage of speakers in the late closure group received a rating of one or higher (indicating more impaired intelligibility) than in the early closure group (35% vs 5%). Debates about the timing and method of primary repair of the palate are likely to continue for some time; the employment of valid and reliable methods for evaluating intelligibility will provide critical information to inform such debates.

Kuehn and Moller (2000) drew attention to the paucity of studies examining the efficacy of speech therapy for individuals with cleft palate. Therefore, it is not surprising that there have been few studies that have employed intelligibility as an *outcome measure for speech therapy* (but see Prins and Bloomer, 1965).

Intelligibility has been used as an *outcome measure for other non-surgical interventions*. Konst *et al.* (2000) compared two groups of toddlers with cleft palate: those who had received pre-surgical infant orthopaedic (PIO) treatment and those who had not. Intelligibility was measured in this prospective randomized study using both listener ratings and transcription. The conclusion was that there was no difference in intelligibility (in terms of percentage of words understood) between the two groups. However, Pinto, Dalben and Pegoraro-Krook (2007) found intelligibility to be significantly better after placement of a prosthesis in a group of speakers with unoperated cleft palate or with VPI following primary palatoplasty, when judged on a six-point interval scale by a group of speech–language pathologists who were blinded to prosthetic status.

16.5   Current and Future Developments

One relatively recent trend is the development of disorder-specific intelligibility tests for speakers with cleft palate. This trend follows the development and application of disorder-specific tests for other populations, such as individuals with dysarthria (Kent et al., 1989). The advantage of such tests is that they target speech sounds or phonemic contrasts known to be vulnerable for the specific population. These tests provide a severity measure and also identify phonemic contrasts that contribute to reductions in intelligibility (and have therefore been termed 'explanatory' tests; Kent et al., 1989). In theory, efficiency of speech therapy could be increased by targeting those contrasts most likely to lead to improvements in intelligibility. However, this hypothesis has yet to be tested empirically.

Whitehill and Chau (2004) designed an intelligibility test for Cantonese speaking children with cleft palate. The test was modified from one originally designed for Cantonese speakers with dysarthria (Whitehill and Ciocca, 2000), to incorporate contrasts known to be vulnerable in speakers with cleft palate (e.g. alveolar versus velar place of articulation for stop consonants). The most problematic contrasts, based on listener choices in the closed-set identification task, were place of articulation of stops and nasals (e.g. alveolar versus velar nasal), stop versus fricative and stop versus affricate. Single-word intelligibility could be predicted with 91% accuracy using three phonetic contrasts. This study was limited by its inability to capture error patterns that could not be characterized phonemically.

Hodge and Gotzke (2007) also employed a phonetic contrast approach in the development of a measure of intelligibility for young, English speaking children with cleft palate. Word pairs were selected to provide opportunities for cleft-related and developmental error patterns expected for these children, based on a review of the literature. Five error categories are represented: manner preference errors, place preference errors, sibilant errors, voicing errors and cluster errors. In this imitative word measure, software records the children's productions directly to computer and plays these back to listeners to complete both open-set and closed-set identification tasks. In the closed-set task, listeners also judge whether the targeted sounds are 'clear' or 'distorted'. Gotzke (2005) assessed the reliability and validity of the measure for 12 children with cleft palate and 12 children of a similar age without cleft palate. In addition to having lower intelligibility scores on both open and closed-set tasks, the children with cleft palate had a higher percentage of correct distorted judgements. Intelligibility scores from the word measure and a 100-word spontaneous speech sample, determined using orthographic transcription, were correlated positively ($r = 0.79$). Further development and evaluation of this measure is underway.

As part of their development of a set of computer based single-word intelligibility tests for use with children with cleft palate, Zajac and colleagues presented a measure that uses a set of 50 phonetically-balanced single words selected randomly from a larger word list, judged using orthographic transcription by naïve listeners (Lloyd et al., 2008; Plante et al., 2008). Future plans for this measure include the development of a closed-set task targeting phonetic contrasts known to be problematic for children with repaired cleft palate (Zajac, 2008). The development of intelligibility tests specific to individuals with cleft palate may facilitate speech therapy intervention that will have the maximum impact on improved intelligibility and communicative function. Computer-mediated recording and judging will greatly increase the clinical feasibility and efficiency of intelligibility measurement.

Another relatively recent development has been the employment of automatic speech recognition systems in the determination of intelligibility in speakers with cleft palate. Currently these efforts are being spearheaded by Maier and colleagues at the University of Erlangen-Nurnberg in Germany (Maier, 2009; Schuster et al., 2006). Schuster et al. (2006) designed and tested an automatic speech recognition system with 31 children with cleft lip and/or palate. Single-word recognition scores varied from 1.2 to 75.8%. Differences were noted between cleft types: scores were highest for children with cleft lip only and lowest for children with isolated cleft palate. There was a significant correlation between the intelligibility scores obtained using the automatic speech recognition system and evaluation of speech intelligibility by a panel of expert listeners. While this approach certainly offers great promise, particularly in terms of time effectiveness, and addresses some of the constraints associated with listener variables, more research and development is needed in this area for it to become feasible. Current automatic speech recognition technology does not appear very effective in modelling or predicting the speech intelligibility of typically-developing children, let alone that of children with speech disorders. Finding innovative, efficient and valid solutions to address the challenge of using human listeners and controlling the multiple listener variables that can influence intelligibility scores is an important area for future development.

Although intelligibility is being increasingly recognized as an important outcome measure for individuals with cleft palate, there is still debate regarding the best method for evaluating intelligibility and this is reflected in current practice. Rating scales remain the most commonly used approach to evaluate intelligibility in speakers with cleft palate, although identification methods (open or closed-set) appear to have better validity. Reaching a consensus on a standardized approach to measuring intelligibility for children with cleft palate is a research priority.

There appears to be an increasing acceptance that speech outcome measures for individuals born with cleft palate should include both individual dimensions of speech (e.g. resonance, articulation, voice) and one or more global measures (e.g. intelligibility, acceptability) (Lohmander et al., 2009). However, the relationship between individual and global measures remains unclear. A number of early studies examined correlations between a variety of speech measures, including intelligibility (McWilliams, 1953, 1954; Moore and Sommers, 1975; Philips, 1954; Subtelny and Subtelny, 1959; Subtelny, Koepp-Baker and Subtelny, 1961; Subtelny, Van Hattum and Myers, 1972; Van Demark, 1966). However, few studies have investigated how well global measures can be predicted, using individual dimensions of disordered speech. One notable exception (Hardin, Lachenbruch and Morris, 1985) employed multiple regression analyses to predict 'speech proficiency' (judged using a rating scale) at age 14, using 16 independent variables (12 speech variables and four non-speech variables) obtained at ages 4–13, in a group of speakers with unilateral cleft lip and palate. Speech proficiency could be predicted with a relatively high degree of accuracy using a small set of predictor variables, although the most efficient set of predictor variables varied by age and gender. For example, the best set of predictors for males ($R^2 = 0.82$) was three variables collected at age five: change in the percentage of glottal stops/pharyngeal fricatives, percentage of oral distortions and percentage of affricates (all based on articulation test results). For females, the best set of predictors ($R^2 = 0.88$) was three variables collected at age 12: percentage of fricatives, age of surgery and percentage of glottal stops/pharyngeal fricatives.

Henningsson *et al.* (2008) recommended further studies to investigate the extent to which the individual speech parameters in their 'universal parameters' protocol correlate with the two global measures of severity (intelligibility and acceptability); they discussed the possibility of a weighted scale system to enhance such correlations. This approach would be similar to that employed in several protocols to predict velopharyngeal status (e.g. Pittsburgh Weighted Speech Scale; McWilliams and Philips, 1979; Lohmander *et al.*, 2009). Identifying the relative contribution of individual speech variables (e.g. articulation, resonance and voice) to measures of intelligibility and acceptability is another important topic for future research. The results of such studies would generate hypotheses to test in experimental studies investigating the effect of intervention focused on each of these variables on global outcome measures of speech ability.

The fifth trend concerns the growth of multicentre studies. The rationale for such studies has been articulated clearly by Shaw *et al.* (2000) and others. Multicentre studies pose particular challenges when more than one language is involved. This issue has been discussed previously (Brøndsted *et al.*, 1994; Hutters and Henningsson, 2004; Lohmander *et al.*, 2009) and is addressed in a separate chapter in this book (Chapter 9). However, most previous discussions have focused on cross-linguistic comparisons of articulation/phonology, usually at the segmental level. The inclusion of intelligibility as an outcome measure in multicentre studies may allow key research questions to be addressed with sufficient power (number of participants) to provide meaningful answers. However, cross-linguistic evaluations of intelligibility may pose a unique set of challenges. Evaluating intelligibility cross-linguistically has rarely been addressed and warrants further attention.

Although an intelligibility score or rating may provide information on the extent to which an individual's speech is understood by a given listener, in a given context, it certainly does not provide a complete picture of that individual's communicative competence, the impact of a speech disorder on an individual's daily life, or a speaker's level of satisfaction with his or her speech. Lohmander *et al.* (2009) suggested that global measures such as speech intelligibility or acceptability represent the level of communicative 'activity and participation', according to the International Classification of Functioning, Disability, and Health (World Health Organization, 2001). There have been several recent efforts to place speech intelligibility (and other speech variables) in a broader context such as that embraced by the ICF framework (Sommerlad *et al.*, 2002; Havstam *et al.*, 2008; Chapter 17). However, a great deal of research is still needed in this area. For example, it is not known the degree to which a statistically significant difference in intelligibility scores (say, before and after intervention, or between two groups of individuals) has a meaningful, functional impact on an individual's life. Adopting the ICF framework to identify relationships between measures of speech intelligibility and communicative effectiveness is another critical area for future research.

16.6   Conclusion

A review of published studies involving speech evaluation in the cleft palate population revealed that intelligibility was included as an outcome measure in only 11 of the 88 articles reviewed (Lohmander and Olsson, 2004). In contrast, 62 articles included resonance as an outcome variable and 56 articles reported results of articulation measures. While measures of articulation and resonance reflect important aspects of speech impairment in this population, intelligibility provides a direct, global index of functional speech outcome.

In our clinical experience, intelligible speech is a particularly important goal for young children born with cleft palate. Once the phonemic contrasts that are so critical to intelligibility have been established, speech therapy can focus on other aspects of the individual's speech, such as articulatory distortions, resonance and voice quality. These latter features have a lesser impact on intelligibility, but negatively affect the acceptability of speech. Whether intelligible or acceptable speech is being targeted, it is important to have a clear understanding of the underlying concepts, of factors that can influence each dimension, and to have reliable and valid methods for measuring (and measuring change in) these variables.

References

Bagnall, A. and David, D. (1988) Speech results of cleft palate surgery: two methods of assessment. *British Journal of Plastic Surgery*, **41**, 488–495.

Brøndsted, K., Grunwell, P., Henningsson, G. *et al.* (1994) A phonetic framework for the cross-linguistic analysis of cleft palate speech. *Clinical Linguistics & Phonetics*, **8**, 109–125.

Fletcher, S.G. (1978) *Diagnosing Speech Disorders from Cleft Palate*, Grune Stratton, New York.

Gotzke, C.L. (2005) Speech intelligibility probe for children with cleft palate, version 3: assessment of reliability and validity. Master's thesis, University of Alberta, Canada.

Hardin, M.A., Lachenbruch, P.A. and Morris, H.L. (1985) Contribution of selected variables to the prediction of speech proficiency for adolescents with cleft lip and palate. *Cleft Palate Journal*, **23**, 10–23.

Havstam, C., Lohmander, A., Dahlgren Sandberg, A. and Elander, A. (2008) Speech and satisfaction with outcome of treatment in young adults with unilateral or bilateral complete clefts. *Scandinavian Journal of Plastic and Reconstructive Surgery and Hand Surgery*, **42**, 182–189.

Henningsson, G., Kuehn, D.P., Sell, D. *et al.* (2008) Universal parameters for reporting speech outcomes in individuals with cleft palate. *Cleft Palate-Craniofacial Journal*, **45**, 1–17.

Hodge, M. and Gotzke, C.L. (2007) Preliminary results of an intelligibility measure for English-speaking children with cleft palate. *Cleft Palate-Craniofacial Journal*, **44**, 163–174.

Hodge, M. and Whitehill, T.L. (2010) Intelligibility impairments, in *Handbook of Speech and Language Disorders* (eds J.S. Damico, M.J. Ball and N. Müller), Wiley-Blackwell Publishers, Chichester, pp. 99–114.

Hutters, B. and Henningsson, G. (2004) Speech outcome following treatment in cross-linguistic cleft palate studies: methodological considerations. *Cleft Palate-Craniofacial Journal*, **41**, 544–549.

Kent, R.D., Weismer, G., Kent, J.F. and Rosenbek, J.C. (1989) Toward phonetic intelligibility testing in dysarthria. *Journal of Speech and Hearing Disorders*, **54**, 482–499.

Keuning, K.H.D., Wieneke, G.H. and Dejonckere, P.H. (1999) The intrajudge reliability of the perceptual rating of cleft palate speech before and after pharyngeal flap surgery: the effect of judges and speech samples. *Cleft Palate-Craniofacial Journal*, **36**, 328–333.

Konst, E.M., Weersink-Braks, H., Rietveld, T. and Peters, H. (2000) An intelligibility assessment of toddlers with cleft lip and palate who received and did not receive presurgical infant orthopedic treatment. *Journal of Communication Disorders*, **33**, 483–501.

Konst, E.M., Rietveld, T., Peters, H.F.M. and Weersink-Braks, H. (2003) Use of a perceptual evaluation instrument to assess the effects of infant orthopedics on the speech of toddlers with cleft palate. *Cleft Palate-Craniofacial Journal*, 40, 597–605.

Kuehn, D.P. and Moller, K.T. (2000) Speech and language issues in the cleft palate population: the state of the art. *Cleft Palate-Craniofacial Journal*, 37, 348–383.

Leeper, H.A., Pannbacker, M. and Roginski, J. (1980) Oral language characteristics of adult cleft-palate speakers compared on the basis of cleft type and sex. *Journal of Communication Disorders*, 13, 133–146.

Lloyd, A., Plante, C., Haley, K. and Zajac, D.J. (2008) Predictors of speech intelligibility in children with cleft lip/palate: preliminary findings. Poster presented at the Annual Convention of the American Speech-Language-Hearing Association, Chicago, USA (November 2008).

Lohmander, A. and Olsson, M. (2004) Methodology for perceptual assessment of speech in patients with cleft palate: a critical review of the literature. *Cleft Palate-Craniofacial Journal*, 41, 64–70.

Lohmander, A., Friede, H., Elander, A. *et al.* (2006) Speech development in patients with unilateral cleft lip and palate treated with different delays in closure of the hard palate after early velar repair: a longitudinal perspective. *Scandinavian Journal of Plastic and Reconstructive Surgery and Hand Surgery*, 40, 267–274.

Lohmander, A., Willadsen, E., Persson, C. *et al.* (2009) Methodology for speech assessment in the Scandcleft project – An international randomized clinical trial on palatal surgery: experiences from a pilot study. *Cleft Palate-Craniofacial Journal*, 46, 347–367.

Maier, A. (2009) Speech of children with cleft lip and palate: automatic assessment. Doctoral dissertation, University of Erlangen-Nurnberg, Germany. http://peaks.informatik.uni-erlangen.de/maier.pdf (accessed 24 March 2011).

McWilliams, B.J. (1953) An experimental study of some of the components of intelligibility of the speech of adult cleft palate patients. Doctoral dissertation, University of Pittsburgh, USA.

McWilliams, B.J. (1954) Some factors in the intelligibility of cleft palate speech. *Journal of Speech and Hearing Disorders*, 19, 524–528.

McWilliams, B.J. and Philips, B.J. (1979) *Velopharyngeal Incompetence. Audio Seminars in Speech Pathology*, W.B. Saunders, Philadelphia.

McWilliams, B.J., Morris, H.L. and Shelton, R.L. (1984) *Cleft Palate Speech*, B.C. Decker Inc, Philadelphia.

Moller, K.T. and Starr, C.D. (1984) The effects of listening conditions on speech ratings obtained in a clinical setting. *Cleft Palate Journal*, 21, 65–69.

Moore, W.H. and Sommers, R.K. (1975) Phonetic contexts: their effects on perceived intelligibility in cleft-palate speakers. *Folia Phoniatrica*, 27, 410–422.

Pannbacker, M. (1975) Oral language skills of adult cleft palate speakers. *Cleft Palate Journal*, 12, 95–106.

Peterson-Falzone, S.J., Hardin-Jones, M.A. and Karnell, M.P. (2001) *Cleft Palate Speech*, 3rd edn. Mosby, St. Louis.

Philips, B.R. (1954) An experimental investigation of the relationship between ratings of speech intelligibility based on auditory and visual cues and on auditory cues alone in a group of cleft palate adults. Masters thesis, University of Pittsburgh, USA.

Pinto, J.H.N., Dalben, G.S. and Pegoraro-Krook, M.I. (2007) Speech intelligibility of patients with cleft lip and palate after placement of speech prosthesis. *Cleft Palate-Craniofacial Journal*, 44, 635–641.

Plante, C., Lloyd, A., Haley, K. and Zajac, D. (2008) Single-word intelligibility testing in children with cleft lip/palate: reliability and validity. Poster presented at the Annual Convention of the American Speech-Language-Hearing Association, Chicago, USA (November 2008).

Podol, J. and Salvia, J. (1976) Effects of visibility of a prepalatal cleft on the evaluation of speech. *Cleft Palate Journal*, 13, 361–366.

Prins, D. and Bloomer, H.H. (1965) A word intelligibility approach to the study of speech change in oral cleft patients. *Cleft Palate Journal*, 2, 357–363.

Purcell, A. (2006) Measuring perceptual speech outcome after surgical intervention for bilateral cleft lip and palate. Doctoral dissertation, University of Sydney, Australia.

Rohrich, R.J., Rowsell, A.R., Johns, D.F. *et al.* (1996) Timing of hard palatal closure: a critical long-term analysis. *Plastic and Reconstructive Surgery*, 98, 236–246.

Samar, V.J. and Metz, D.E. (1988) Criterion validity of speech intelligibility rating-scale procedures for the hearing-impaired population. *Journal of Speech and Hearing Research*, 31, 307–316.

Schiavetti, N., Metz, D.E. and Sitler, R.W. (1981) Construct validity of direct magnitude estimation and interval scaling of speech intelligibility. *Journal of Speech and Hearing Research*, 24, 441–445.

Schuster, M., Maier, A., Haderlein, T. *et al.* (2006) Evaluation of speech intelligibility for children with cleft lip and palate by means of automatic speech recognition. *International Journal of Pediatric Otorhinology*, 70, 1741–1747.

Sell, D. (2005) Issues in perceptual speech analysis in cleft palate and related disorders: a review. *International Journal of Language and Communication Disorders*, 40, 103–121.

Sell, D., Grunwell, P., Mildinhall, S. *et al.* (2001) Cleft lip and palate care in the United Kingdom – The Clinical Standards Advisory Group (CSAG) Study. Part 3: speech outcomes. *Cleft Palate-Craniofacial Journal*, 38, 30–37.

Shaw, W.C., Semb, G., Nelson, P. *et al.* (2000) *The Eurocleft Project 1996–2000. Standards of Care for Cleft Lip and Palate in Europe*, European Commission Biochemical and Health Research. IOS Press, Amsterdam, The Netherlands.

Sommerlad, B.C., Mehendale, F.V., Birch, M.J. *et al.* (2002) Palate repair revisited. *Cleft Palate-Craniofacial Journal*, 39, 295–307.

Southwood, M.H. and Weismer, G. (1993) Listener judgements of the bizarreness, acceptability, naturalness and normalcy of dysarthria associated with amyotrophic lateral sclerosis. *Journal of Medical Speech-Language Pathology*, 1, 151–161.

Subtelny, J. and Subtelny, J.D. (1959) Intelligibility and associated physiological factors of cleft palate speakers. *Journal of Speech and Hearing Research*, 2, 353–360.

Subtelny, J., Koepp-Baker, H. and Subtelny, J.D. (1961) Palatal function and cleft palate speech. *Journal of Speech and Hearing Disorders*, 26, 213–224.

Subtelny, J.D., Van Hattum, R.J. and Myers, B.B. (1972) Ratings and measures of cleft palate speech. *Cleft Palate Journal*, 9, 18–27.

Tonz, M., Schmid, I., Graf, M. *et al.* (2002) Blinded speech evaluation following pharyngeal flap surgery by speech pathologists and lay people in children with cleft palate. *Folia Phoniatrica et Logopaedica*, 54, 288–295.

Van Demark, D.R. (1966) A factor analysis of the speech of children with cleft palate. *Cleft Palate Journal*, 6, 31–37.

Van Lierde, K.M., De Bodt, M., Van Borsel, J. *et al.* (2002) Effect of cleft type on overall speech intelligibility and resonance. *Folia Phoniatrica et Logopaedica*, 54, 158–168.

Van Lierde, K., Monstrey, S., Bonte, K. *et al.* (2004) The long-term speech outcome in Flemish young adults after two different types of palatoplasty. *International Journal of Pediatric Otorhinolaryngology*, 68, 865–875.

Weismer, G. and Laures, J.S. (2002) Direct magnitude estimates of speech intelligibility in dysarthria. *Journal of Speech, Language, and Hearing Research*, 45, 421–433.

Whitehill, T.L. (2002) Assessing intelligibility in speakers with cleft palate: a critical review of the literature. *Cleft Palate-Craniofacial Journal*, 39, 50–58.

Whitehill, T.L. and Chau, C.H.-F. (2004) Single-word intelligibility in speakers with repaired cleft palate. *Clinical Linguistics & Phonetics*, 18, 341–355.

Whitehill, T.L. and Chun, J.C. (2002) Intelligibility and acceptability in speakers with cleft palate, in *Investigations in Clinical Phonetics and Linguistics* (eds F. Windsor, M.L. Kelly and N. Hewlett), Lawrence Erlbaum Associates, Inc, Mahwah, NJ, pp. 405–415.

Whitehill, T.L. and Ciocca, V. (2000) Perceptual-phonetic predictors of single-word intelligibility: a study of Cantonese dysarthria. *Journal of Speech, Language, and Hearing Research*, **43**, 1451–1465.

Witt, P.D., Berry, L.A., Marsh, J.L. *et al.* (1996) Speech outcome following palatoplasty in primary school children: do lay peer observers agree with speech pathologists? *Plastic & Reconstructive Surgery*, **98**, 958–965.

Witzel, M.A. (1995) Communicative impairment associated with clefting, in *Cleft Palate Speech Management: A Multidisciplinary Approach* (eds R.J. Shprintzen and J. Bardach), Mosby, St. Louis, pp. 137–166.

World Health Organization (2001) International Classification of Functioning, Disability and Health (ICF), World Health Organization, Geneva, Switzerland.

Zajac, D.J. (2008) Translating principles of speech science to clinical practice: current and future trends in craniofacial disorders. *Perspectives on Speech Science and Orofacial Disorders*, **18**, 31–40.

17

Communicative Participation

Christina Havstam[1] and Anette Lohmander[2]

[1] Sahlgrenska University Hospital, Division of Speech and Language Pathology, SE 413 45
Gothenburg, Sweden
[2] Karolinska Institutet, Department of Clinical Science, Intervention and Technique,
Division of Speech and Language Pathology, SE 141 86, Stockholm, Sweden

17.1   Introduction

As people born with clefts of the palate are often later than their peers in uttering their
first words and often less intelligible during early childhood, they could be at risk of
experiencing greater communicative frustration and developing a less positive attitude
to communication compared to those without cleft. Often their speech is increasingly
normalized during their later childhood and adolescence, and both children and parents
have reported increasing satisfaction with speech as the children grow older (Broder,
Smith and Strauss, 1992). Some individuals, however, continue to have a speech disorder
as adults. Since studies of speech in adults are scarce, it is difficult to estimate the exact
numbers. The few studies that have been published have mostly compared different
surgical techniques for repairing the palate (Becker et al., 2000; Van Lierde et al., 2004;
Farzaneh et al., 2008, 2009). They have reported quite different speech results but signs
of velopharyngeal incompetence constitute the most common disorder and have been
reported in up to 60% of the investigated individuals. Some have found more speech
impairments in bilateral than unilateral complete clefts (Farzaneh et al., 2008, 2009),

whereas others have found similar results regardless of cleft extension (Havstam *et al.*, 2008).

Whether a lasting or transient speech impairment has an impact on a person's self-image or will to communicate is not really known, but most speech–language therapists are well aware of the large variation in how people deal with their speech impairments. The same type and degree of speech impairment can have very different effects on different individuals, and different types or degrees of impairment can result in almost the same restrictions for an individual's participation in society. It seems clear that there are other factors that influence how much people's lives will be influenced by their speech impairment. The International Classification of Functioning, Disability and Health (ICF) (World Health Organization (WHO) 2001) offers a framework that can make these factors easier to define and overview. This chapter deals with the communicative participation of individuals born with a cleft involving the palate by describing the ICF, issues related to communicative participation and how to measure it, studies of communicative participation and clinical implications.

17.2   ICF

To broaden the perspective when describing health and health-related states, the ICF was introduced by the World Health Organization in 2001 (Figure 17.1) as a sequel to the previous International Classification of Impairment, Disability and Handicap (ICIDH).

The ICF attempts to integrate the different perspectives of health from biological, individual and social angles, and complements the International Classification of Diseases (ICD). The ICF focuses on the impact rather than the cause of a disorder and aspires to introduce a 'common metric' for reporting the individual experience of disability. It is a classification system consisting of two parts, where part one relates to a person's functioning and disability, and part two to contextual factors. The first part is classified in a more elaborate way and consists of two main components. The first component relates to body functions and structures, and the second to activities and participation

	Part 1: Functioning and Disability		Part 2: Contextual Factors	
Components	Body Functions and Structures	Activities and **Participation**	Environmental Factors	Personal Factors
Domains	Body functions Body structures	Life areas (tasks, actions)	External influences on functioning and disability	Internal influences on functioning and disability

Figure 17.1   Overview of ICF (© World Health Organization (WHO), 2001).

in different life areas. The second part consists of two components, environmental factors and personal factors. The environmental factors that interact with the components activity and participation are listed and can be qualified as barriers or facilitators. The personal factors are mentioned but not listed in the ICF, as they are considered to be dependent on the cultural context in which the person lives and are, therefore, difficult to qualify and compare between different cultural contexts.

On basis of the ICF it can be inferred that the same impairment of body functions and structures can have different consequences for activities and participation for different individuals, depending on their individual contextual factors.

17.3   Communicative Participation

17.3.1   Definition

The Participation component of ICF is defined as 'involvement in a life situation'. The construct Communicative Participation has been defined by Eadie *et al.* (2006) as 'taking part in life situations where knowledge, information, ideas, or feelings are exchanged. It may take the form of speaking, listening, reading, writing, or nonverbal means of communication… and must involve a communicative exchange' (p. 309). Thus, the scope is broad and communicative participation can be studied and described in many different ways, from the individuals' own satisfaction with their speech and communication, observational studies of their social interaction, and investigations of how people in their environment react to their speech, to surveys of demographic data such as their education level, employment and marital status.

17.3.2   Related Issues

17.3.2.1   Satisfaction with Outcome of Treatment   There seems to be a growing consensus that a person's own satisfaction with the treatment he or she has received is an important factor, if not the most important, when the health care is evaluated (Semb *et al.*, 2005). The timing of the assessments of treatment satisfaction has varied. A number of studies have approached young adults after their treatment has been terminated to get a final subjective evaluation of treatment outcome (Becker *et al.*, 2000; Havstam *et al.*, 2008; Farzaneh *et al.*, 2008, 2009). Other studies have investigated satisfaction with outcome in children and adolescents both among the individuals with cleft themselves and their parents (Strauss, Broder and Helms, 1988; Broder, Smith and Strauss, 1992; Semb *et al.*, 2005; Hunt *et al.*, 2006; Noor and Musa, 2007). A majority of both individuals with cleft and their parents report that they are satisfied with their speech outcome, and satisfaction increases as the children grow older (Broder, Smith and Strauss, 1992). It should be noted that a few remain dissatisfied with their speech into adulthood. However, dissatisfaction with appearance is more common and has been found to correlate with factors related to quality of life (Marcusson, Paulin and Ostrup, 2002; Sinko *et al.*, 2005; Oosterkamp *et al.*, 2007). Most of the research dealing with quality of life has focused on the associations with dissatisfaction with appearance and, at present, there is no proof of dissatisfaction with speech being associated with lower quality of life.

Another question has been whether children or adolescents agree with their parents in how satisfied they are with treatment outcome. Broder, Smith and Strauss (1992) compared satisfaction with appearance and speech in five-to-eighteen-year-olds, and found that parents of females expressed more concern about their daughters' appearance than parents of males, who were more concerned with their sons' speech. Another study of thirteen-to-eighteen-year-olds (Strauss, Broder and Helms, 1988) found that 9% of the patients thought their main problem was speech and 13% their appearance. When their parents were asked about their teenagers' main problems, the areas were reversed; 10% thought it was their speech and 6% their appearance. It seems plausible that teenagers are particularly critical of their own appearance, and it is possible that their speech would become a concern in later years. An investigation of communication attitude in 10-year-olds born with a cleft involving the palate showed that there were significant correlations between the children's total score on the Swedish version of the Communication Attitude Test (CAT-S) and their parents' answers to the question 'Do you feel satisfied with the way your child speaks?' (Havstam, Sandberg and Lohmander, 2011). Whether the parents' feelings of satisfaction influenced their children's communication attitude or if the parents' satisfaction was shaped by how they perceive their children's communication attitude is not known.

17.3.2.2 *Listeners' Impressions*   Since communication presupposes at least one other person participating in the communicative exchange, the environmental factors in terms of the communication partners involved are important to study. It is also a common belief that our self-concept is shaped by the feedback we receive from people in our environment, particularly significant people in our nearest family during our early years (Erikson, 1968). There have been a few investigations on how individuals with cleft palate are perceived by people outside their family. Richman (1978) studied the effects of facial disfigurement on teachers' perception of how intelligent the children were. Teachers tended to rate cleft children with facial disfigurement less accurately; highly intelligent children were underestimated whereas less intelligent children were overestimated. Berry *et al.* (1997) compared the personality characteristics attributed to speech samples of a group of children with a cleft to a group of unaffected children and found no differences. The majority of the children in the cleft group, however, were assessed to have normal speech and no comparisons based on different speech status were carried out. This makes it difficult to infer if impaired speech was perceived in a negative way as individual differences are obscured in the group comparisons, which is typical for many group comparisons of individuals with clefts due to the large individual variations in speech outcome. The participants with speech impairments are rarely identified for separate analysis, and often the ones with pronounced speech disorders are not included at all.

A study that did single out speakers with speech impairments was carried out by Blood and Hyman (1977). They investigated how hypernasal children's speech was perceived by peers, using audio samples of four girls assessed to have normal, mild, moderate and severe hypernasality, respectively. The samples were played to 120 children from kindergarten to second grade, who subsequently answered five questions about the person speaking, for example 'Did you like the person talking?'. The researchers classified the answers as positive, negative or neutral, and found that listeners responded more negatively to the voice samples as hypernasality increased. The youngest children were not as negative to the moderately hypernasal voice, but all children were negative to the severely hypernasal voice. Numbers were very small in this study, but there is an indication that hypernasality is perceived in a negative way.

Research of other types of speech disorders has found similar tendencies. Lass *et al.* (1993) asked 13-year-olds with normal speech to listen to tape recordings of 16 children aged 6–11 years. Eight of the children had dysarthric speech and eight normal. The listeners then rated probable personality traits for each speaker on 22 scales containing polarized adjective pairs, for example 'not smart–smart' and 'mean–nice'. The children with dysarthria were rated less favourably on all 22 scales, compared to the children with normal speech, and the differences were statistically significant. The same design was used with eight children with voice disorder compared to eight children with normal speech (Lass *et al.*, 1991). The children with voice disorders were perceived in a significantly more negative way on twelve of the 22 scales. This indicates that children with a speech impairment can be met with negative attitudes from peers. However, in order to reflect a situation representative of their actual communicative participation, more holistic and naturalistic types of study designs need to be employed, since listening to isolated audio recordings disregards the personal interaction between the children and people in their environment.

There has been some concern that speech–language therapists who are specialized in cleft palate speech have become 'overtrained' in noting minor deviations in speech, and hence would not be representative of the people a person meets in a natural environment. In an effort to create more naturalistic listener situations, Brunnegård, Lohmander and van Doorn (2009) exposed untrained listeners to audio recordings of speech impairments of various degrees. The speech ratings made by the untrained listeners roughly agreed with speech assessments made by specialized speech–language therapists, although the untrained listeners did not always note minor signs of velopharyngeal incompetence.

Another question has been whether individual satisfaction with speech agrees with speech assessments made by trained speech–language therapists. The answer is that they do not correlate for the adolescents and young adults that have been studied so far (Semb *et al.*, 2005; Havstam *et al.*, 2008). This is similar to comparisons of satisfaction with appearance with professional or instrumental evaluations of treatment outcome, where no correlations have been found (Semb *et al.*, 2005; Sinko *et al.*, 2005; Meyer-Marcotty and Stellzig-Eisenhauer, 2009; Mani, Semb and Andlin-Sobocki, 2010). This lack of agreement is an indication that there are other factors that influence how satisfied one feels with oneself, and if a higher quality of life is what treatment aims for, a 'perfect' result from the viewpoint of the specialist may not be the most important target. The concept of *burden of care* is also of importance to a young person's quality of life, and the impact of having to go through treatment for which one is not personally motivated could be as negative as living with impaired speech or appearance.

17.3.2.3 Interaction   Studies of communicative interaction in persons born with cleft are scarce and the impact of a speech impairment has not often been studied specifically. Richman (1997) studied speech and ratings of facial appearance in individuals born with cleft in relation to different types of behaviour at 6, 9 and 12 years of age. Minor speech problems were found to be associated with behavioural inhibition at age 9 years but not at ages 6 or 12 years. More pronounced speech difficulties, however, were not associated with inhibition at any age. An observational study of interaction patterns was made by Slifer *et al.* (2004), who studied communicative behaviour experimentally in 34 eight-to-fifteen-year-olds and 34 controls. Unfortunately, children with severe speech impairments were excluded based on a review of their clinical records. Social encounters were set up with 'trained peers' acting as potential communication partners, approaching the participants in similar ways. Comparisons between children with oral clefts and controls revealed statistically significant differences; children with cleft made fewer choices and more often failed to respond to questions from peers. Parents of children with cleft reported greater dissatisfaction with the child's facial appearance and rated them as less socially competent. There were also within-group associations; parents' perception of their child's social competence and the child's self-perception of social acceptance were positively correlated for both groups. Children with clefts who felt more socially accepted more often looked a peer in the face. The authors interpreted these findings as indicating a need for interventions to enhance social skills in children with clefts. More research is needed if we are to know if and how a cleft-related speech disorder influences interaction between individuals.

17.3.3   Measurement Issues

If the guidelines provided by the WHO in the ICF-model are to be followed, there is a current need for instruments measuring communicative participation, since most of the available instruments within speech–language therapy measure speech function (Eadie *et al.*, 2006). There is a limited number of instruments measuring communicative participation designed for primarily adults with communication disorders (ASHA QL, BOSS) and voice disorders (VAPP, VHI, VoiSS, V-RQOL) (Eadie *et al.*, 2006). About forty years ago, Lanyon (1967) and Erickson (1969) designed questionnaires about attitudes to communication for adults who stammer, and in 1984 Brutten designed a communication attitude test for children (the CAT; Brutten and Dunham, 1989). These questionnaires cover feelings about one's own speech as well as how one perceives interpersonal communication at large. Some of the items are universal, but a number of them relate to experiences largely specific to people who stammer. The SPAA-C (Speech Participation and Activity of Children; McLeod, 2004) is a questionnaire designed for children with any type of speech impairment according to the structure of the ICF, with the emphasis on the categories of Activity and Participation, Environmental and Personal Factors. It is directed not only at the individual child but also at significant others in the child's environment, such as parents, siblings, peers and teachers. The authors themselves note that asking a child's friends about their impression of the child's speech involves a risk of increasing their friends' awareness of the child's speech impairment in a negative way and should be used with caution.

At present, there is a need for an instrument adapted to the more specific needs of those born with a cleft involving the palate, adapted to different ages. Such an instrument or questionnaire would be an important complement both for research and clinical purposes.

17.3.4   Studies of Communicative Participation

A person's communicative participation can be influenced by many factors other than the quality of his or her speech. This is particularly evident when one's focus of interest is a person born with a cleft, as the cleft can affect facial appearance, and hearing, as well as causing regurgitation of food or drink, and all of these things can be seen as potential risk factors for social exclusion and reduced communicative participation.

Large surveys investigating various variables related to quality of life in adults born with clefts have found a number of differences compared to individuals without cleft, although the findings are sometimes contradictory. No clear differences in educational level, income or employment have been found (McWilliams and Paradise, 1973; Ramstad, Ottem and Shaw, 1995a), but men born with cleft palate have been found to have lower intelligence scores compared to controls (Nopoulos et al., 2002; Persson, Becker and Svensson, 2008). Fewer individuals with cleft marry, and when they do so it is later (McWilliams and Paradise, 1973; Ramstad, Ottem and Shaw, 1995a), and anxiety, depression, and palpitations are twice as common among young adults born with cleft (Ramstad, Ottem and Shaw, 1995b).

One study found that young adults born with cleft rated themselves lower for quality of life in terms of social contacts and family life (Marcusson, Akerlind and Paulin, 2001). Another study of adolescents born with cleft found no signs of introversion and the adolescents with cleft scored their overall self-concept higher than controls (Persson et al., 2002). Leonard et al. (1991) found average or above average self-concept in children with cleft, lower self-concept in teenage girls and higher in teenage boys. These studies have used different methodology and inclusion criteria, and studied different age groups in their comparisons, and this makes it difficult to draw clear conclusions. However, based on the majority of the studies that have been conducted previously, most researchers have agreed that there is no such thing as a 'cleft palate personality' or that a cleft has any predictable consequences for an individual's adjustment in life (Clifford, 1983; Richman, 1983; Strauss and Broder, 1991; Bradbury, 2001).

Efforts to clarify possible causality between cleft-related factors, such as poor speech or deviant appearance, and psychosocial problems have not resulted in any clear connections. It is probably safe to say that a majority of the individuals born with cleft participate normally in society if they live in the western world, where most studies have been performed. An interview study conducted in South Africa (Patel and Ross, 2003), however, reported that the participants had been greatly affected by negative societal ideas and myths about the cleft. This points to the importance of the environmental factors for an individual's participation in society. Another study identified the experience of having been teased as a predictor of poor psychological functioning (Hunt et al., 2006). The Eurocleft study reported that, on average, 65% of the children had been teased about different features related to the cleft, and it was most common when the child was 8–11 years old (Semb et al., 2005). Alas, no data on children without cleft were given for comparison. In a Malaysian study both adolescents and their parents reported that teasing was common and the parents thought that it had influenced their children's self-confidence (Noor and Musa, 2007). Hence, it is not unlikely that a child born with a cleft will receive unwanted comments or questions about the cleft and/or their speech at some point.

Another study, using an instrument designed for children who stammer (the Communication Attitude Test), found a significantly more negative communication attitude in 10-year-olds with clefts compared to 10-year-olds without clefts (Havstam, Sandberg and Lohmander, 2011). The children's attitudes were significantly correlated to parents' satisfaction with speech and to speech status as assessed by trained listeners, but the correlations were not very strong and explained only a part of the variance. As often with investigations of people with cleft palate, the group was heterogeneous. The majority of the group had attitudes within a normal range and about a third had more negative attitudes.

An interview study about the experience of growing up with cleft palate and a cleft-related speech impairment indicated that insight into reduced intelligibility, rather than hindering communication, can be an incentive for a person to take more responsibility for the communicative situation at large (Havstam *et al.*, 2010). Another study found that adolescent dissatisfaction with appearance was linked to psychosocial adjustment problems only when it was part of a negative overall view of the self (Bilboul, Pope and Snyder, 2006), indicating that people with a positive self-image can cope with their impairments without letting them influence their participation in society.

17.4   Conclusions and Clinical Implications

Given the difference between professional assessments of speech made by speech–language therapists and how satisfied the individuals themselves are with their speech, it is important that we do not continue to treat speech disorders that do not constitute a problem for the affected individual. Communication is a complex phenomenon that includes more than just speech quality, and sometimes a person's communicative participation may be best improved by other types of interventions than speech training. To assess the experienced communicative participation of the person born with cleft alongside the assessment of speech status, which is already routinely performed at most cleft centres, would provide a valuable contribution to the understanding of the person's communicative situation at large, and give important indications for intervention.

A speech impairment may involve a risk of being met with prejudice, at least when it comes to first impressions. To provide information about the cleft and cleft-related speech disorders to people who meet children with clefts can be one way of overcoming misconceptions, as can providing a young child with a model of how to deal with curiosity and comments from people in their environment. Since teasing has been found to influence a person's psycho-social functioning, and it has been established that cleft-related teasing is quite common, it is important to be attentive to such tendencies in a child's environment, and, if needed, help them with strategies to deal with unwanted comments and questions about the cleft.

References

Becker, M., Svensson, H., Sarnas, K.V. and Jacobsson, S. (2000) Von Langenbeck or Wardill procedures for primary palatal repair in patients with isolated cleft palate – speech results. *Scandinavian Journal of Plastic and Reconstructive Surgery and Hand Surgery*, 34, 27–32.

Berry, L.A., Witt, P.D., Marsh, J.L. *et al.* (1997) Personality attributions based on speech samples of children with repaired cleft palates. *Cleft Palate-Craniofacial Journal*, 34, 385–389.

Bilboul, M.J., Pope, A.W. and Snyder, H.T. (2006) Adolescents with craniofacial anomalies: psychosocial adjustment as a function of self-concept. *Cleft Palate-Craniofacial Journal*, 43, 392–400.

Blood, G.W. and Hyman, M. (1977) Children's perception of nasal resonance. *Journal of Speech and Hearing Disorders*, 42, 446–448.

Bradbury, E. (2001) Growing up with a cleft: the impact on the child, in *Management of Cleft Lip and Palate* (eds A.C.H. Watson, D.A. Sell and P. Grunwell), Whurr Publishers, London, pp. 365–378.

Broder, H.L., Smith, F.B. and Strauss, R.P. (1992) Habilitation of patients with clefts: parent and child ratings of satisfaction with appearance and speech. *Cleft Palate-Craniofacial Journal*, 29, 262–267.

Brunnegård, K., Lohmander, A. and van Doorn, J. (2009) Untrained listeners' ratings of speech disorders in a group with cleft palate: a comparison with speech and language pathologists' ratings. *International Journal of Language and Communication Disorders*, 44, 656–674.

Brutten, G.J. and Dunham, S.L. (1989) The communication attitude test. A normative study of grade school children. *Journal of Fluency Disorders*, 14, 71–77.

Clifford, E. (1983) Why are they so normal? *Cleft Palate Journal*, 20, 83–84.

Eadie, T.L., Yorkston, K.M., Klasner, E.R. *et al.* (2006) Measuring communicative participation: a review of self-report instruments in speech-language pathology. *American Journal of Speech-Language Pathology*, 15, 307–320.

Erickson, R.L. (1969) Assessing communication attitudes among stutterers. *Journal of Speech and Hearing Research*, 12, 711–724.

Erikson, E.H. (1968) *Identity, Youth and Crisis*, W.W. Norton, New York.

Farzaneh, F., Becker, M., Peterson, A.M. and Svensson, H. (2008) Speech results in adult Swedish patients born with unilateral complete cleft lip and palate. *Scandinavian Journal of Plastic and Reconstructive Surgery and Hand Surgery*, 42, 7–13.

Farzaneh, F., Becker, M., Peterson, A.M. and Svensson, H. (2009) Speech results in adult Swedish patients born with bilateral complete cleft lip and palate. *Scandinavian Journal of Plastic and Reconstructive Surgery and Hand Surgery*, 43, 207–213.

Havstam, C., Sandberg, A.D. and Lohmander, A. (2011) Communication attitude and speech in 10-year-old children with cleft (lip and) palate: an ICF-perspective. *International Journal of Speech-Language Pathology*, 13 (2), 156–164.

Havstam, C., Laakso, K., Lohmander, A. and Ringsberg, K.C. (2010) Taking charge of communication: adults' descriptions of growing up with a cleft-related speech impairment. *Cleft Palate-Craniofacial Journal*, in press.

Havstam, C., Lohmander, A., Dahlgren Sandberg, A. and Elander, A. (2008) Speech and satisfaction with outcome of treatment in young adults with unilateral or bilateral complete clefts. *Scandinavian Journal of Plastic and Reconstructive Surgery and Hand Surgery*, 42, 182–189.

Hunt, O., Burden, D., Hepper, P. *et al.* (2006) Self-reports of psychosocial functioning among children and young adults with cleft lip and palate. *Cleft Palate-Craniofacial Journal*, 43, 598–605.

Lanyon, R.I. (1967) The measurement of stuttering severity. *Journal of Speech and Hearing Research*, 10, 836–843.

Lass, N.J., Ruscello, D.M., Stout, L.L. and Hoffmann, F.M. (1991) Peer perceptions of normal and voice-disordered children. *Folia Phoniatrica*, 43, 29–35.

Lass, N.J., Ruscello, D.M., Harkins, K.E. and Blankenship, B.L. (1993) A comparative study of adolescents' perceptions of normal-speaking and dysarthric children. *Journal of Communication Disorders*, 26, 3–12.

Leonard, B.J., Brust, J.D., Abrahams, G. and Sielaff, B. (1991) Self-concept of children and adolescents with cleft lip and/or palate. *Cleft Palate-Craniofacial Journal*, 28, 347–353.

Mani, M., Semb, G. and Andlin-Sobocki, A. (2010) Nasolabial appearance in adults with repaired unilateral cleft lip and palate: relation between professional and lay rating and patients' satisfaction. *Journal of Plastic Surgery and Hand Surgery*, 44, 191–198.

Marcusson, A., Akerlind, I. and Paulin, G. (2001) Quality of life in adults with repaired complete cleft lip and palate. *Cleft Palate-Craniofacial Journal*, 38, 379–385.

Marcusson, A., Paulin, G. and Ostrup, L. (2002) Facial appearance in adults who had cleft lip and palate treated in childhood. *Scandinavian Journal of Plastic and Reconstructive Surgery and Hand Surgery*, 36, 16–23.

McLeod, S. (2004) Speech pathologists' application of the ICF to children with speech impairment. *Advances in Speech-Language Pathology*, 6, 75–81.

McWilliams, B.J. and Paradise, L.P. (1973) Educational, occupational, and marital status of cleft palate adults. *Cleft Palate Journal*, 10, 223–229.

Meyer-Marcotty, P. and Stellzig-Eisenhauer, A. (2009) Dentofacial self-perception and social perception of adults with unilateral cleft lip and palate. *Journal of Orofacial Orthopedics*, 70, 224–236.

Noor, S.N. and Musa, S. (2007) Assessment of patients' level of satisfaction with cleft treatment using the Cleft Evaluation Profile. *Cleft Palate-Craniofacial Journal*, 44, 292–303.

Nopoulos, P., Berg, S., VanDemark, D. *et al.* (2002) Cognitive dysfunction in adult males with non-syndromic clefts of the lip and/or palate. *Neuropsychologia*, 40, 2178–2184.

Oosterkamp, B.C., Dijkstra, P.U., Remmelink, H.J. *et al.* (2007) Satisfaction with treatment outcome in bilateral cleft lip and palate patients. *International Journal of Oral and Maxillofacial Surgery*, 36, 890–895.

Patel, Z. and Ross, E. (2003) Feflections on the cleft experience by South African adults: use of qualitative methodology. *Cleft Palate-Craniofacial Journal*, 40, 471–480.

Persson, M., Aniansson, G., Becker, M. and Svensson, H. (2002) Self-concept and introversion in adolescents with cleft lip and palate. *Scandinavian Journal of Plastic and Reconstructive Surgery and Hand Surgery*, 36, 24–27.

Persson, M., Becker, M. and Svensson, H. (2008) General intellectual capacity of young men with cleft lip with or without cleft palate and cleft palate alone. *Scandinavian Journal of Plastic and Reconstructive Surgery and Hand Surgery*, 42, 14–16.

Ramstad, T., Ottem, E. and Shaw, W.C. (1995a) Psychosocial adjustment in Norwegian adults who had undergone standardised treatment of complete cleft lip and palate. I. Education, employment and marriage. *Scandinavian Journal of Plastic and Reconstructive Surgery and Hand Surgery*, 29, 251–257.

Ramstad, T., Ottem, E. and Shaw, W.C. (1995b) Psychosocial adjustment in Norwegian adults who had undergone standardised treatment of complete cleft lip and palate. II. Self-reported problems and concerns with appearance. *Scandinavian Journal of Plastic and Reconstructive Surgery and Hand Surgery*, 29, 329–336.

Richman, L.C. (1978) The effects of facial disfigurement on teachers' perception of ability in cleft palate children. *Cleft Palate Journal*, 15, 155–160.

Richman, L.C. (1983) Self-reported social, speech, and facial concerns and personality adjustment of adolescents with cleft lip and palate. *Cleft Palate Journal*, 20, 108–112.

Richman, L.C. (1997) Facial and speech relationships to behavior of children with clefts across three age levels. *Cleft Palate-Craniofacial Journal*, 34, 390–395.

Semb, G., Brattstrom, V., Molsted, K. *et al.* (2005) The Eurocleft study: intercenter study of treatment outcome in patients with complete cleft lip and palate. Part 4: relationship among treatment outcome, patient/parent satisfaction, and the burden of care. *Cleft Palate-Craniofacial Journal*, 42, 83–92.

Sinko, K., Jagsch, R., Prechtl, V. *et al.* (2005) Evaluation of esthetic, functional, and quality-of-life outcome in adult cleft lip and palate patients. *Cleft Palate-Craniofacial Journal*, 42, 355–361.

Slifer, K.J., Amari, A., Diver, T. *et al.* (2004) Social interaction patterns of children and adolescents with and without oral clefts during a videotaped analogue social encounter. *Cleft Palate-Craniofacial Journal*, **41**, 175–184.

Strauss, R.P. and Broder, H. (1991) Directions and issues in psychosocial research and methods as applied to cleft lip and palate and craniofacial anomalies. *Cleft Palate-Craniofacial Journal*, **28**, 150–156.

Strauss, R.P., Broder, H. and Helms, R.W. (1988) Perceptions of appearance and speech by adolescent patients with cleft lip and palate and by their parents. *Cleft Palate Journal*, **25**, 335–342.

Van Lierde, K.M., Monstrey, S., Bonte, K. *et al.* (2004) The long-term speech outcome in Flemish young adults after two different types of palatoplasty. *International Journal of Pediatric Otorhinolaryngology*, **68**, 865–875.

World Health Organization (WHO) (2001) International Classification of Functioning, Disability and Health (ICF), World Health Organization, Geneva, Switzerland.

18

Evaluation and Evidence-Based Practice

Linda D. Vallino-Napoli

Alfred I. duPont Hospital for Children, Center for Pediatric Auditory and Speech Sciences (CPASS), Wilmington, DE 19803-3616, USA

18.1 Introduction

Clinical experience has shown that there are many children with cleft palate who will not require intervention after cleft palate repair. Others will exhibit abnormal speech in the presence of adequate velopharyngeal (VP) closure or as a function of velopharyngeal inadequacy (VPI) and will need intervention. Based on the literature, it is estimated that at least 50% of children with repaired cleft palate will require speech therapy some time in their life (Albery, 1989; Peterson-Falzone, Karnell and Hardin-Jones, 2010). About 20% of children following palatoplasty will present with hypernasal speech as a result of VPI; for these additional surgical intervention (e.g. pharyngoplasty) to improve VP function will be required. In some few cases, surgery may improve nasal speech but does not result in an immediate correction of cleft-related articulation error patterns (e.g. compensatory errors), so speech therapy will be necessary.

Decisions for selecting a particular approach to intervention have often been dependant on strategies described in papers and textbooks, or on what was once taught, 'years of clinical experience', an opinion or fad. There is, in fact, a disparity between the clinical

Cleft Palate Speech: Assessment and Intervention, First Edition. Edited by Sara Howard, Anette Lohmander.

© 2011 John Wiley & Sons, Ltd. Published 2011 by John Wiley & Sons, Ltd.

practices to improve speech in those with cleft palate and the evidence to support their effectiveness; and, because of this, therapy progress can be slow or ineffective resulting in high costs and resource allocation. The literature is scant and insufficient in providing convincing evidence of the direct effects of various intervention strategies on speech and resonance. For example, eight primary studies published over the past 35 years have focused on the outcomes of articulation treatment and six primary research studies have been concerned with outcomes of pharyngoplasty on speech and resonance.

Evidence-based practice (EBP) is a mechanism for providing quality care by using the best available research and integrating it into clinical practice and patient preferences or values (Sackett *et al.*, 1997). It is a move away from, not a negation of, a practice that is solely experience based, tradition based or eminence based (Law, 2002; Reilly, Douglas and Oates, 2004; McCarthy, Collins and Pusic, 2008). In EBP, the research study design and the quality of the study are key features in determining the strength of the evidence that can be used to facilitate treatment planning. Using the conceptual framework of EBP, we ask, 'Does the intervention work, is there a better and more effective intervention, and who are the individuals who will best benefit from the intervention?'

We are amidst changes in health care regulation, health care delivery and health care financing. Consumer health care rights are inducing clinicians to provide scientific evidence to support treatment recommendations (Enderby and Emerson, 1995; McCarthy, Collins and Pusic, 2008) or demonstrate the success of one treatment compared to another. McCarthy, Collins and Pusic (2008) posit that in the current climate, the expert opinions and habit-based practices that 'we have relied on in the past will be insufficient to carry us successfully into the future of healthcare.' (p. 1942).

EBP links the available evidence and scientific research with clinical practice. The clinical benefits of controlled research designs and systematic reviews in supporting relevant and effective treatment cannot be overlooked. The purpose of this chapter is to introduce the concepts of EBP, using them to examine the effectiveness of interventions for speech disorders associated with cleft palate.

18.2   Intervention for Speech Disorders

In previous chapters we learned the aetiology of cleft associated speech disorders. Treatment programmes focus on correcting articulation and resonance disorders. Intervention can be non-surgical, including behavioural speech therapy, or surgical, or a combination of both. Behavioural speech therapy (Chapters 13 and 15) refers to the method that directly modifies a targeted speech sound error using a progression hierarchy to establish the sound in isolation, and continues sequentially until the sound is established in words, phrases, sentences, conversation (Peterson-Falzone, Karnell and Hardin-Jones, 2010). For some patients, conventional strategies to correct abnormal articulatory patterns or modify hypernasality have been unsuccessful and so clinicians have used biofeedback techniques. These include electropalatography (EPG) (Chapter 12) to correct posterior articulation placement, nasometry (Chapter 11) to reduce hypernasality and nasopharyngoscopy (Chapter 8) to achieve velopharyngeal closure. Others (Kuehn, 1991; Kuehn *et al.*, 2002) have explored the possible utility of velopharyngeal muscle strengthening to improve hypernasal speech using continuous positive airway pressure (CPAP).

When hypernasality occurs following palatoplasty further surgery may be required to correct velopharyngeal inadequacy (VPI). Pharyngoplasties, such as pharyngeal flap or sphincter pharyngoplasty, or other types of pharyngoplasties are the most common techniques used. Other non-speech cleft associated problems such as malocclusion may require maxillary advancement, which may affect speech. The effectiveness of these interventions can be examined using EBP principles; this is discussed in the following section.

18.3   Evidence-Based Practice

The focus of this chapter is intervention, but it is important to realize that EBP is a process relevant to other aspects of care in cleft palate, including assessment, diagnosis, prognosis and health care economics. The activities of EBP involve six essential steps: develop a clear clinical question, access the most relevant and best evidence, appraise the evidence, integrate the evidence to clinical practice, evaluate the usefulness of this evidence in your clinical practice (Sackett et al., 2000) and, finally, disseminate findings (Schlosser, 2003).

An integral aspect of EBP is rating the quality or strength of the evidence using an evidence hierarchy (Table 18.1). Hierarchies are used to assess the evidence about intervention studies but can be suitably applied to non-treatment studies as well. Common to all hierarchies (Appendix 18.A) is the ranking of levels of evidence from high to low depending on study design. Within this conceptual framework, a higher ranked level of evidence is generally interpreted as holding more 'authority' than a study considered having a lower level of evidence. The randomized clinical trial (RCT) is ranked highest and considered 'best' evidence, whereas the lower ranked case report is considered 'weaker' evidence. Albeit seemingly the case in theory, it should be recognized that the hierarchy is not absolute (Guyatt et al., 2002a). A study ranked as having a low level of evidence does not mean that it is always least useful to the practitioner. Not all research questions can be answered using RCT, nor is the RCT always appropriate or practical for a given clinical problem; and in some cases an RCT is not possible for ethical reasons (Reilly, Douglas and Oates, 2004). Thus, a lower level study may provide the best evidence needed for quality care if it affords a better understanding about a condition or intervention. Although it is acknowledged that not all levels of evidence are equal, it cannot be ignored that for any given level of evidence there may be value; a philosophy adopted in this chapter.

Another aspect of EBP is that practice recommendations are graded (e.g. good, fair, poor or A, B, C) based on a level of evidence. Table 18.2 shows the grading scale, corresponding study quality along with implications for practice. A high quality Level I evidence providing consistent treatment recommendations is assigned a Grade A, suggesting that a clinician should adopt the superior treatment. At the other end, studies (level IV) in which there is insufficient evidence for or against a type of intervention suggests that a clinician might consider other treatment options while always keeping a watchful eye out for new evidence.

An excellent way of imparting knowledge about effective practice to clinicians while avoiding information overload is by published review. Reviews provide a comprehensive analysis and synthesis of the literature addressing a topic. They are popular among clinicians to guide their clinical practice. There are two types of reviews, narrative and

Table 18.1 Levels of Evidence (ranked from high to low) for evaluating the effectiveness of intervention studies[a].

Evidence level	Types of studies	Descriptors of study types
I	Systematic review of published randomized control trials (RCT)	Systematic review uses explicit methods to locate primary studies and explicit criteria to assess them. The RCT is used to compare interventions or to compare an intervention with no intervention. Participants are randomly assigned to a treatment group or non-treatment group
II	One properly designed RCT	
III.1	Well controlled studies without randomization	A study that is a well designed controlled study but without the randomization because ethical or practical reasons preclude randomization
III.2	Well designed cohort or intervention-comparison study,[a] preferably from one or more centres	Cohort studies are those that follow a participant over time. Intervention-comparison studies refer to research that compares an intervention group with a comparison group.
III.3	Multiple time series with or without intervention Single case or single subject	Single case or single subject involves an experimental design to examine the effects of an intervention in one or two individuals.
IV	Expert opinion/Reports of committees Case report/Case series Clinical example Descriptive study Studies of poor methodological quality	Expert opinion refers to a consensus of experience from 'experts' without empirical evidence to support the opinion. Case report refers to a report of an intervention outcome in 1–2 individuals. Case series refers to a descriptive study that follows a group of individuals having a similar condition or receiving the same treatment over a given period. There is no experimental protocol group allocation. Note: Studies at Level IV do not test hypotheses or treatment effectiveness

[a]Adapted from the Joanna Briggs Institute for Evidence Based Practice (The Joanna Briggs Institute. http://www.joannabriggs.edu.au/pubs/approach_history.php). For the purpose of this chapter, intervention-comparison study replaced the conventional term case-control study to more accurately describe the constructs of the intervention studies used in cleft palate. Case-control studies typically are used in epidemiology studies to refer to comparisons of persons with specific conditions (cases) to those without the condition (controls).

Table 18.2 Scale (ranked from high to low) for grading recommendations and implications for practice.

Grade	Recommendations	Qualifying evidence	Implications for practice
A	Strong recommendation	Consistent level I evidence Consistent findings from multiple studies of levels II, III or IV	Clinicians should follow a strong recommendation unless a clear and compelling rationale for an alternative approach is present.
B	Recommendation	Levels II, III or IV evidence with consistent findings	Clinicians should generally follow a recommendation but be watchful for new information and consider patient preferences.
C	Option[a]	Levels II, III or IV evidence, but inconsistent findings	Clinicians should be flexible in their decision making regarding appropriate practice, consider patient preferences.
D	Option[a]	Level IV evidence in which there is little or no systematic empirical evidence or troubling inconsistent or inconclusive studies of any level[b]	Clinicians should consider all options in their decision making, be watchful of newly published evidence, consider benefit vs no benefit or even harm, and consider patient preferences.

[a]Option refers to the fact that the evidence does not allow for a recommendation to be made for or against a given intervention. Adapted from http://www.plasticsurgery.org/Medical_Professionals/ Health_Policy_and_Advocacy/Health_Policy_Resources/Evidence-based_GuidelinesPractice_ Parameters/Description_and_Development_of_Evidence-based_Practice_Guidelines/ASPS_Grade_ Recommendation_Scale.html (accessed 19 October 2009).
[b]From the Oxford Centre for Evidence Based Practice (http://www.cebm.net/).

systematic, each distinctly different in objective and methodology. These differences, summarized in Table 18.3, are detailed in the following sections.

18.3.1 Narrative Review

The narrative review is a 'summary of evidence' based on an assembly of studies written by experts in a speciality (Akobeng, 2005) and for many years has been considered the anchor for evidence-based practice (Enderby and Emerson, 1995). Relative to intervention for cleft related speech disorders, the narrative review has predominated the literature (Starr, 1993; Enderby and Emerson, 1995; Kuehn and Moller, 2000; Peterson-Falzone, Karnell and Hardin-Jones, 2010).

Table 18.3 Differences between narrative review and systematic review.

Features	Narrative review	Systematic review
Quality	Often broad in scope	Often a focused clinical question
Sources and search	Not usually specified; potentially biased	Comprehensive sources and explicit search strategy
Selection	Not usually specified, potentially biased	Criterion-based selection, uniformly applied
Appraisal	Variable	Rigorous critical appraisal
Synthesis	Often a qualitative summary	Quantitative summary (One that includes a statistical synthesis is a meta-analysis)
Inferences	Sometimes evidence based	Usually evidence based

Adapted from Cook et al. (1997).

The narrative review is an overview of a topic of interest with the data often interpreted based on the reviewer's experience or theoretical constructs (Kirkevold, 1997). It is generally conducted without explicitly stated questions or search criteria, with less focus on a quantitative answer to a tailored clinical question (Cook, Mulrow and Haynes, 1997); and as a result runs the risk of bias (Guyatt et al., 2002b). Hence, treatments may be underestimated or overestimated. Accepting the narrative review as evidence for an intervention can be tenuous or unreliable and may result in an endorsement or use of a treatment that fails to do any good (Neilhouse and Priske, 1989; Antman et al., 1992; Cook, Mulrow and Haynes, 1997). In an effort to keep current and maintain best practice, clinicians need to search for the evidence using strategies that permit a more meticulous approach. A promising means by which this can be accomplished is the systematic review (Oxman, Cook and Guyatt, 1994).

18.3.2 Systematic Review

The systematic review is a rigorous and efficient approach in identifying and summarizing the results of multiple original studies (Mulrow, 1994; Cook, Mulrow and Haynes, 1997). It is considered to be one of the highest forms of evidence for answering a clinical question (McCauley and Hargrove, 2004; Dollaghan, 2007) and the means by which a clinician can stay current and maintain best practice. Mulrow (1994) calls the systematic review a 'fundamental activity' that serves to 'establish whether scientific findings are consistent and can be generalized across populations, settings, and treatment variations ...' The process of the systematic review addresses the shortfalls of a narrative review by explicitly identifying the inclusion and exclusion criteria, undertaking a comprehensive search for the evidence, and summarizing the results according to explicit rules (Guyatt et al., 2002b).

By way of critical examination of primary studies, the systematic review allows clinicians to understand consistencies (or inconsistencies) among the varied pieces of research evidence (Cook, Mulrow and Haynes, 1997) and to draw conclusions about the validity and relevance of findings to their own practice (Reilly, Douglas and Oates, 2004). For example, the findings of the review may help clinicians learn about which type of articulation therapy may be better suited to treat a subgroup of patients exhibiting a particular type of articulation error. The utility of the systematic review exceeds that of a narrative review in that it reveals what is known and not known about treatment, what intervention may benefit the patient and what warrants further research (Irwin, Pannbacker and Lass, 2008). It is the basis upon which practice guidelines are developed. It can be used to justify insurance payments and provide a rationale for programme cost allocations.

In health care, the most useful database of systematic reviews, known as Cochrane Reviews, provides summaries of evidence of the effects of intervention. Currently, the Cochrane Library contains systematic reviews related to cleft palate for three topics: feeding intervention (Glenny *et al.*, 2004), surgical management for submucous cleft palate (Nasser *et al.*, 2008) and electropalatography (EPG) for the treatment of articulation errors (Lee, Law and Gibbon, 2009). To date, there are none relevant to behavioural or instrumental speech intervention or secondary surgery for speech and resonance related to cleft palate. However, more recently, the American Speech-Language-Hearing Association (ASHA) has initiated a series of evidence-based systematic reviews (EBSRs) related to intervention and diagnosis for a number of topics in communication and swallowing disorders, none of which have targeted intervention for speech disorders related to cleft palate.

18.4 The Systematic Review Process

The strength of and professional advocacy for the systematic review in identifying best evidence has prompted its use in this chapter to examine the effectiveness of intervention used to modify speech disorders associated with cleft palate. This section provides a brief overview of the process and is illustrated in Figure 18.1.

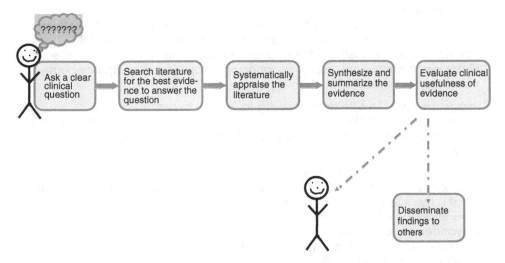

Figure 18.1 Systematic review process.

18.4.1   Developing a Clinical Question

An appropriate and efficient literature search for the best evidence regarding treatment requires the development of well designed clinical questions having three or four essential components: population or problem of interest, specific intervention of interest, comparative intervention (relevant but not always an option) and outcomes relative to the patient. For this chapter questions (Table 18.4) were developed using three elements: the population of interest was children with cleft palate; the types of intervention were behavioural speech therapy, visual feedback and surgery (pharyngoplasty, orthognathic); and the outcomes evaluated were changes in articulation and resonance.

18.4.2   Searching for Best Evidence

Electronic databases are the most common place to start searching for published literature, including the Cochrane Library. Reference lists from key journals are hand searched to identify papers not located electronically. 'Grey' literature referring to papers, reports or technical notes may be reviewed but these documents are not peer reviewed and often

Table 18.4   Clinical questions under review for treatment effectiveness.

Clinical question – Behavioural speech therapy
1. For individuals with cleft palate who require speech therapy, what is the effect of articulation therapy?

Clinical questions – Visual feedback therapy
2. For individuals with cleft palate who require intervention, what is the effect of visual feedback therapy using electropalatography in correcting compensatory articulation errors?
3. For individuals with cleft palate who require intervention, what is the effect of visual feedback therapy using nasometry in reducing nasal speech?
4. For individuals with cleft palate who require intervention, what is the effect of visual feedback therapy using nasopharyngoscopy in achieving adequate velopharyngeal closure?

Clinical question – Muscle strengthening to reduce hypernasality
5. For individuals with cleft palate who require intervention, what is the effect of continuous positive airway pressure (CPAP) therapy in reducing hypernasal speech?

Clinical questions – Secondary surgery to correct VPI
6. For individuals who have persistent hypernasality after primary palate repair, what is the effect of pharyngoplasty on speech?
7. For individuals who have cleft palate, what is the effect of maxillary advancement on resonance?
8. For individuals who have cleft palate, what is the effect of maxillary advancement on articulation?

---

hard to locate. Search terms are used to identify study designs, subject samples, intervention types and therapy outcomes.

Studies considered for systematic review are generally primary studies published in peer-reviewed journals containing original data. For the purpose of this chapter, these studies had to incorporate an intervention of interest applied to at least one person with a cleft palate and include subject description, research methodology, report of outcomes and had to be written in English.

In systematic reviews, preference is given to the randomized clinical trial (RCT). However, for intervention studies in cleft palate the RCT is not common and other research designs such as intervention-comparison, case series and single subject designs are considered for review if they meet specified criteria. The inclusion of retrospective studies in a systematic review warrant careful consideration because they rely on the accuracy of the medical record in which important information may not be available and are subject to selection bias (Hess, 2004). Narrative review articles, book chapters, theses and dissertations, and opinion papers are usually excluded because they are not published in peer-reviewed literature.

18.4.3   Evaluating and Synthesizing the Evidence

Studies are identified based on explicit inclusion/exclusion criteria. Details of each selected study are extracted (e.g. study design, interventions, outcomes and quality), ranked and graded using one of the evidence hierarchies (Appendix 18.A). In this chapter, the levels of evidence from The Joanna Briggs Institute for Evidence-based Practice (Joanna Briggs Institute, 2008) and the American Society of Plastic Surgeons (ASPS) Grades of Recommendation Scale were adopted (American Society of Plastic Surgeons, 2010). The final synthesis of the evidence has been summarized and placed into tables (Tables 18.5–18.9).

18.5   Evidence Findings Establishing Therapy Effectiveness

The focus of this section is to answer the questions posed in Table 18.4 in order to determine best evidence for the intervention undertaken to treat speech and resonance disorders associated with cleft palate. As shown within the text and in Tables 18.5–18.9, most studies were consistent with evidence levels III–IV. There were few RCTs, only one meeting the ASPS criteria for level I evidence.

18.5.1   Speech Therapy – Question 1

Eight studies met the inclusion criteria (Table 18.5). This includes three RCTs, two non-randomized intervention-comparison studies, one case study and two case series; all for which pre- and post-treatment data were reported. The measureable outcomes reported in six studies were changes in articulation or phonologic patterns with one commenting but not measuring speech intelligibility (Hodson *et al.*, 1983) and another (Van Demark

Table 18.5 Evidence of effectiveness using articulation therapy to improve sound production.

Source	Study design	Subjects	Speech characteristics	Intervention	Intervention duration	Assessments	Measured outcome(s)	Post-treatment findings	Evidence level/ Quality
Chisum et al. (1969) (USA)	Intervention-comparison	Intervention group: N = 11 (8 cleft palate, 3 ncvpi[a]: 6 repaired cleft palate, 2 wore speech appliance and 3 with ncvpi wore speech appliance Comparison group: N = 12 (9 cleft palate, 3 ncvpi: 7 repaired cleft palate of which 1 had pharyngeal flap, others wore speech appliance) Age: 6–12 years	Resonance: all participants had either hypernasality, nasal emission or both VP function: all subjects –'borderline vpi' Articulation: 'mild to moderate articulation problems' affecting plosives, fricatives, glides	Intervention group: Motor learning emphasizing response-shaping-with focus on /s/ and 'additional fricatives' Comparison group: no treatment	Intervention group: 30 minute individual treatment twice weekly for minimum 30 lessons within a 6 month period or 48 lessons within 9 month period (mean instruction period 7.18 months) Control group: mean control period – 6.83 months	223 – item articulation test administered before and 6 months after speech therapy	Change in articulation scores	Intervention group: Significant (p<0.05) decrease in articulation error scores in the intervention group compared to controls: number of pre-treatment errors on sibilants and fricatives significantly reduced Comparison group: As a group, no significant reduction in articulation scores after 6 months of no treatment	III.2/C

						IV/D
Hodson et al. (1983) (USA)	Case study pre- and post-treatment comparison	N = 1 (repaired cleft palate) Age: 5 years	VP function: adequate Articulation: velar deviations, cluster reduction and deletion, liquid deviations, glottal stops	Phonology remediation programme in order to increase intelligibility	4 cycles of therapy over 13 months 36 weekly 60–90 minute sessions, 20 minutes twice weekly at school plus home programme (65 total hours over 13 weeks)	The Assessment of Phonological Processes administered before and 13 months after treatment	Change in phonological patterns	After four cycles of therapy over 13 months, participant improved articulatory production eliminating nasal additions/replacements and use of glottal stop only 3 times. Upon dismissal of therapy, participant was judged to be 'generally intelligible.'

(Continued)

Table 18.5 (Continued)

Source	Study design	Subjects	Speech characteristics	Intervention	Intervention duration	Assessments	Measured outcome(s)	Post-treatment findings	Evidence level/ Quality
Albery and Enderby (1984) (UK)	Randomized control trial (RCT)	Participants were randomly allocated to one of two groups: Intervention Group: $N = 25$ Comparison Group: $N = 21$ Mean age: 8:7 years All subjects had repaired cleft palate	VP function: Intervention group: adequate or borderline adequate Comparison group: conventional speech therapy Articulation: errors noted on fricatives, alveolars, velar plosives	Intervention group: received intensive conventional speech therapy Control group received weekly conventional speech therapy	Intervention group: 3 sessions of speech therapy daily (2 individual 30-minute sessions and 1 group session) for 6 weeks Control group: conventional weekly sessions	Edinburgh Articulation Test and Frenchay Articulation Test administered before treatment and 6, 12, 18, and 24 months after treatment in both groups Intervention group not concealed from clinician evaluating the participant	Change in number of articulation errors	Intervention group: significant ($p < 0.01$) and improvement in articulation immediately post-therapy with maintenance throughout 2 year follow-up Comparison group: slight improvement in articulation immediately post-therapy with continued improvement noted at the 2 year follow-up period Despite improvement in articulation in both groups, intervention group continued to exhibit better articulation than control group after 2 years	II/B

| Van Demark and Hardin 1986 (USA) | Case series pre- and post-treatment comparison | N = 13 (repaired cleft palate) Age: 6;8–12;0 years | VP function: competent (n = 10) or marginally competent (n = 3) Articulation: oral distortions, nasal distortions, glottal stops, pharyngeal fricatives substitutions | Systematic multiple sound approach | 6-week intensive programme consisting of 4 1-hour sessions per day for 26 days for total of 104 hours – half of the sessions were individual and other half with another child | Iowa Cleft Palate Articulation Test administered before and immediately after therapy with follow-up 9 months after post-treatment | Change in percentage of articulation errors, nasality, and VP competence | Percentage of errors (substitutions and omissions) decreased immediately after therapy and most participants maintained post-therapy level 9 months later. Some participants continued to make gains with speech therapy at school and few regressed. Average ratings for nasality decreased post treatment VP function did not change in 3 participants (marginal) and changed in one (normal to marginal) immediately after treatment. At the 9 month follow-up, marginal VP function was noted in 1 participant. | IV/D |

(Continued)

Table 18.5 (Continued)

Source	Study design	Subjects	Speech characteristics	Intervention	Intervention duration	Assessment	Measured outcome(s)	Post-treatment findings	Evidence level/ Quality
Broen et al. (1993) (USA)	Case study pre-and post-treatment comparison	N = 1 Age: 3 years (repaired cleft lip and palate) Wearing prosthetic applicance	Articulation: glottal stop, /h/ substitutions, omitted obstruent consonants	Clinician designed speech programme carried out by the parent at home and monitored by clinician	Home intervention programme scheduled 10 minutes twice daily 5 days per week (records suggested that sessions averaged 18 minutes with sessions offered twice daily 50% of the time and once daily 50% of the time)	Percentage of sounds produced via spontaneous speech sample Speech samples obtained before intervention and at 2–3 month intervals and after the final fitting of a speech bulb at 3;9 years	Percentage of sounds produced at correct place of articulation	By the end of treatment, nasal and glottalized oral productions disappeared but glottal stops persisted	IV/D

Pamplona, Ysunza and Espinosa (1999) (Mexico)	Prospective, randomized trial (RT)	Phonologic intervention: N = 14 Conventional Articulation intervention: N = 15 Age: 3–7 years	Articulation: all subjects had compensatory errors (glottal stops, pharyngeal fricatives, pharyngeal stops, mid-dorsum contacts) VP function: all participants had VPI	Phonologic intervention Conventional articulation therapy	Participants in both intervention groups received 1-hour sessions twice weekly until participants achieved normal articulation	Independent rates blind to the interventions assessed speech before and after the completion of treatment Method used to assess articulation not reported	Mean total time of speech therapy (to reach normal articulation)	Phonologic intervention: mean total time in therapy: 14.5 months (range: 6–22 months) Conventional therapy: mean total time in therapy: 30.07 months (range: 14–46 months) Speech therapy time was significantly reduced for participants receiving phonologic treatment to correct compensatory errors than than those receiving conventional therapy	II/B

(Continued)

Table 18.5 (Continued)

Source	Study design	Subjects	Speech characteristics	Intervention	Intervention duration	Assessment	Measured outcome(s)	Post-treatment findings	Evidence level/Quality
Pamplona et al. (2004) (Mexico)	Prospective, randomized trial (RT)	Phonologic intervention: N = 15 Naturalistic intervention: N = 15 Age range: 3–7 years All participants had repaired cleft palate	Articulation: all subjects had compensatory errors (glottal stops pharyngeal fricatives, pharyngeal stops, mid-dorsum contacts) VP function: all participants had VPI‡	Phonologic intervention: speech therapy based on phonologic rules and modification of groups of sounds Naturalistic approach: speech therapy based on whole language principles	Participants in both intervention groups received 1-hour sessions twice weekly until participants achieved normal articulation as judged by the clinician	Independent rates blind to the interventions assessed speech every three months until the compensatory errors were corrected Method used to assess articulation not reported	Mean total time in speech therapy (to reach normal articulation)	Phonologic approach: mean total time in therapy: 14.5 months (range 4–27 months) Naturalistic approach: mean total time in speech therapy: 16.2 months (range: 4–27 months) No significant difference in the mean total time in therapy to improve articulation between the two groups	II/B

| Pamplona et al. (2005) (Mexico) | Intervention-comparison | Intervention group: summer programme $N = 45$ Matched control group: conventional therapy $N = 45$ All participants had repaired cleft palate Age range: 3–10 years | Articulation: participants in both groups exhibited compensatory articulation errors (glottal stops, pharyngeal fricatives) ranging in degree from mild to severe) VP function: all participants had VPI‡ | Therapies based on phonological principles, naturalistic, and whole-language approaches | Intervention group: intensive therapy provided 4 hours/day, 5 days per week for 3 weeks Control group: therapy provided 1 hour twice weekly for 1 year | Speech sampling obtained during play and story telling Severity of compensatory articulation errors judged at the end of summer camp (3 weeks) in the intervention group and at one year in the control group | Change in severity of compensatory articulation errors | Both study groups showed significant reduction in the severity of compensatory errors ($p < 0.05$) There was no significant difference in the severity of compensatory errors between the study groups at the completion of their treatment period | III.2/C |

‡ncvpi: non-cleft velopharyngeal inadequacy.

Table 18.6 Evidence for use of electropalatography (EPG) to treat articulation disorders in children with cleft palate.

Citation	Study design	Subjects	Speech characteristics	Intervention	Intervention schedule	Assessments	Outcomes measured	Post-treatment findings	Evidence level/ Grade
Michi et al. (1986) (Japan)	Single subject before before and after treatment	N = 1 Age: 6 years Dx: cleft lip and palate	Articulation: Lateral misarticulation and palatalized articulation on sibilants and affricates VP function: adequate	Basic training to establish correct articulatory placement for error sound followed by visual articulation therapy using EPG to identify palatograph patterns and sensations of tongue placement and to discriminate misarticulations	49 1-hour sessions for 12 months	Audio recording of articulation before and after treatment EPG pattern monitored during treatment with definitive comparisons made before and after treatment	Qualitative change in EPG lingual patterns and perceptual judgements of speech	Articulation was normal or nearly normal at the end of training as judged by naïve listeners Palato-lingual contact on /s/, /t/, /l/, /ʃ/ (shi) was almost equivalent to that of a speaker with normal articulation	IV/D
Gibbon and Hardcastle (1989) (UK)	Single subject before before and after	N = 1 Age: 13 years Dx: bilateral cleft lip and palate	Articulation: posterior patterns of articulation including palatal fricatives, velar consonants for alveolar plosives and nasals, posterior nasal frication VP function: Adequate at word level, less so during conversational speech	Visual articulation feedback using EPG to eliminate labial-velar double-articulations, establish anterior tongue placement for alveolar plosives and nasals – details of treatment programme provided	14 weekly 1-hour sessions	Narrow transcription of a word list before and after treatment EPG progress assessed during each session while in use with definitive comparisons made before and after treatment	Changes in EPG patterns of palato-lingual contacts for sound errors Changes in articulation based on phonetic transcription	Changed aberrant tongue postures resulting in perceived accuracy of alveolar sound, some palatalizations persisted when compared to normal speaker. Perceptually normal productions of all alveolar, bilabial, velar, and lateral consonants with some palatalization detected in alveolar grooved fricatives	IV/D

Michi et al. (1993) (Japan)	RCT-parallel group	N = 6 Age: 4–6 years Dx: cleft lip and palate	Resonance: normal in 5 and intermittent hypernasality and nasal emission in 1 Articulation: 6 subjects with palatalized /s/ errors with 2 also displaying lateralizations on /s/	Participants randomly assigned to 3 treatment conditions: EPG and friction display method (n = 2) EPG therapy (n = 2) No visual feedback – traditional articulatory placement (n = 2) Baseline data obtained in all groups	Weekly 60-minute individual therapy sessions Total sessions: 8 sessions (2 months)	10 repeated presentations of /s/ at different levels before, during, and after treatment to monitor progress for each treatment group.	Qualitative change in EPG lingual pattern of /s/	Progress of patients with slight posterior tongue elevation was the same with or without visual feedback Patients with excessive posterior or slight tongue elevation progressed rapidly in using EPG in learning the correct placement for /s/ II/B
Whitehill, Stokes and Man (1996) (China)	Single subject multiple baseline	N = 1 Age: 18 years Dx: cleft lip and palate	Resonance: moderate hypernasal speech and nasal emission Articulation: posteriorly placed plosives, fricatives, affricates	Targeted at /s/ and /t/ at word level and conversational speech	23 1-hour sessions over 4 months	Phonetic transcription of targeted phonemes in single words and conversational speech before and after treatment EPG progress assessed during each session while in use with definitive comparisons made before and after treatment	Changes in EPG articulatory patterns documented by mean percent of palatal contact Perceptual changes in target phonemes in words and conversation	EPG showed more anterior placement on /s/ and /t/ which were also perceived as accurate with a transfer of the normal pattern on non-targeted EPG changes reflected in perceptual judgments of improved production of the error phonemes Nasal emission eliminated but no reduction in hypernasal speech III.3/B

(Continued)

Table 18.6 (Continued)

Citation	Study design	Subjects	Speech characteristics	Intervention	Intervention schedule	Assessment	Outcomes measured	Post-treatment findings	Evidence level/ Grade
Stokes et al. (1996) (China)	Single subject[a] multiple baseline	N = 2 Ages: 5:08 and 7:08 years Dx: cleft lip and palate	Deviant fricatives and affricates	EPG integrated with traditional articulation therapy focusing on /s/ to facilitate self monitoring on this sound	1-hour weekly sessions for 7 weeks	Whole word phonetic transcription using standard Cantonese phonology test Data collected at baseline, probe, and 4 months after treatment	Qualitative change in EPG lingual patterns Progress measured as percentage of accuracy of target sound	After therapy, EPG patterns showed maximal palatal contact and target phonemes were perceptually acceptable	III.3/C
Gibbon et al. (2001) (UK)	RCT-crossover	N = 12 Age: 15–18 years (M: 10;05 years) Dx: cleft palate +/– cleft lip	VP function: Adequate Articulation: compensatory errors	Subjects randomly assigned to one of two treatment regimes: Regime1: 5 subjects receiving 4 EPG sessions followed by 4 non-EPG sessions Regime 2: 7 subjects receiving 4 non-EPG sessions followed by 4 EPG sessions Target for all sessions: anterior placement for /t/ and /s/ and groove formation for (sh)	8 30–45 minute individual sessions	Data collected at baseline, and after 4 and 8 sessions	Changes in EPG lingual patterns for target phoneme Change in CoG[b] index	9/12 showed positive change in articulation with more anterior placement recorded CoG values increased indicating a more forward placement on /t/ and /s/ following EPG therapy	II/C

Study	Design	Participants	Assessment	Intervention	Duration	Outcome measures	Measures	Results	Level
Fujiwara (2007) (Japan)	Case series	N = 5 Age: 8–13 years (M: 10:75) Dx: cleft lip and palate	VP function: adequate in 4/5 when the study started. One participate received a pharyngeal flap during the study. Articulation: palatalized (t, ts, s) and lateralized sibilants (sh, ch)	EPG home training using a portable training unit (PTU) Initial EPG training sessions took place at the speech clinic demonstrating target pattern after which participants used PTU at home to continue the treatment program	30 minutes/ day for 7 to 8 months	EPG recordings were made during monthly follow up visits in the speech clinic	Change in the EPG lingual patterns for the target sound /t/ Change in CoG index	All 5 participants showed marked changes in EPG patterns and increased CoG values demonstrating maximal palatal contact for the correct anterior production of /t/ in all 5 participants	IV/C
Lohmander, Henriksson and Havstam (2010) (Sweden)	Single subject multiple baseline with ABA design	N = 1 Age: 11 years Dx: cleft palate	VP function: marginal Articulation: retracted /s/ and /t/ Intelligibility: slight to moderately reduced	The intervention design included baseline and no treatment (A), treatment period using EPG (B), and follow-up after treatment was terminated (A). Initial EPG and sound placement training took place in the speech clinic after which all therapy took place at home with the participant using a portable EPG training unit. Follow up visits were made in the speech clinic	8 months During the treatment phase, the participant practised her target consonants 10 minutes 1–2 times daily for 5 days for a total of 20 hours of training	Standardized articulation testing Intelligibility ratings	Change in the EPG lingual pattern amd CoG Changes in speech of the targeted phonemes	Participant showed normal EPG articulatory patterns on /s/ and /t/ after 2 months (8 hours) and increased CoG values Articulation of the targeted sounds improved after treatment but transfer from single words to conversational speech was difficult and there was no significant change in intelligibility	III.2/B

[a]For the purpose of this systematic review single subject will include 1–2 subjects and case series to refer to 3 or more subjects.

[b]CoG refers to 'centre of gravity' an index that represents the concentration of electrodes in anterior-posterior dimension and is valuable in evaluating progress for sounds made from an incorrect posterior position to a more correct anterior position (Gibbon et al., 2001; Fujiwara, 2007; Lohmander, Henriksson and Havstam, 2010).

Table 18.7 Evidence for the effectiveness of biofeedback using videonasopharyngoscopy to improve velopharyngeal closure for speech.

Citation	Study design	Subjects	Speech characteristics	Intervention	Intervention schedule	Assessments	Measured outcome(s)	Post-treatment findings	Evidence level/ Grade
Yamaoka et al. (1983) (Japan)	Case series pre-post treatment	N = 59 Age: 8–45 years All had cleft palate and VPI	Persistent VPI No description of speech reported	Video nasopharyngoscopy biofeedback therapy	1 hour session bimonthly for a year	Nasopharyngoscopy	Qualitative report of changes in VP function	59% achieved 'improved velopharyngeal function' within one year	IV/D
Kawano et al. (1985) (Japan)	Observational pre-post treatment	N = 5 Age: over 9 years All participants had repaired cleft palate	All participants exhibited laryngeal fricatives on (sh) and /s/ Persistent VP opening during the production of laryngeal fricatives	Video nasopharyngoscopy biofeedback therapy	Case 1: Treatment provided 4 times in two months Cases 2–5: Treatment schedule and duration not reported	Perceptual speech ratings Nasopharyngoscopy	Qualitative report of changes in VP function and speech	After one year of treatment, participants achieved normal articulation and adequate VP function	IV/D
Witzel, Tobe and Salyer (1988) (Canada)	Case study pre-post treatment	N = 1 Age: 10 years old Repaired cleft lip and palate Posterior nasal fricative	Audible nasal emission on /s/ and inadequate VP closure on this error sound	Video nasopharyngoscopy biofeedback therapy_	One session	Perceptual speech ratings Nasopharyngoscopy	Qualitative report of changes in VP function and speech Change in articulation	Eliminated pharyngeal fricative and referred to speech therapy for maintanence of place and manner for sibilant-fricative phonemes VP closure occurred during correct /s/ production and maintained after one year	IV/D

Witzel, Tobe and Salyer (1989) (Canada)	Case studies pre-post treatment	$N = 3$ Age: 34–50 years All had cleft lip and palate with pharyngeal flap	All patients had persistent hypernasality with compensatory articulation errors including glottal stops and pharyngeal fricatives	Video nasopharyngoscopy biofeedback therapy	Subject 1: 30 minute feedback sessions at monthly intervals and received weekly conventional speech therapy Subject 2: 2 30-minute sessions Subject 3: 4 sessions at 1–2 intervals with weekly conventional speech therapy	Perceptual speech ratings Nasopharyngoscopy	VP closure	Subject 1: Normal resonance and articulation post treatment; glottal stop eliminated Follow-up at 2.5 months and 1 year showed normal resonance, adequate velopharyngeal function, articulation improvement on sibilants and /k/ Subject 2: At end of session, resonance and articulation were normal; improved velopharyngeal closure Subject 3: Improved velopharyngeal closure and articulation but did not continue treatment	IV/D

(Continued)

Table 18.7 (Continued)

Citation	Study design	Subjects	Speech characteristics	Intervention	Intervention schedule	Assessments	Measured outcome(s)	Post-treatment findings	Evidence level/ Grade
Ysunza et al. (1997) (Mexico)	Intervention-comparison	N = 17 Group 1: N = 9 Median age: 11;9 years Group 2: N = 8 Median age: 11;11 years	All had compensatory articulation errors All had negative medial movement of the lateral pharyngeal walls	Both groups received 3 weeks of conventional speech therapy and eventually sessions were introduced in 1 group using video nasopharyngoscopy biofeedback therapy	Group 1: 60-minute sessions 3 times per week aimed at correcting compensatory errors Group 2: 60-minute sessions 3 times per week aimed at correcting compensatory errors + addition 25 minute biofeedback therapy twice weekly	Perceptual speech ratings Nasopharyngoscopy	Qualitative report of changes in lateral pharyngeal wall movement and correction of compensatory errors	Group 1: After 12 weeks 8/9 subjects continued to show outward displacement of the lateral pharyngeal walls Group 2: after 12 weeks, negative movement of the lateral pharyngeal walls had been modified Difference between groups significant p < 0.05 After 6 months, all 17 subjects underwent pharyngeal flap which corrected VPI in all but 2 cases who then received biofeedback therapy. After 18 months, all patients had normal resonance and articulation	III.2/C

Table 18.8 Evidence for the effectiveness of pharyngoplasty to improve velopharyngeal function for resonance and speech.

Citation	Study Design	Subjects	Intervention	Interval between surgery and post-op evaluations	Assessment	Measured Outcome(s)	Post-treatment Findings	Evidence Level/ Grade
Witt et al. (1994) (USA)	Case series Pre-post treatment	N = 20 Age: 3–17 years (M: 11.8 years) Repaired cleft palate (3) SMCP (3) Noncleft VPI (4)	Sphincter pharyngoplasty	Mean: 5 months (range: 2–9 months)	Perceptual rating of resonance, nasal emission, speech quality, intelligibility Nasopharyngoscopic ratings of VP closure, VP closure pattern, and estimated % of orifice closure during speech	Change in resonance, nasal emission, speech quality, intelligibility VP closure and pattern of closure, % VP closure	Nasal resonance: improved in 79% but only 18 % showed complete resolution in of hypernasality and nasal emission: 23.5% were hyponasal Nasal emission: improved in 79% Speech quality and intelligibillity: improvement in 42% and 21%, respectively 75% showed quantativie decrease in VP orifice size with 35% showing complete VP closure 18% showed complete resolution of hypernasality, nasal emission 65% were considered candidates for additional surgery	IV/D

(Continued)

Table 18.8 (Continued)

Citation	Study Design	Subjects	Intervention	Interval between surgery and post-op evaluations	Assessments	Measured Outcome(s)	Post-treatment Findings	Evidence Level/ Grade
Ysunza et al. (2002) (Mexico)	Randomized trial (RT)	Total N = 50 Group 1: N = 25 Age: 4–7; 7 years (Median: 4; 7 years) Group 2: N = 25 Age: 4–7; 4 years (Median: 4; 5 years)	Group 1: Pharyngeal flap Group 2: Sphincter pharyngoplasty	4 months	Blinded perceptual ratings Qualitative nasopharyngoscopy ratings Multiview videofluoroscopy Multiview videofluoroscopy – pre operatively only	Improved VP closure	Group 1: Complete VP closure in 88% Group 2: Complete VP closure in 84% For both groups, the remaining subjects showed reduced gap size with bubbling through VP port during speech Nonsignificant difference (<0.05) between the mean size of VP closure gap between the two surgical groups No speech results reported	III.2/C
Tönz et al. (2002) (Switzerland)	Case series Pre-post treatment	N = 23 Mean age: 9.7 years at time of surgery	Pharyngeal flap	<1 year (0.89 years) Range: 0.4–5.3 years	Perceptual rating scale – assessors blinded to pre and post operative taperecordings Lay assessors used binary scale to answer questions about nasality and intelligibility	Change in resonance, articulation, intelligibility	Hypernasality improved in 87% No cases of hyponasality Articulation improved in 87% Intelligibility improved in 83% Overall improvement by SLPs: 87% Overall improvement by lay assessors: 83% No participant was judged to have normal speech after pharyngeal flap surgery	IV/D

Åbyholm et al. (2005) (USA, UK, Norway)	Randomized trial (RT) Multicenter	N = 97 Age: 3–25 years	Group 1: Pharyngeal flap Group 2: Sphincter pharyngoplasty	3 months post-op and 12 months post-op	Blinded perceptual evaluations Nasopharyngoscopy Nasometry Allocation to groups concealed	Change in resonance and nasalance	At 1 year, both pharyngoplasty and sphincter pharyngoplasty eliminated hypernasality in about 85% of patients. At 3 months, almost twice as many participants eliminated hypernasality with pharyngeal flap than sphincter pharyngoplasty, but this difference was not evident at 12 months. No significant differences in nasalance between the groups. There was no statistical difference between the two groups	II/C
Van Lierde et al. (2008) (Belgium)	Case series Pre-post treatment	N = 7 Age: 4.7–9.1 years (mean: 6.9 years)	Pharyngeal flap	6 months and 1 year post-op	Perceptual evaluations Nasometry	Change in articulation, resonance, voice, intelligibility and nasalance scores	Errors on /r/ and the fricatives /s/ and /sch/ persisted at one year. Improvement in resonance noted at 6 week post-op period from a median score of 3 (range 1–3) suggestive of moderate hypernasality to a median score of 2. Voice: essentially normal. Intelligibility improved both at 6 weeks and 1 year after surgery, but still slightly impaired. Nasalance scores improved up to 1 year and were commensurate with normative values; scores on /i/ an /a/ continued to be elevated	IV/D

Table 18.9 Evidence for orthognathic surgery to alter resonance and speech in patients with cleft palate.

Citation	Study Design	Subjects	Pre-operative speech characteristics	Intervention	Interval between surgery and post-op evaluations	Assessments	Outcomes Measured	Post-treatment findings	Evidence Level/ Grade
Schwarz and Gruner (1976) (Switzerland)	Non-random group comparison pre-post treatment	N = 40 Group 1: 31 participants with cleft lip and palate Group 2: 9 participants without cleft and maxillary hypoplasia	Not clearly stated and difficult to ascertain	Maxillary advancement	4 months	Qualitative descriptions of articulation impairment	Changes in articulatory impairment and VP function	Articulation improved in 31 participants with cleft palate VP function deteriorated with an increase in forward movement of the maxilla	IV/D
Witzel & Munroe (1977) (Canada)	Case report: Pre-post treatment	N = 1 Age: 16 years Bilateral cleft lip and palate	Normal resonance and sibilant distortions	Maxillary advancement	2 months	Perceptual speech ratings	Changes in resonance and speech	Marked hypernasality Improved sibilant production	IV/D
McCarthy, Coccaro and Schwartz (1979) (USA)	Non-random group comparison pre-post treatment	N = 40 Group 1: 14 with cleft palate (one with pharyngeal flap) Group 2: 25 without cleft and maxillary hypoplasia	Unreported	Maxillary advancement	Unreported			Improved /s/ productions in all participants No changes in VP orifice size in any group Nasopharyngeal height and depth, velar length, and angle hard/soft palate increased in participants with cleft palate	IV/D

Study	Study design	Participants		Intervention	Follow-up	Outcome measures	Outcomes	
Poole, Robinson and Nunn (1986) (UK)	Case series: Pre-post treatment	N = 7 Mean age: 18.6 years (range: 7–21 years) All subjects had cleft palate +/– cleft lip	Unreported	Maxillary advancement	4 months	Perceptual speech ratings Nasopharygoscopy	Changes in resonance, speech, and VP function	Resonance was unchanged and articulation improved in 6; no alterations in VP function In one, resonance deteriorated, articulation remained unchanged, and nasopharyngoscopy showed a VP gap	IV/D
Kummer et al. (1989) (USA)	Case series: Pre-post treatment	N = 16 Mean age: 22 years (range: 14–35 years) Cleft lip/ palate (7) – two with pharyngeal flap Cleft lip (1) Noncleft (8)	11/16 showed articulation errors on /s/ and 7/16 on (sh)	Maxillary advancement	3–6 months	Templin-Darley Test of Articulation Perceptual ratings of resonance and nasal emission Videofluoroscopy	Changes in articulation Qualitative changes in resonance, nasal emission and VP function	Articulation improvement: 7 Articulation deterioration: 0 Nasal emission: mild and inconsistent in 2 Resonance: change from hyponasality to normal resonance in 1 and from normal to slight hypernasality in 1 – noncleft participants VP function: 9 showed 'diminished contact', 8 'apparent decrease in velar height', 3 'decrease in velar thickness', and 4 'increase in velar length'	IV/D

(Continued)

Table 18.9 (Continued)

Citation	Study Design	Subjects	Pre-operative speech characteristics	Intervention	Interval between surgery and post-op evaluations	Assessments	Outcomes Measured	Post-treatment findings	Evidence Level/ Grade
Okzaki et al. (1993) (Japan)	Case series: Pre-post treatment	N = 10 Age: 16–20 years All subjects had cleft palate +/- cleft lip, one of which had a pharyngeal flap	Articulation: palatalized articulation and pharyngeal fricative 1, not reported in remaining 9 Hypernasality: None (1), slight (4), mile (1), moderate (4) Nasal emission: Absent (3), mild (5), severe (2)	Maxillary advancement	1 year	Perceptual speech ratings Nasopharyngoscopy Lateral cephalogram	Changes in articulation, resonance, nasal emission and VP function	After surgery, resonance deteriorated in 8/10 patients 5 patients were slight to mildly hypernasal before surgery, and 3 were moderately hypernasal Articulatory improvement – none Nasal emission: essentially unchanged Cehphalometric results: Increased distance between velum and PPW in 6 VP function: changes in 3 (fair to poor), others remained unchanged from pre-op function	IV/D

Study	Design	Sample	Results	Intervention	Timepoints	Outcome measures	Findings	Level of evidence
Haapanen et al. (1997) (Finland)	Case series: Pre-post treatment	N = 15 Mean Age: 23.3 years (range: 18–41 years) All subjects had repaired cleft lip and palate	Hypernasality in 27% (4) Audible nasal emission 13% (2) VP function: competent in 93% (14)	Maxillary advancement	2, 6, 12 months	Perceptual speech ratings Nasometry Pressure-Flow	Changes in resonance, nasalance scores, and VP areas	At one year post-op 27% (4/15) of the patients experienced deterioration in speech and were hypernasal Nasalance scores increased in 4 patients VP function deteriorated in 27% (4) VP orifice areas did not change Although not the focus of the study, some patients reported that it was easier to produce sibilants	IV/D
Chua et al. (2010) (People's Republic of China)	Randomized Trial (RT)	N = 22 N = 11 Intervention: Maxillary distraction (DO) N = 11 Comparison: Conventional maxillary advancement (CO) Age: 16–22 years All subjects had cleft lip/palate	Resonance: normal in 20/22 (2 hypernasal in DO group) Nasal emission: present in one from CO group, none in DO group Nasalance: Within normative range for all participants VP function: Normal: 13 Borderline touch closure: 5 Mild VPI: 1 Moderate VPI: 1	Maxillary distraction vs Conventional maxillary advancement	Before surgery and 3–8 months (mean 4 months) and 12–29 months (mean 17 months)	Perceptual rating of resonance and nasal emission Nasometry VP function using nasoendoscopy using a rating scale	Changes in resonance (hypernasality), nasal emission, nasalance, and VP gap size	No significant differences in measured outcomes between participants receiving DO or CO DO is no better than CO at preventing VPI and speech disorders	II/B

and Hardin, 1986) reporting on changes in nasality and VP competence. In two other studies (Pamplona, Ysunza and Espinosa, 1999; Pamplona et al., 2004), mean total time in speech therapy was the measureable outcome. Most of these papers reported positive outcomes in articulation following speech therapy but the evidence to support this was weak.

There are few studies comparing treatment regimes for correction of articulation errors to draw a definitive conclusion about which approach is best. Two randomized control studies (level II) used time in treatment as the main outcome. One (Pamplona, Ysunza and Espinosa, 1999) showed that time needed to eliminate compensatory errors was significantly reduced when a phonologic approach was used compared to conventional articulation therapy. The other (Pamplona et al., 2004) showed no difference between a phonological approach and naturalistic approach in the time needed to correct compensatory misarticulations. Although it was said that the speech samples were randomly assigned to examiners for transcription, it is somewhat questionable as to whether group allocation was actually concealed from the examiners. This would challenge the strict regime of an RCT and the level of evidence suggested by these studies.

Evidence supporting studies on the effect of treatment intensity is conflicting. Two studies (Albery and Enderby, 1984; Pamplona et al., 2005) compared the effects of a more intensive therapy schedule to weekly treatment sessions. Using an RCT (level II), Albery and Enderby (1984) reported that regardless of the intensity schedule, children exhibit a reduction in articulation errors following therapy, but those having more intensive treatment showed more immediate and significant changes than those receiving weekly treatment and maintained these skills after two years. Using an intervention-comparison design (level III.2), Pamplona et al. (2005) reported no difference in the severity of compensatory articulation between either group. The case series (level IV) by Van Demark and Hardin (1986) showed that articulation improved following treatment. At nine months, the majority of children maintained their post-treatment level, few made gains with speech therapy continued at school, and some regressed. These investigators also reported changes in nasality and VP competence as a function of articulation therapy, showing that nasality decreased and persistence of marginal VP function in one participant. In this study 10/13 participants exhibited normal VP function and three marginal function, so it is difficult to make any generalizations about the direct effect of treatment on these variables.

Using intelligibility as an outcome, Hodson et al. (1983) reported a case study (level IV) using a phonological approach to modify articulation. After one year, the child could best be described as 'generally intelligible.'

From these studies, which generally report positive outcomes, it is not possible to conclude that any one intervention is better than another. Although speech therapy to correct articulation disorders associated with cleft palate is supported, clinicians should be watchful of newly published evidence for treatment effectiveness that is supported by well developed research methodology.

Criteria in future studies that would strengthen the evidence include: specification of subject inclusion and exclusion criteria, description of randomization procedures for RCTs, blinding of researchers and evaluators, clearly stated measureable outcomes, accurate reporting of articulation errors, resonance, classification of velopharyngeal function, clear descriptions of treatment regimens, intervention schedules and intervention delivery, and long term follow-up after treatment cessation beyond one year. Consistency in design would make study replication possible and comparisons possible.

18.6 Instrumentation – Visual Feedback

18.6.1 Electropalatography (EPG) – Question 2

Eight primary studies (Table 18.6) and one systematic review of an RCT met the criteria for inclusion. As shown in the table, all studies using EPG to modify treat intractable speech errors report positive outcomes. Lee, Law and Gibbon (2009) published in the Cochrane Review Library a systematic review of RCTs focusing on the effectiveness of EPG to treat articulation errors associated with cleft palate. Using comprehensive search criteria, the authors were only able to identify one study (Michi *et al.*, 1993) that met the specified inclusion standard for this appraisal. Based on their findings, they concluded that that the current level of evidence to support the efficacy of EPG is not strong.

Notwithstanding the conclusions reached by Lee, Law and Gibbon (2009), it is necessary to acknowledge that they were derived from one study and the moderate evidence (level II) from other controlled studies (Lohmander, Henriksson and Havstam, 2010; Gibbon *et al.*, 2001) (Table 18.6) cannot be ignored showing the efficiency with which individuals modify their maladaptive articulatory patterns using EPG; changes in patterns that have not responded to traditional speech therapy. From these studies, the evidence strength for the use of EPG for treatment of cleft related articulation errors is low but suggest that patients experience positive articulatory gains within a fairly short time. Long term benefits are unknown.

Although continued investigation into the use of EPG in speech intervention is supported, high quality prospective controlled studies are needed before EPG can be considered a routine therapeutic tool for articulation errors associated with cleft palate.

18.6.2 Nasometry Therapy – Question 3

Despite the popularity of the nasometer (Kay Pentax, Lincoln Park, NJ) for clinical practice, the evidence to support its therapeutic use is very weak. Studies of the effectiveness of nasometry therapy are dated (Fletcher, 1972; Fletcher, 1978; Burrell, 1989). One primary study by Fletcher (1972) met the inclusion criteria for this systematic review. In a report of two adults who wore speech bulbs, Fletcher (1972) described treatment using TONAR II to reduce hypernasality. Although the results showed that both participants were able to reduce nasality to successful criteria of 15% or below within the session, information regarding the treatment programme and long term outcome was not provided. Further study is required to support its routine use as a treatment tool to manage hypernasal speech.

18.6.3   Nasopharyngoscopy – Question 4

The studies on nasopharyngoscopy as a biofeedback tool to obtain velopharyngeal closure are few. Five studies met the eligibility for inclusion (Table 18.7). Three studies (Kawano et al., 1985; Witzel, Tobe and Salyer, 1988; Witzel, Tobe and Salyer, 1989) reported complete velopharyngeal closure, normal resonance and resolution of speech errors after nasopharyngoscopy biofeedback while Yamaoka et al. (1983) reported improved velopharyngeal closure in 60% of patients. Ysunza et al. (1997) showed that negative lateral pharyngeal wall movement associated with compensatory errors could be modified using biofeedback and articulation therapy compared to speech therapy alone, thereby potentially improving the outcome of pharyngeal flap surgery.

In these studies, little was learned about the details of the intervention programme, patient selection, patient tolerance, treatment duration, measureable outcomes, qualitative and/or quantitative evaluation of progress, or maintenance of any long term improvement. At this time, the evidence for use of nasopharyngoscopy as a biofeedback tool for routine use is weak but it may be useful in selected clinical situations.

18.6.4   Continuous Positive Air Pressure (CPAP) – Question 5

There is limited evidence on the use of CPAP to treat hypernasal speech or that it is more effective than other intervention approaches to treat this condition. The evidence for this technique is relatively low (Level IV) and comes from a case series report (Kuehn, 1991) and a non-randomized pre-post intervention case series study (Kuehn et al., 2002). Results in this latter study of 43 subjects showed a net reduction in hypernasality using CPAP; however, responses to treatment were variable across subjects and clinical sites, the reasons for which were unstated. The factors limiting the strength of evidence for routine use of CPAP in managing hypernasality include lack of adequately defined subject selection, information regarding VP function and nasality of subjects and limited follow-up in addition to the lack of a control group in the study by Kuehn et al. (2002). The results of a well designed randomized control trial are necessary to provide conclusive evidence.

18.7   Surgery

In this chapter, the term pharyngoplasty is used to describe operations on the velopharyngeal structures. These include sphincter pharyngoplasty (SP) and superior based pharyngeal flap (SBPF).

18.7.1   Pharyngoplasty – Question 6

There have been numerous studies examining outcomes of pharyngoplasty to improve velopharyngeal function for speech (Chapter 5), the majority of which were retrospective and only five studies met inclusion criteria (Table 18.8). All studies reviewed reported improvement in speech following pharyngoplasty. The best evidence comes from the results of a double blinded RCT (Åbyholm *et al.*, 2005), which showed improvement in approximately 85% of the cases regardless of the surgery performed (SBPF or SP). Until the results of future well controlled studies suggest otherwise, it can be said that the evidence supports improved resonance after surgery in the majority of cases and that the results for SBPF and SP are comparable in achieving adequate speech.

Lack of standard assessments, subject selection, blinding of evaluators, long term follow-up and clear outcome criteria decrease the value of the lower ranked studies.

18.7.2   Orthognathic Surgery (Maxillary Advancement) – Questions 7 and 8

Eight studies met the eligibility criteria for inclusion (Table 18.9): one randomized trial, two non-random group comparisons before and after maxillary advancement, and five case series. With one exception (Chua *et al.*, 2010), the evidence for changes in speech (including resonance, nasal emission and articulation) and VP function following maxillary advancement is conflicting, coming from the low (IV) level of evidence in seven reported studies. As shown in the table, there were more individuals in the group who did not experience any adverse effects in nasality than who did following surgery.

Up to this point, all reported studies were those that addressed the effects of the conventional orthognathic (CO) surgery to advance the maxilla. Participants were not randomized into groups and there were no comparisons between types of treatment. More recently, distraction osteogenesis (DO) has become an alternative option for correcting maxillary hypoplasia, receiving the attention of Chua *et al.* (2010). In their randomized trial, these investigators compared the effects of DO and CO on speech and VP function. This good quality study (level II) included appropriately blinded group allocation and raters as well as qualitative and quantitative assessments. Their findings convincingly suggest that DO is no more advantageous than CO in preventing speech disorders and VPI.

The evidence that maxillary advancement has a negative effect on resonance or a positive effect on articulation is not strong, thus making it difficult to draw firm conclusions about its effect on speech. On the other hand, the evidence that is stronger and most convincing is that which suggests no differences in the effects of DO and CO in producing changes speech and VP function.

18.8   Comments about Intervention Effectiveness

Does speech therapy work? The positive outcomes reported here suggest that it does but guidelines regarding these interventions are not yet well established. The evidence for biofeedback therapy to correct compensatory errors (EPG), modify hypernasality (nasometry and CPAP) and achieve velopharyngeal closure (nasoendoscopy) is not strong, and in great need of continuing investigation. Until evidence is provided that suggests otherwise, these might be best used as experimental or adjuncts to speech therapy for which progress in treatment require close and diligent record keeping.

The evidence for pharyngoplasty to improve velopharyngeal function is stronger than the other types of intervention for hypernasal speech but normal speech postoperatively was not achieved in every person studied. The evidence for the effects of maxillary surgery on altering speech is inconclusive.

Regardless of the type of intervention, the paucity of evidence rated as strong or moderately strong underscores the necessity for well designed studies evaluating the effectiveness of speech, visual feedback and surgical intervention.

18.9   Intervention and the International Classification of Function (ICF)

The measured outcomes in the studies of intervention discussed in this chapter are impairment based. They provide an understanding of the effects of the cleft condition and treatment. The effect of the speech disability on other areas of one's life, such as education, social interactions, opportunities to engage in activities and employment opportunities, has not been adequately addressed in our literature. If the objective of intervention is to optimize communication and improve the quality of life, both impairment and social factors need to be integrated into a carefully developed treatment plan and it effectiveness evaluated. This is a concept that is covered by Havstam and Lohmander (Chapter 17) and very relevant in planning future studies on intervention.

18.10   Research Designs for Intervention Studies

'*Reviews of the literature often end with a call for more research.*' (Law *et al.*, 2000). The results of research or systematic review often generate more questions than answers. This chapter is no exception. EBP has an effective role in bridging the gap between the available evidence and directing future research and best practice. Based on the available evidence for treatment, premium prospective research trials are needed. Table 18.10 summarizes some of the questions warranting further study and the research designs that might be considered suitable for answering them.

18.11   Conclusions

Speech impairment related to cleft palate is complex. More than 25 years ago McWilliams, Morris and Shelton (1984) wrote, 'The empirical research literature on articulation training for patients with cleft palate is scanty.' (p. 316). While there still may be too few studies and their limitations obvious, they have been valuable in serving as a guide to treatment thus far, and have raised our awareness about the need for improvements in research design and patient care. It is expected that EBP in the ICF framework will bridge the gap between available evidence, research and clinical application and enhance the lives of our patients.

Table 18.10 Questions for future studies of treatment effectiveness for speech disorders associated with cleft palate and suggested research designs for answering them.

Questions	Suggested research designs
What treatment is most effective for correcting compensatory articulation errors?	• Properly designed RCT • Well controlled intervention-comparison without randomization • Well controlled single or several subjects (multiple baseline)
Who are the appropriate candidates for a given type of intervention recommended (e.g. conventional speech therapy, visual feedback, CPAP)?	• Case series • Mixed research methods – qualitatively identify speech symptoms and administer treatment plan. Using quantitative analyses (e.g. logistics regression) to examine the relationship among the factors in the treatment outcome • Well developed case study before and after treatment
What treatment is most effective for correcting compensatory articulation errors?	• Properly designed RCT • RCT parallel • Well controlled intervention-comparison without randomization • Well controlled single or several subjects (multiple baseline)
With regard to service delivery, how often should therapy be applied and for how long?	• Properly designed RCT • Well controlled intervention-comparison without randomization
What outcome measures can be identified to evaluate the effects of speech therapy?	• Properly designed RCT • Well controlled intervention-comparison without randomization
Can customization of surgical technique selection improve the overall speech outcome?	• Properly designed RCT • Well controlled intervention-comparison without randomization • Rigorously designed case study
Which surgical technique for primary palate repair gives the best speech outcome?	• Properly designed RCT • Well controlled intervention-comparison without randomization
What are the long term effects of children with cleft lip and palate with respect to education, occupation and social relationships?	• Qualitative study using focus group design and questionnaires that can be analysed quantitatively • QOL scales that can be quantitatively analysed
What are the social outcomes of improved speech?	• Qualitative study using focus group design and questionnaires that can be analysed quantitatively • Interviewing • Case study

Appendix 18.A Commonly Used Evidence Hierarchies for Intervention Studies

Agency for Healthcare Research and Quality. http://www.ahrq.gov/CLINIC/ptsafety/chap3.htm

[a]Oxford Centre for Evidence Based Medicine Levels of Evidence (2009). http://www.cebm.net/index.aspx?o=1025

American Society of Plastic Surgery. Scales for Rating Evidence. http://www.plasticsurgery.org/Medical_Professionals/Health_Policy_and_Advocacy/Health_Policy_Resources/Evidence-based_GuidelinesPractice_Parameters/Description_and_Development_of_Evidence-based_Practice_Guidelines/ASPS_Evidence_Rating_Scales.html

American Society of Plastic Surgery. Scales for Grading Practice Recommendations. http://www.plasticsurgery.org http://www.plasticsurgery.org/Medical_Professionals/Health_Policy_and_Advocacy/Health_Policy_Resources/Evidence- based_GuidelinesPractice_Parameters/Description_and_Development_of_Evidence-based_Practice_Guidelines/ASPS_Evidence_Rating_Scales.html

American Speech-Language-Hearing Association (2004). Evidence-Based Practice in Communication Disorders: An Introduction [Technical Report]. http://www.asha.org/policy

[a]Joanna Briggs Institute (2008)
http://www.joannabriggs.edu.au/Documents/JBI%20Approach%20to%20%20of%20Recommendation.pdf

[a]The National Health and Medical Research Council. http://www.nhmrc.gov.au/_files_nhmrc/file/guidelines/levels_grades05.pdf

[a]Includes grades of recommendations.

References

Åbyholm, F., D'Antonio, L. and Davidson Ward, SL., *et al.* VPI Surgical Group (2005) Pharyngeal flap and sphincterplasty for velopharyngeal insufficiency have equal outcome at 1 year postoperatively: results of a randomized trial. *Cleft Palate-Craniofacial Journal*, **42**, 501–511.

Akobeng, A.K. (2005) Understanding systematic reviews and meta-analysis. *Archives of Disease in Childhood*, **90**, 845–848.

Albery, L. (1989) Approaches to the treatment of speech problems, in *Cleft Palate: The Nature and Remediation of Communication Problems* (ed. J. Stengelhofen), Churchill Livingstone, Edinburgh, pp. 97–110.

Albery, L. and Enderby, P. (1984) Intensive speech therapy for cleft palate children. *British Journal of Disorders of Communication*, **19**, 115–124.

American Society of Plastic Surgeons (2010) Scale for grading practice recommendations. http://www.plasticsurgery.org/Medical_Professionals/Health_Policy_and_Advocacy/Health_Policy_Resources/Evidence-based_GuidelinesPractice_Parameters/Description_and_Development_of_Evidence-based_Practice_Guidelines/ASPS_Grade_Recommendation_Scale.html (accessed 4 November 2010).

American Speech-Language-Hearing Association (2004) Evidence-Based Practice in Communication Disorders: An Introduction [Technical Report]. http://www.asha.org/policy (accessed 25 March 2011).

Antman, E.M., Lau, J., Kupelnick, B. *et al.* (1992) A comparison of results of meta-analysis of randomized control trials and recommendations of clinical experts. *Journal of the American Medical Association*, 268, 240–248.

Broen, P.A., Doyle, S.S. and Bacon, C.K. (1993) The velopharyngeally inadequate child: phonologic change with intervention. *Cleft Palate Journal*, 30, 500–507.

Burrell, K. (1989) The modification of nasality using nasometer feedback. Thesis, University of Minnesota, Minneapolis.

Chisum, L., Shelton, R.I., Andt, W.B. and Elbert, M. (1969) The relationship between remedial speech instruction activities and articulation change. *Cleft Palate Journal*, 6, 57–64.

Chua, H.D.P., Whitehill, N., Samman, L.K. and Cheung, L.K. (2010) Maxillary distraction vs orthognathic surgery in cleft lip and palate patients: effects on speech and velopharyngeal function. *International Journal of Oral Maxillofacial Surgery*, 39, 633–640.

Cook, D.J., Mulrow, C.D. and Haynes, R.B. (1997) Systematic reviews: synthesis of best evidence for clinical decisions. *Annals of Internal Medicine*, 126, 376–380.

Dollaghan, C.A. (2007) *The Handbook for Evidence-Based Practice in Communication Disorders*, Paul H. Brookes Publishing Company, Baltimore.

Enderby, P. and Emerson, J. (1995) *'Does Speech and Language Therapy Work?' A Review of the Literature*, Whurr Publishing, London.

Fletcher, S.G. (1972) Contingencies for bioelectronic modification of nasality. *Journal of Speech Hearing Disorders*, 37, 329–346.

Fletcher, S.G. (1978) *Diagnosing Speech Disorders from Cleft Palate*, Grune and Stratton, New York.

Fujiwara, Y. (2007) Electropalatography home training using a portable training unit for Japanese children with cleft palate. *Advances in Speech-Language Pathology*, 9, 66–72.

Gibbon, F.E. and Hardcastle, W.J. (1989) Deviant articulation in a cleft palate child following late repair of the hard palate: a description and remediation procedure using electropalatography (EPG). *Clinical Linguistics & Phonetics*, 3, 93–110.

Gibbon, F.E., Hardcastle, W.J., Crampin, L. *et al.* (2001) Visual feedback therapy using electropalatography (EPG) for articulation disorders associated with cleft palate. *Asia Pacific Journal of Speech Language and Hearing*, 6, 53–58.

Glenny, A.M., Hooper, L., Shaw, B.C. *et al.* (2004) Feeding interventions for growth and development in infants with cleft lip, cleft palate or cleft lip and palate. *Cochrane Database of Systematic Reviews*, (3).

Guyatt, G., Haynes, B., Jaeschke, R. *et al.* (2002a) Introduction: the philosophy of evidence-based medicine, in *Users' Guides to the Medical Literature: A Manual for Evidence-Based Clinical Practice* (eds G. Guyette and D. Rennie), American Medical Association Press, Chicago, IL, pp. 3–12.

Guyatt, G., Hayward, R., Richardson, W.S. *et al.* (2002b) Moving from evidence to action, in *Users' Guides to the Medical Literature: A Manual for Evidence-Based Clinical Practice* (eds G. Guyette and D. Rennie), American Medical Association Press, Chicago, IL, pp. 175–199.

Haapanen, M.L., Kalland, M., Heliövaara, A. *et al.* (1997) Velopharyngeal function in cleft patients undergoing maxillary advancement. *Folia Phoniatrica et Logopaedica*, 49, 42–47.

Hess, D.R. (2004) Retrospective studies and chart reviews. *Respiratory Care*, 49, 1171–1174.

Hodson, B.W., Chin, L., Redmond, B. and Simpson, R. (1983) Phonological evaluation and remediation of speech deviations of a child with a repaired cleft palate: a case study. *Journal of Speech Hearing Research*, 48, 93–98.

Irwin, D.L., Pannbacker, M. and Lass, N.J. (2008) *Clinical Research Methods in Speech-Language Pathology and Audiology*, Plural Publishing, San Diego.

Joanna Briggs Institute. (2008) http://www.joannabriggs.edu.au/Documents/JBI%20Approach%20 to%20EBP%20Levels%20of%20Evidence%20Grades%20of%20Recommendation.pdf: (accessed 27 October 2010).

Kawano, M., Isshiki, N., Harita, Y. and Tanokuchi, F. (1985) Laryngeal fricative in cleft palate speech. *Acta Otolaryngology (Stockh)*, **419** (Suppl.):180–188.

Kirkevold, M. (1997) Integrative nursing research-an important strategy to further the development of nursing science and practice. *Journal of Advanced Nursing*, **25**, 977–984.

Kuehn, D.P. (1991) New therapy for treating hypernasal speech using positive airway pressure (CPAP). *Plastic Reconstructive Surgery*, **88**, 959–966.

Kuehn, D.P. and Moller, K.T. (2000) Speech and language issues in the cleft palate population: the state of the art. *Cleft Palate-Craniofacial Journal*, **37**, 1–34.

Kuehn, D.P., Imrey, P.B., Tomes, L. *et al.* (2002) Efficacy of Continuous positive airway pressure for treatment of hypernasality. *Cleft Palate-Craniofacial Journal*, **39**, 267–275.

Kummer, A.W., Strife, J.L., Grau, W.H. *et al.* (1989) The effects of Le Fort I osteotomy with maxillary movement on articulation, resonance, and velopharyngeal function. *Cleft Palate Craniofacial Journal*, **29**, 152–156.

Law, M. (2002) *Evidence-Based Rehabilitation: A Guide to Practice*, Slack Inc, Thoroughfare, NJ.

Law, J., Boyle, J., Harris, F. *et al.* (2000) Prevalence and natural history of primary speech and language delay: findings from a systematic review of the literature. *International Journal of Language Communication Disorders*, **35**, 165–188.

Lee, A.S.Y., Law, J. and Gibbon, F.E. (2009) Electropalatography for articulation disorders associated with cleft palate. *Cochrane Database of Systematic Reviews*, 3 (Art. No.: CD006854). doi: 10.1002/14651858.CD006854.pub2.

Lohmander, A., Henriksson, C. and Havstam, C. (2010) Electropalatography in home training of retracted articulation in a Swedish child with cleft palate: effect on articulation pattern and speech. *International Journal of Speech Language Pathology*, **12**, 483–496.

McCarthy, C.M., Collins, E.D. and Pusic, A.L. (2008) Where do we find the best evidence? *Plastic Reconstructive Surgery*, **122**, 1942–1947.

McCarthy, J.G., Coccaro, P.J. and Schwartz, M.D. (1979) Velopharyngeal function following maxillary advancement. *Plastic Reconstructive Surgery*, **64**, 180–189.

McCauley, R. and Hargrove, P. (2004) A clinician's introduction to systematic reviews in communication disorders: the course review paper with muscle. *Contemporary Issues in Communication Science and Disorders*, **31**, 173–181.

McWilliams, B.J., Morris, H.L. and Shelton, R.L. (1984) *Cleft Palate Speech*, Decker, Philadelphia PA.

Michi, K., Suzuki, N., Yamshita, Y. and Imai, S. (1986) Visual training and correction of articulation disorders by use of dynamic palatography: serial observation in a case of cleft palate. *Journal of Speech and Hearing Disorders*, **51**, 226–238.

Michi, K.-I., Yamashita, Y., Imai, S. *et al.* (1993) Role of visual feedback treatment for defective /s/ sounds in patients with cleft palate. *Journal of Speech Hearing Research*, **36**, 277–285.

Mulrow, C.D. (1994) Systematic reviews: rationale for systematic reviews. *British Medical Journal*, **309**, 597–599.

Nasser, M., Fedorowicz, Z., Newton, T. and Nouri, M. (2008) Interventions for the management of submucous cleft palate. *Cochrane Database of Systematic Reviews* 1 Art. No.: CD006703. doi: 10.1002/14651858.CD006703.pub2.

Neilhouse, P.F. and Priske, S.C. (1989) Quotation accuracy in review articles. *DICP*, **23**, 594–596.

Okazaki, K., Satoh, K., Kato, M. *et al.* (1993) Speech and velopharyngeal function following maxillary advancement in patients with cleft lip and palate. *Annals of Plastic Surgery*, **30**, 304–311.

Oxford Centre for Evidence Based Medicine Levels Evidence (2009) http://www.cebm.net (accessed March 2009).

Oxman, A.D., Cook, D.J. and Guyatt, G.H. (1994) Users' guides to the medical literature. VI. How to use an overview. Evidence-based medicine working group. *Journal of the American Medical Association*, **272** (17), 1367–1371.

Pamplona, M.C., Ysunza, A. and Espinosa, J. (1999) A comparative trial of two modalities of speech intervention for compensatory articulation in cleft palate children, phonologic approach versus articulatory approach. *International Journal of Pediatric Otorhinolaryngology*, **49**, 21–26.

Pamplona, M.C., Ysunza, A., Patiño, C. and Ramírez, E. (2004) Naturalistic intervention in cleft palate children. *International Journal of Pediatric Otorhinolaryngology*, **68**, 75–81.

Pamplona, M.C., Ysunza, A., Patiño, C. et al. (2005) Speech summer camp for treating articulation disorders in cleft palate patients. *International Journal of Pediatric Otorhinolaryngology*, **69**, 351–359.

Peterson-Falzone, S.J., Karnell, M.P. and Hardin-Jones, M. (2010) *Cleft Palate Speech*, 4th edn. Elsevier, St. Louis, MO.

Poole, M.D., Robinson, P.P. and Nunn, M.E. (1986) Maxillary advancement in cleft palate patients. A modification of the Le Fort I osteotomy and preliminary results. *Journal Maxillofacial Surgery*, **14**, 123–127.

Reilly, S., Douglas, J. and Oates, J. (2004) *Evidence Based Practice in Speech Pathology*, Whurr Publishers, London.

Sackett, D., Richardson, W., Rosenberg, W. and Haynes, R. (1997) *Evidence-Based Medicine: How to Practice and Teach EBM*, Churchill Livingstone, New York.

Sackett, D.L., Strauss, S.E., Richardson, W.S. et al. (2000) *Evidence-Based Medicine: How to Practice and Teach EBM*, 2nd edn. Churchill Livingstone, London.

Schlosser, R.W. (2003) *The Efficacy of Augmentative and Alternative Communication: Toward Evidence-Based Practice*, Academic Press, San Diego, CA.

Schwarz, C. and Gruner, E. (1976) Logopaedic findings following advancement of the maxilla. *Journal Maxillofacial Surgery*, **4**, 40–55.

Starr, C.D. (1993) Behavioral approaches to treating velopharyngeal closure and nasality, in *Cleft Palate: Interdisciplinary Issues and Treatment* (eds K.T. Moller and C.D. Starr), Pro-ED, Austin, TX, pp. 337–356.

Stokes, S.F., Whitehill, T.L., Yuen, K.C.P. and Tsui, A.M.Y. (1996) EPG treatment of sibilants in two Cantonese-speaking children with cleft palate. *Clinical Linguistics & Phonetics*, **10**, 265–280.

Tönz, M., Schmid, I., Graf, M. et al. (2002) Blinded speech evaluation following pharyngeal flap surgery by speech pathologists and lay people in children with cleft palate. *Folia Phoniatrica et Logopaedica*, **54**, 288–295.

Van Demark, D.R. and Hardin, M.A. (1986) Effectiveness of intensive articulation therapy for children with cleft palate. *Cleft Palate Journal*, **23**, 215–224.

Van Lierde, K.M., Bonte, K., Baudonck, N. et al. (2008) Speech outcome regarding overall intelligibility, articulation, resonance and voice in Flemish children a year after pharyngeal flap surgery. A pilot study. *Folia Phoniatrica et Logopaedica*, **60**, 223–232.

Whitehill, T.L., Stokes, S.F. and Man, Y.H.Y. (1996) Electropalatography treatment in an adult with late repair of cleft palate. *Cleft Palate-Craniofacial Journal*, **33**, 160–168.

Witt, P.D., D'Antonio, L.L., Zimmerman, G.J. and Marsh, J.L. (1994) Sphincter pharyngoplasty: a preoperative and postoperative analysis of perceptual speech characteristics and endoscopic studies of velopharyngeal function. *Plastic Reconstructive Surgery*, **93**, 1154–1168.

Witzel, M.A. and Munro, I.R. (1977) Velopharyngeal insufficiency after maxillary advancement. *Cleft Palate Journal*, **14**, 176–180.

Witzel, M.A., Tobe, J. and Salyer, K. (1988) The use of nasopharyngoscopy biofeedback therapy in the correction of inconsistent velopharyngeal closure. *International Journal Pediatric Otolaryngology*, **15**, 137–142.

Witzel, M.A., Tobe, J. and Salyer, K. (1989) The use of nasopharyngoscopy biofeedback therapy in adults after pharyngeal flap surgery. *Cleft Palate Journal*, **26**, 129–134.

Yamaoka, M., Matsuya, T., Miyazki, T. *et al.* (1983) Visual training for velopharyngeal closure in cleft palate patients; a fibrescopic procedure (preliminary report). *Journal of Maxillofacial Surgery*, **11**, 191–193.

Ysunza, A., Pamplona, C., Femat, T. *et al.* (1997) Videonasopharyngoscopy as an instrument for visual feedback during speech in cleft palate patients. *International Journal of Pediatric Otorhinolaryngology*, **41**, 291–298.

Ysunza, A., Pamplona, C., Ramírez, E. *et al.* (2002) Velopharyngeal surgery: a prospective randomized study of pharyngeal flaps and sphincter pharyngoplasties. *Plastic Reconstructive Surgery*, **110**, 1401–1407.

Index

Cleft Palate Speech: Assessment and Intervention, First Edition. Edited by Sara Howard,
Anette Lohmander.
© 2011 John Wiley & Sons, Ltd. Published 2011 by John Wiley & Sons, Ltd.

Printed in the United States
By Bookmasters